Eleanor Gittens

A CONCISE INTRODUCTION TO MENTAL HEALTH IN CANADA

A CONCISE INTRODUCTION TO MENTAL HEALTH IN CANADA

Third Edition

Emily Jenkins, Allie Slemon, and Dan Bilsker with Elliot M. Goldner

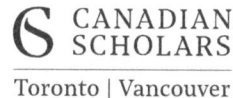

Toronto | Vancouver

A Concise Introduction to Mental Health in Canada, Third Edition
Emily Jenkins, Allie Slemon, and Dan Bilsker with Elliot M. Goldner

First published in 2022 by
Canadian Scholars, an imprint of CSP Books Inc.
425 Adelaide Street West, Suite 200
Toronto, Ontario
M5V 3C1

www.canadianscholars.ca

Copyright © 2011, 2016, 2022 Emily Jenkins, Allie Slemon, Dan Bilsker, Elliot M. Goldner, and Canadian Scholars.

All rights reserved. No part of this publication may be reproduced, stored in a retrieval system, or transmitted, in any form or by any means, without the prior written permission of Canadian Scholars, under licence or terms from the appropriate reproduction rights organization, or as expressly permitted by law.

Every reasonable effort has been made to identify copyright holders. Canadian Scholars would be pleased to have any errors or omissions brought to its attention.

Library and Archives Canada Cataloguing in Publication

Title: A concise introduction to mental health in Canada / Emily Jenkins, Allie Slemon, and Dan Bilsker with Elliot M. Goldner.
Names: Goldner, Elliot M. (Elliot Michael), 1953- author. | Jenkins, Emily (Emily K.), 1981- author. | Slemon, Allie, author. | Bilsker, Dan, author.
Description: Third edition. | Revision of: Goldner, Elliot M. (Elliot Michael), 1953-. A concise introduction to mental health in Canada. | Includes bibliographical references and index.
Identifiers: Canadiana (print) 20220234094 | Canadiana (ebook) 20220234108 |
    ISBN 9781773382524 (softcover) | ISBN 9781773382531 (PDF) |
    ISBN 9781773382548 (EPUB)
Subjects: LCSH: Mental health—Canada—Textbooks. | LCSH: Mental illness—Canada—Textbooks. | LCSH: Mental health services—Canada—Textbooks. | LCGFT: Textbooks.
Classification: LCC RA790.7.C3 G65 2022 | DDC 362.20971—dc23

Page layout by S4Carlisle Publishing Services
Cover design by Em Dash
Cover image by Shutterstock/BABAROGA

Printed and bound in Ontario, Canada

Canada

Contents

Foreword vii
    Jonathan Morris, Chief Executive Officer of the Canadian Mental Health Association, British Columbia Division

Preface ix

Chapter 1
What Is Mental Health? 1

Chapter 2
Understanding Mental Health through the Physical Sciences 27

Chapter 3
Mental Health Examined through the Social Sciences 49

Chapter 4
The Spectrum of Mental Health Challenges 73

Chapter 5
Substance Use, Dependence, and Addictive Behaviour 95
Emma Garrod

Chapter 6
Trauma, Violence, and Mental Health 125
Nancy Clark, Allie Slemon, and Emily Jenkins

Chapter 7
Sex, Gender, and Sexuality 143

Chapter 8
Culture, Ethnicity, and Mental Health 163
Victoria Smye

Chapter 9
Mental Health and Illness in Children and Youth 189
Skye Barbic

Chapter 10
Mental Health and Illness in Older Adults 215

Chapter 11
Responding to Mental Health Crisis, Emergency, and Disaster 233

Chapter 12
Mental Health and the Criminal Justice System 251
Amanda Butler, Katherine Rossiter, and Tonia Nicholls

Chapter 13
Mental Health Legislation and Patients' Rights 287
Iva W. Cheung

Chapter 14
Treatment Approaches for Mental Health and Substance Use Challenges 309
Courtney Devane, Allie Slemon, and Emily Jenkins

Chapter 15
Mental Health Services in Canada 339
Erin Michalak and Rebecca Zappelli

Chapter 16
Canada's Role in Global Mental Health 357
Jill Murphy and Leena Chau

Chapter 17
Population Perspectives on Mental Health and Substance Use 375

Copyright Acknowledgements 399
Index 405

Foreword

> Mental health is the capacity of each and all of us to feel, think, and act in ways that enhance our ability to enjoy life and deal with the challenges we face. It is a positive sense of emotional and spiritual well-being that respects the importance of culture, equity, social justice, interconnections, and personal dignity.
> —Public Health Agency of Canada

Like many who work, advocate, or practice in the space of mental health and substance use care, I bring the perspective of an "insider" with lived experience of depression in my twenties during university, and the perspective of having a loved one living with severe and persistent mental illness.

My first experiences of working in the field were as a youth crisis line volunteer in the United Kingdom, where I learned about the sacredness of listening to understand and the privilege of bearing witness to pain, strength, struggle, and hope. My latest experiences include the excitement of being a public servant amidst the development of the country's first provincial Ministry of Mental Health and Addictions before my current role leading a provincial office of the Canadian Mental Health Association.

As I look back on 25 years of a career in mental health, the challenges, opportunities, perspectives, and learning I've experienced reflect the breadth and depth of the issues covered in this book. This updated text will serve as an important repository of interdisciplinary knowledge for someone starting their career in mental health, or for someone like me, who still has much to learn!

As I write this, Canada and the global community continue to be immersed in the unpredictable and far-reaching consequences of the COVID-19 pandemic. By November 2021, this worldwide health emergency had seen almost 250 million cases and 5 million deaths. Global leaders gathered at a critical summit designed to manifest commitments to mitigate the certainty of a drastically changed and much less liveable world ravaged by climate change. Indigenous communities continue to respond to the grief and trauma of repeated confirmations of unmarked graves at former residential school sites. And closer to home, British Columbia continues to lose almost six lives per day due to the ongoing drug poisoning crisis.

While this is not an exhaustive list of the complex and intersecting challenges gripping our world, the crises listed above have brought the issue of our mental health and well-being into stark relief. I am grateful for the words of Louise Bradley, former President and CEO of the Mental Health Commission of Canada, who wrote the foreword for the last edition of this book, and who described the surging effort to respond to the pandemic as having "risen from a collective will mobilized by the eye-opening realization that protecting our bodies from harm is only half the battle."

Arguably, the present moment is an important reckoning for the state of individual and collective mental health and well-being, with the chapters in this book being essential reading. This updated text continues to bring a multi-perspectival examination of mental health in Canada and beyond. Comprised of interdisciplinary knowledge, written by researchers, practitioners, advocates, and people with lived experience, this book now provides an expanded framework for understanding mental health today and into the future.

The book allows for a treatment of some of the most pressing issues related to mental health and substance use. For example, after decades of advocacy by organizations like the Canadian Mental Health Association, there is a deepening focus on the disproportionate representation of people living with mental illness in conflict with the law and incarcerated in the criminal justice system. The interface between mental health legislation and patients' rights is becoming a more prominent concern in the aftermath of systemic investigation reports calling for improvements in how the legislation is applied when people are at their most vulnerable. This is against a backdrop of rising rates of people apprehended and detained under mental health legislation. Further, the book takes a close look at culture, ethnicity, and mental health, disrupting taken-for-granted assumptions and underscoring the opportunity to take up decolonizing approaches to research and practice. All of these are topics covered in this impressive volume.

The foundational and leading-edge content of this book will provide a comprehensive and rich survey of the current context of mental health in Canada. This will help the reader engage with more texts about mental health, including best practices, innovative policy, pioneering technologies, and more. Despite the need for much more investment in mental health and substance use care research, our understanding continues to grow, and this book will help you keep pace with some of the latest thinking and approaches. I agree with Louise Bradley's comments in the last foreword for this book. The text remains ideal for students, practitioners, people living with mental illness, and it continues to deserve a much broader audience. Improving policy and practice continues to require comprehension and vision across many constituencies, and this book helps to take things an important stride further.

My dear friend and colleague The Right Honourable Sir Norman Lamb from the UK describes the "moral imperative" of putting mental health on a more equal footing with physical health care. This book is a compassionate, cogent, and strong foundation to help us all respond to this moral imperative, pushing back stigma and making change one step at a time.

—*Jonny Morris, Chief Executive Officer,*
Canadian Mental Health Association, BC Division

Preface

The writing of this third edition of our textbook has been bittersweet. In 2016, we experienced the sudden and unexpected death of our dear friend, colleague, and mentor, Dr. Elliot Goldner. This loss has been felt far and wide in mental health and substance use circles—and beyond. Elliot was a passionate and committed clinician, scientist, and advocate who made profound contributions to the field, both nationally and internationally. This new edition of our textbook serves as a tribute to Elliot's legacy. It features several chapters that have been written or updated by close friends, colleagues, and students whom he mentored and who continue to push the boundaries and advance science and practice in the mental health and substance use field. It also includes the addition of a new primary co-author, Allie Slemon, currently a doctoral student at the University of British Columbia, School of Nursing. This reflects an effort to "pay it forward," to create an opportunity like the one that Elliot initially provided, for student co-authorship and capacity building.

Since the publication of the second edition of the textbook in 2016, there have been several changes that have impacted the mental health and substance use landscape, both in Canada and internationally. The International Classification of Diseases (11th revision) was published with substantial modification to mental disorder classification categories, as well as changes to enhance diagnostic accessibility among clinicians globally. We continue to witness dramatic shifts in our understandings of mental health and illness. Research and technological advancements over the last several decades have contributed to new medications and treatment options that have altered the experiences of people living with mental health challenges. A focus on mental *health* (in addition to mental *illness*) has continued to gain momentum within the population and public health field, resulting in a strengthened focus on mental health promotion and illness prevention, with the goal of improving the health and well-being of our societies. In 2018, Canada became the second country in the world to legalize the possession and use of non-medical cannabis—a historic and welcome event for many, including those who advocate for a public health approach to substance use, as opposed to the traditional "war on drugs."

Despite these advancements, the Canadian mental health care system remains fragmented and under-resourced, and widespread stigma towards individuals experiencing mental health and substance use challenges endures. Harmful drug policies have contributed to the continuation of the drug poisoning crisis, which has claimed the lives of over 24,600 people in Canada since 2016. We are also currently living in the midst of the COVID-19 pandemic, which has had substantial adverse impacts on population mental health, particularly for those living with pre-existing mental health or substance use challenges. In this edition of our textbook, we continue our mission to bring these issues to the forefront of awareness and motivate readers to become agents of change.

This third edition of *A Concise Introduction to Mental Health in Canada* continues to represent a unique contribution to the mental health literature. It incorporates a broad range of perspectives to explore mental health and illness in Canada "from synapse to society." This edition includes important updates to terminology, highlights advances in the mental health field, and presents more recent scientific data. Careful attention was made to craft a reader-friendly book that includes timely and relevant "real world" examples of mental health–related issues, success stories, and thought-provoking insights. As in our last editions, we have included a personal mental health toolkit, which offers readers evidence-informed strategies and skills to promote and maintain their own mental health and well-being.

The writing of the first edition of this book involved an unusual collaboration between faculty members and graduate students, each from distinct disciplinary backgrounds. This third edition, with contributions from Elliot Goldner's network, furthers the diversity of perspectives and provides for a truly interdisciplinary book. We believe that this partnership enhances the quality and relevance of this text for readers.

Providing foundational knowledge about mental health and illness in Canada, we want this book to inspire the mental health leaders of tomorrow. We hope that readers will enjoy this book as much as we enjoyed writing it.

Chapter 1

◆

What Is Mental Health?

The mind is its own place, and in itself
Can make Heaven of Hell, and a Hell of Heaven.
—John Milton (English poet and civil servant)

Introduction

Let us imagine that you and a good friend agree to try and make a determination of each other's mental health, choosing one of the following five ratings. How might you go about doing so?

EXCELLENT   VERY GOOD   GOOD   FAIR   POOR

Unfortunately, you won't be able to rely on a blood test, brain scan, or other measurement. No laboratory test or physiological measure has been discovered that can produce a rating of a person's overall mental health, despite the strong links that exist between mental states and the physiological function of various organs of the body. Although changes in heart rate and respiration, as well as alterations in levels of hormones and nervous system activity, may occur with anxiety, depression, or other mental states, they are too non-specific to be used for diagnosis. Possibly, laboratory measures, brain imaging techniques, or other technological tools will be developed to assist with determinations of overall mental health in the future. At present, we must rely on individuals' self-reported mental health, observations, historical information, and inference (i.e., applying logical reasoning to draw conclusions).

To help you make an accurate rating, you might want to have a good definition of mental health; however, this is not as simple a task as you might think. In fact, the World Health Organization (WHO) states that no single definition of mental health is widely accepted; cultural differences and competing professional theories may lead to the adoption of different definitions of mental health in various contexts and cultures. However, for the most part, good mental health is now regarded as not only the absence of mental distress or emotional challenges but also the presence of factors such as the ability to enjoy oneself and the capacity to participate meaningfully in daily life. Moreover, while people often use the term "mental health" synonymously with "mental illness," mental health is actually a separate, strengths-oriented (as opposed to deficit-oriented) concept. The Two Continua Model of mental health and illness, for example, features prominently in the work of various mental health organizations and governments and provides a helpful introduction to this idea. It "holds that both [mental health and mental illness] are related, but distinct dimensions: one continuum indicates the presence or absence of mental health, the other the presence or absence of mental illness" (Westerhof & Keyes, 2010; see Figure 1.1). Importantly, it also acknowledges that mental health and illness intersect and are

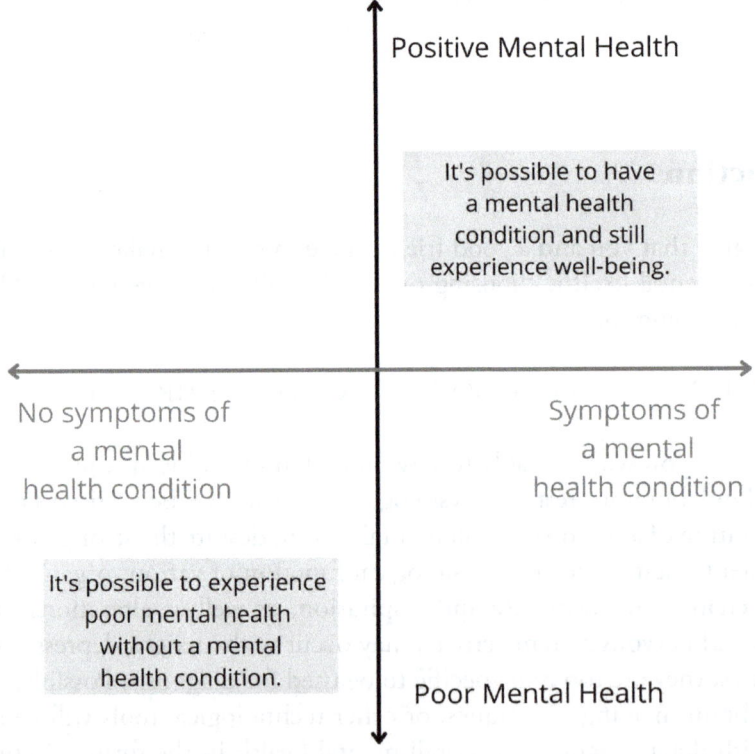

Figure 1.1: This is the Two Continua Model of mental health and illness. This model depicts the relationship between the distinct but related concepts of mental health and mental illness and shows that people who experience mental illnesses can simultaneously experience good mental health. Likewise, people can experience poor mental health without having a diagnosable mental illness.

Source: Adapted from the Canadian Mental Health Association.

What Is Mental Health?

experienced to varying degrees simultaneously—with fluctuations over time and in response to life circumstances.

A reasonable definition of mental health is given below.

> **Mental health** can be defined as "a state of well-being in which every individual realizes [their] own potential, can cope with the normal stresses of life, can work productively and fruitfully, and is able to make a contribution to [their] community." (WHO, 2014)

As noted in the landmark report on mental health from the Canadian Senate's Standing Committee on Social Affairs, Science and Technology (Kirby & Keon, 2004), "Mental health [infers] various capacities including the ability to: understand oneself and one's life; relate to other people and respond to one's environment; experience pleasure and enjoyment; handle stress and withstand discomfort; evaluate challenges and problems; pursue goals and interests; and, explore choices and make decisions." The Senate report also notes that good mental health is associated with positive self-esteem, happiness, interest in life, work satisfaction, mastery, and sense of coherence, and enables individuals to realize their potential and contribute to society. However, in recent years, these conceptualizations of mental health have been critiqued by some scholars and advocates for their individualistic emphasis. Indeed, mental health is best understood from a **socioecological perspective**, which acknowledges health as a product of the interactions between an individual and their broader family, community, and societal contexts. The Public Health Agency of Canada has produced a conceptual model depicting a socioecological understanding of positive mental health (see Figure 1.2).

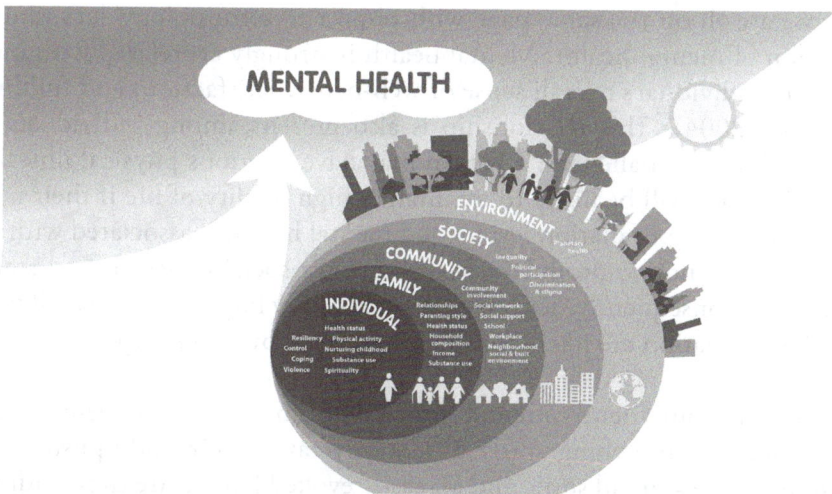

Figure 1.2: The Positive Mental Health Conceptual Framework for Surveillance was developed by the Public Health Agency of Canada and adapted by Agenda Gap. It reflects a socioecological understanding of mental health.

Source: Adapted from the Government of Canada.

Now that you have a solid understanding of mental health, including how it is distinct from mental ill health, let's briefly explore the meaning of other terms commonly used in this text (and out in the real world!), including "mental health challenges," as well as "mental illnesses" and "disorders." What are the differences anyway? The answer lies in the degree of functional impairment experienced. The following definitions provide further clarification.

> **Mental health problems [or challenges]** refer to diminished capacities—whether cognitive, emotional, attentional, interpersonal, motivational, or behavioural—that interfere with a person's enjoyment of life or adversely affect interactions with society and the environment. Feelings of low self-esteem, frequent frustration or irritability, burnout, feelings of stress, excessive worrying, are examples of common mental health problems. Over the course of a lifetime, every individual will be likely, at some time, to experience some mental health problems such as these. Usually, they are normal, short-term reactions that occur in response to difficult situations (e.g., school pressures, work-related stress, marital conflict, grief, changes in living arrangements) … Mental health problems that resolve quickly, do not recur and do not result in significant disability do not meet the criteria required for diagnosis of a mental illness. **Mental disorders or illnesses** refer to clinically significant patterns of behavioural or emotional function that are associated with some level of distress, suffering (even to the point of pain and death), or impairment in one or more areas of functioning (e.g., school, work, social and family interactions). (Kirby & Keon, 2004)

Now that we are all on the same page with respect to terminology, let's return to our discussion of mental health. Mental health is strongly correlated with quality of life (i.e., an individual's overall sense of well-being, satisfaction, and fulfillment in life; WHO, 2004). This relationship is also present among individuals with major physical health challenges; a person may have a serious physical illness that causes disability but will be likely to maintain a high quality of life if their mental health is good. At the population level, good mental health is associated with good physical health, economic productivity, and greater social cohesion and stability (WHO, 2004). Consequently, actions that successfully improve the overall mental health of the population are likely to be accompanied by other important benefits to society.

In considering your friend's mental health, you note that they seem calm and comfortable and are breathing softly at a steady rate. Their body posture is relaxed, and they have a broad smile and an easily evoked laugh. Are these indicators of good mental health? Yes, they are! When health care professionals undertake an examination of an individual's mental health, they generally begin by simply observing the person's overall behaviour, psychomotor activity, speech, and general demeanour.

However, the observation that someone appears to be calm and relaxed is not enough to assume good mental health. If a careful evaluation of a person's mental health is called for, health care professionals may undertake a **mental status examination**, which involves a series of observations, structured questions, and tests of concentration, memory, and other mental functions. For example, a common component of the examination is to ask the person being interviewed to subtract 7 from the number 100, then subtract 7 from the answer, then subtract 7 once again, and to continue doing so (as a mental exercise without paper or pencil). This is meant to test a number of functions, including the person's ability to concentrate on a task, use certain memory functions, and apply arithmetic calculations. Properly done, a mental status examination will account for an individual's cultural and educational background and examine a wide range of mental activity, including the person's capacity to think clearly, express emotions, and make rational judgments.

More detailed and rigorous approaches to assessing mental function have been developed in the form of psychological testing. Thousands of psychological tests have been created, evaluating a range of mental abilities, personality traits, and individual characteristics. Many have been designed to test specific functions, such as short-term memory in those who have experienced brain injury or disease; others examine broad mental functions, such as intelligence or personality, and these are typically designed for use with specific groups, such as children or adults within a designated age range.

But even rigorous mental status examination or detailed psychological testing may be insufficient to provide a meaningful picture of a person's mental health. A cross-sectional view (i.e., examining only one brief point in time) is often inadequate to provide a valid understanding because a person's mental health must be considered over a span of time, taking into account the fluctuations that occur in various facets of their mental life. Some features of our mental lives may fluctuate markedly, including mood states and more transient emotions, such as happiness, sadness, fear, hopefulness, and hopelessness. One "snapshot" may not provide an accurate view of the larger landscape or experience. Transient states of mind across the lifespan may be influenced profoundly by various factors, including one's environment, the existence or absence of stressors, the occurrence of significant life events, and the use of psychoactive substances (i.e., substances that alter the functioning of the brain), including consumption of alcohol and other drugs.

Although mental status examination and psychological testing are valuable tools, they will not provide the full picture of an individual's mental health or the presence of mental illnesses. Furthermore, anthropologists and sociologists have questioned

Brief Mental Status Exam (MSE) Form

1. Appearance	☐ casual dress, normal grooming and hygiene ☐ other (describe):
2. Attitude	☐ calm and cooperative ☐ other (describe):
3. Behavior	☐ no unusual movements or psychomotor changes ☐ other (describe):
4. Speech	☐ normal rate/tone/volume w/out pressure ☐ other (describe):
5. Affect	☐ reactive and mood congruent ☐ normal range ☐ labile ☐ depressed ☐ tearful ☐ constricted ☐ blunted ☐ flat ☐ other (describe):
6. Mood	☐ euthymic ☐ anxious ☐ irritable ☐ depressed ☐ elevated ☐ other (describe):
7. Thought Processes	☐ goal-directed and logical ☐ disorganized ☐ other (describe):
8. Thought Content	**Suicidal** ideation: **Homicidal** ideation: ☐ None ☐ passive ☐ active ☐ None ☐ passive ☐ active If *active*: yes no If *active*: yes no plan ☐ ☐ plan ☐ ☐ intent ☐ ☐ intent ☐ ☐ means ☐ ☐ means ☐ ☐ ☐ delusions ☐ obsessions/compulsions ☐ phobias ☐ other (describe):
9. Perception	☐ no hallucinations or delusions during interview ☐ other (describe):
10. Orientation	Oriented: ☐ time ☐ place ☐ person ☐ self ☐ other (describe):
11. Memory/Concentration	☐ short term intact ☐ long term intact ☐ other (describe): ☐ distractable/inattentive
12. Insight/Judgement	☐ good ☐ fair ☐ poor

Practitioner Signature   **Date**

Patient Name   **ID#**

http://www.apshealthcare.com/provider/documents/brief_mental_status.pdf

Figure 1.3: Mental Status Examination—Rapid Record Form
This form illustrates the various domains commonly assessed through a mental status examination. The terminology used to describe various characteristics of mental status may, at first, feel like a new language. However, these terms quickly become familiar to those working in mental health settings.

Source: APS Healthcare

the validity of such methods when used in certain circumstances, arguing that they may be biased by their social and cultural context. We will return to the important question of whether such assessments are valid in Chapter 4, when we discuss the diagnosis of mental illnesses.

Health of the Human Mind

Brain versus Mind

Mental health literally means "health of the *mind*." Although the various functions of the mind are produced by the brain, the mind and the brain are not equivalent. The brain is the physical organ of the body that produces mental activity; the mind is a set of functions and experiences resulting from a combination of brain activity and the environment in which it operates. Cultural, historical, and educational influences play a large role in shaping the mind. The brain has been compared to computer hardware; in contrast, the mind has been compared to the overall function of the computer with various software programs operating. Whereas the brain is an actual physical object, the mind is a *construct*, that is to say, a concept for which there is not a single visible referent and which cannot be directly observed. We develop constructs in order to organize our thoughts and ideas and attach meaning to our internal and external environments. The mind is an example of a construct that is used by many of us to make sense of our experiences. Other examples of constructs are intelligence, love, and fear.

There are multiple influences on the development of the human mind, as depicted earlier in Figure 1.2. Although individual factors, including biological characteristics (e.g., genetics, neurophysiological processes) and personal health behaviours, play an important role, many social, psychological, and environmental elements also have a profound influence on the mind and experiences of mental health. This combination of factors operates across various domains from the individual level through to the societal level. The factors depicted in Figure 1.2 do not work in isolation; they interact with each other. For example, a stable political environment and economic conditions will contribute to an environment in which society can prosper and flourish, supporting families in providing healthy environments for their children's growth and development. In contrast, unstable political and economic environments, such as those that might accompany times of war, can create havoc, leading to loss and separation of family members, emotional suffering, and food shortages. This social disorder can have a negative impact on our emotional lives, with particularly detrimental consequences for children, who are still developing their unique mental and physical health characteristics.

Pendulum Swings: Physical Sciences and Social Sciences

In recent history, mental health and illness have often been viewed from one of two contrasting perspectives. One is the perspective of the physical sciences, such as biology, chemistry, physics, and neuroscience. From this perspective, there is an emphasis on the function of the brain, neurotransmitters, and endocrine system (e.g., hormones, such as adrenaline, estrogen, and testosterone), and on factors that may affect the function of these biological systems, such as genetic influences and the use of pharmaceutical agents.

The other perspective focuses on factors identified by the social sciences, including the disciplines of anthropology, sociology, psychology, criminology, economics, geography, history, and political science. These factors encompass the effects of family life, culture, society, and political and economic environments.

During different eras, one or the other of these two perspectives has dominated. For example, in the 19th century, scientists tended to hold a biological perspective and explained mental health and illness in terms of brain function. At the time, it was thought that a better understanding of mental health and illness could be derived through study of the brain's intricate structure and function. However, by the middle of the 20th century, social and psychological explanations of human behaviour and mental function dominated, thus shifting the focus of scientific exploration away from the physical sciences. During the second half of the 20th century, there was a strong resurgence of interest in biological explanations of mental function, precipitated by exciting discoveries about the actions of neurotransmitters and the impact of pharmacological agents on brain function (Blows, 2016).

These shifts back and forth between these two perspectives have been described as pendulum swings. These swings have created problems because they lead to reductionistic thinking, that is, a tendency to analyze problems in simplistic terms while ignoring relevant knowledge outside of a narrow view. One of the reasons these pendulum swings occur is that reductionistic thinking is very common. In fact, we all have a tendency to think in this fashion and it requires substantial effort to apply more complex ways of conceptualizing the world around us. Lawrence Kohlberg and other scientists have found that children are likely to use reductionistic thinking and reasoning, whereas some adolescents and adults develop more complex approaches to problem solving (Kohlberg et al., 1983).

Mental health and mental illness are complex topics and, consequently, reductionistic explanations are likely to create misunderstanding. Let us consider the example of depression. As mentioned above, there was a pendulum swing towards biological explanations of mental health and illness during the second half of the 20th century, and when a physician made a diagnosis of depression, it was common practice for the doctor to explain to the patient that "depression results from a chemical imbalance of the brain." However, this biological explanation is inadequate because there are so many different factors associated with depression. As well as biological antecedents, there are many other precipitants for depression, such as difficulties in relationships, loss of loved ones, isolation and loneliness, exclusion and discrimination, challenges at work, and economic strain.

Therefore, the simplistic explanation that depression is caused by a chemical imbalance of the brain is erroneous and does not reflect the many factors that may trigger depressive conditions. However, some might argue that defining depression as a neurochemical imbalance describes the ultimate physical manifestation of depression, no matter the various pathways that lead to it. Even if this were so, we maintain that a description of depression as a chemical imbalance of the brain is an inapt simplification. It risks narrowing our treatment options to include only the prescription of medication or other biological interventions to alter the brain's chemistry. Although the use of medications or other somatic treatments may offer benefits to many people with depression, it is important to recognize the benefits of approaches that stem from beyond the physical sciences to respond to this and other mental health challenges.

While considering both the physical and social science perspectives are helpful in informing a comprehensive understanding of mental health, these perspectives reflect a particular type of knowledge—that is, that which is derived through scientific methods. However, scientific evidence is not the only form of knowledge that can offer useful insights about mental health and illness. It is also important to recognize the expertise that comes from living with mental health or substance use challenges. This notion is captured by the term "lived experience," which signifies the unique perspectives that are gained through first-hand experience of conditions or events that most people do not encounter. Such knowledge can be applied to broaden our understandings, to enhance the relevance of interventions, and to help others with less experience. Another group of people with lived experience are family members of those with mental health challenges. Often, family members and other caregivers provide the lion's share of support and assistance to a person who is unwell; in many instances, the provision of necessary support may become the full-time occupation of a family member. They may become the principal holder of information about the history, treatment response, medication regimen, allergies, sensitivities, or other facets of clinical care. Yet family members often feel excluded, unrecognized, and unsupported by health care professionals. It's important to seek out perspectives of people with lived experience, and there is a growing emphasis on better incorporating this knowledge into our understandings, as well as treatment and intervention approaches.

One of the goals of this book is to help you, the reader, strengthen your ability to utilize multiple perspectives and theories simultaneously when you seek to understand mental health and illness. To help you build this capacity, we have integrated and melded streams of knowledge that have emerged from a variety of disciplinary and intellectual traditions. We include examples of a wide range of approaches, going "from synapse to society," in our discussions of mental health and illness. This book includes an overview of many topics, often providing only basic, introductory information; therefore, further studies and readings are encouraged. At the end of each chapter, you will find the following features: Glossary (these terms appear in boldface where they are first defined in the text); Critical Thinking Questions; Recommended Readings; and Recommended Websites. These are meant to assist you as you continue to expand your knowledge beyond the covers of this book.

A Historical View of Mental Health in Canada

In addition to the definition of "mental health" provided earlier in the chapter, the term is also used widely to refer to the entire field, including the various efforts by societies to address mental health and illness. This involves a wide range of formal and informal services and supports, such as counselling and psychotherapy services provided by a wide range of health care professionals, emergency and hospital-based psychiatric treatment services, social services for people with mental health challenges, and initiatives aimed at promoting good mental health instituted by governments and non-profit agencies. In this section, we examine societal approaches to mental health from a historical perspective and consider the evolution of mental health practices in Canada.

Traditional Mental Health and Spiritual Practices

Long before this land was known as Canada, First Nations, Inuit, and Métis people developed practices to address mental and spiritual health and wellness. It is important to keep in mind that the Indigenous populations in Canada comprise many hundreds of different nations, each with their own practices and traditions. Practices have been passed down through many generations by oral tradition, and some persist to this day. Traditional practices that are relevant to mental health and spirituality among Indigenous peoples include ritual chants, ceremonial dances, drumming, ritual journeys, communal sweats, and other spiritual rites (Howell et al., 2016; Sasakamoose et al., 2016).

An example is the sweat lodge ritual, which is still regularly practised by Indigenous peoples in many parts of Canada. As a purification ceremony, it can be performed by itself or in combination with other ceremonial activities. Generally, the ritual involves the careful selection of a site for the sweat lodge, which is then created by first digging a firepit in which specially chosen rocks are heated. A dome is then built to encompass the firepit and form the lodge, often constructed of saplings that are then covered with layers of blankets or other materials. For some, the dome represents the womb of Mother Earth. Once built, the sweat lodge is used by a group of people for the purposes of purification and improvement of

What Is Mental Health?

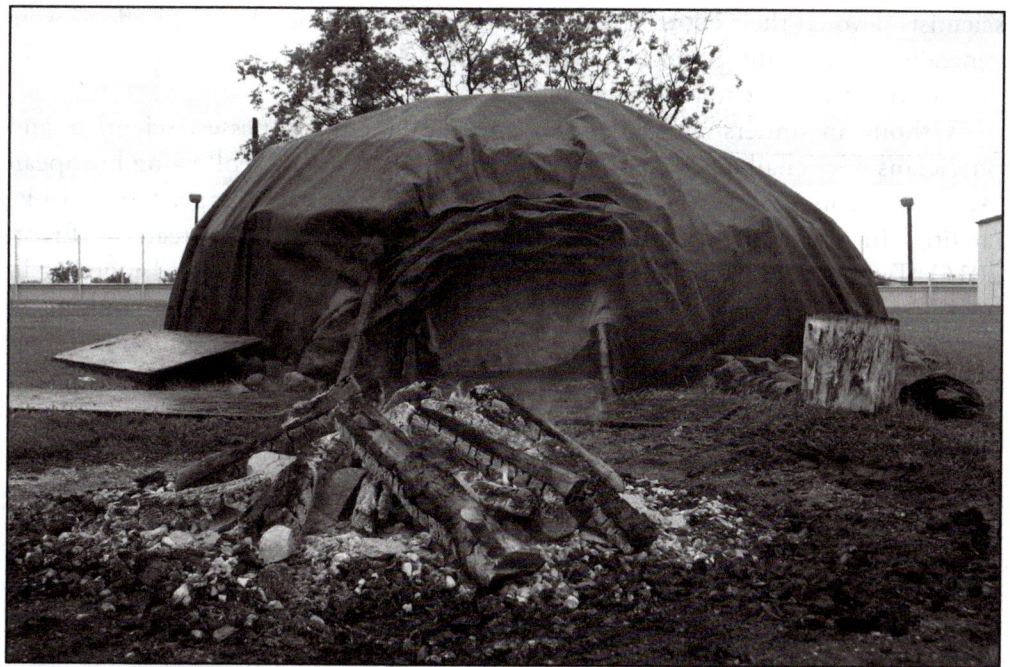

Figure 1.4: Sweat lodge in St. Norbert, Manitoba.

Source: GetStock/Judy Waytiuk

their mental and spiritual health. What is it like to go through the sweat lodge ritual? Many people describe a meditative response in which one's senses seem to be tuned differently, invoked by the communal experience and the sensory effects of the intense heat from the rocks. Those who complete a sweat lodge ritual often describe emerging with a new perspective on important issues or challenges they have been encountering.

Other examples of rituals and practices have been developed around the world for the purpose of promoting spiritual and mental well-being. Often, these exist within religious contexts and include communal or individual prayer and meditation.

Treatment of Mental Illnesses in Canada

Since colonization of North America by European settlers and the establishment of the nation of Canada, the societal approach to mental health has focused on the treatment of individuals considered to be "mentally ill." At the time of Confederation, it was presumed that mental illnesses were caused by physical disease or damage to the brain, although the specific structures or problems could not be identified. Medical scientists devoted their efforts to finding brain abnormalities, but their efforts were generally unsuccessful. Abnormal brain structure could rarely be identified, even in people with severe mental illnesses.

Without an understanding of the causes of mental illnesses, scientists and physicians were challenged to devise appropriate treatments. Following European examples, residential asylums were established. These were large, hospital-like facilities in which people experiencing mental illnesses were "treated" (Ernst, 2016). Typically, hundreds or thousands of individuals were housed together in institutional settings where they were tended to by physicians, nurses, and orderlies. The stated purpose of these residential asylums was to provide safe settings for physical and spiritual care and to shield individuals from the harm and peril that commonly befell people with mental illnesses. However, a contrary view ascribes less humanitarian motivations for asylum development. This view asserts that members of society were concerned primarily with the segregation of those with mental illnesses, as they did not want the discomfort of eccentric behaviour in their midst.

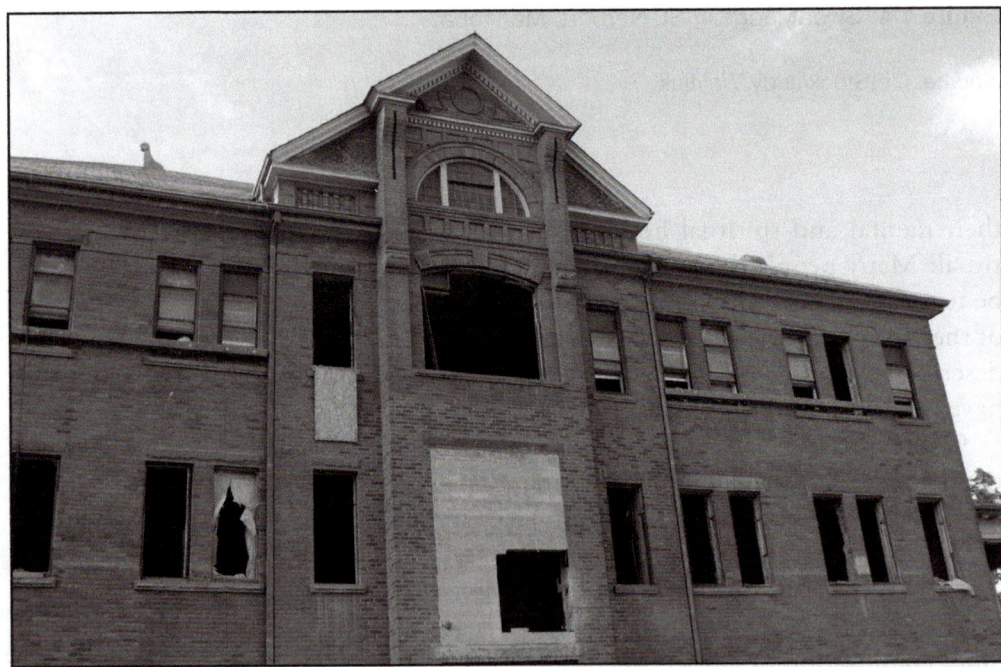

Figure 1.5: Building K of the historic Mimico Lunatic Asylum of the 1880s has been renovated by Humber College in Toronto.

Source: GetStock/Charline Xia

Whatever motivations may have been in play within Canadian society, a policy of institutionalization led to the proliferation of these large asylums, also known as psychiatric hospitals, across the country beginning in the mid- to late- 1800s and continuing until the 1960s. Over the first century of Canada's nationhood, there were few treatments that effectively reduced the suffering of people affected by severe mental illnesses. Historical accounts of Canadian asylums indicate that many tended to be custodial (i.e., providing "protective" supervision) rather than caring. A large proportion of those admitted to these institutions experienced profound trauma and abuse and ended up as inmates for decades of their lives; removed from friends, family, and society. Due to this situation,

> institutions experienced severe overcrowding and had little more than food, clothing, pleasant surroundings, and perhaps some means of employment and exercise to offer. Limited resources made life in institutions difficult. Although a medical superintendent usually directed an institution, overcrowded wards, and few resources created rowdy, dangerous, and unbearable situations. (Austin & Boyd, 2010)

Current wisdom indicates that there is a relatively small group of individuals who do appear to need long-term residential care because the seriousness of their symptoms exceeds the skill sets and capacities of even the most intensive community services and supports. However, such individuals are best served in smaller facilities that are more home-like and less institutional in their design and approach. Most people, even those with relatively severe mental illnesses, can be supported in community settings (Kilian et al., 2016).

Increased Use and Acceptance of Psychotherapy

By the 1950s, while many people with mental illnesses were being placed in large residential asylums, a new development in psychiatry began to have a substantial impact. Psychoanalysis, a form of treatment developed by the Viennese psychiatrist Sigmund Freud in the early 1900s, had become popular in North America as a treatment for less severe and more common mental health challenges (Scull, 2018). Psychoanalysis was based on a complicated set of theories developed by Freud that postulated people's mental health challenges were a result of deep-seated emotional conflicts that people were not even aware of. Psychoanalytic treatment consisted of frequent sessions in which *psychoanalysts* probed into the inner thoughts and conflicts of their clients, who stretched out on the couch and agreed to share their every thought. Psychoanalytic treatment, which could continue for months or even years, aimed to help clients resolve long-standing emotional difficulties. Freud's imaginative theories and ideas captured the interest of artists, writers, and playwrights, who popularized psychoanalysis as a way to explore the depths of the human psyche.

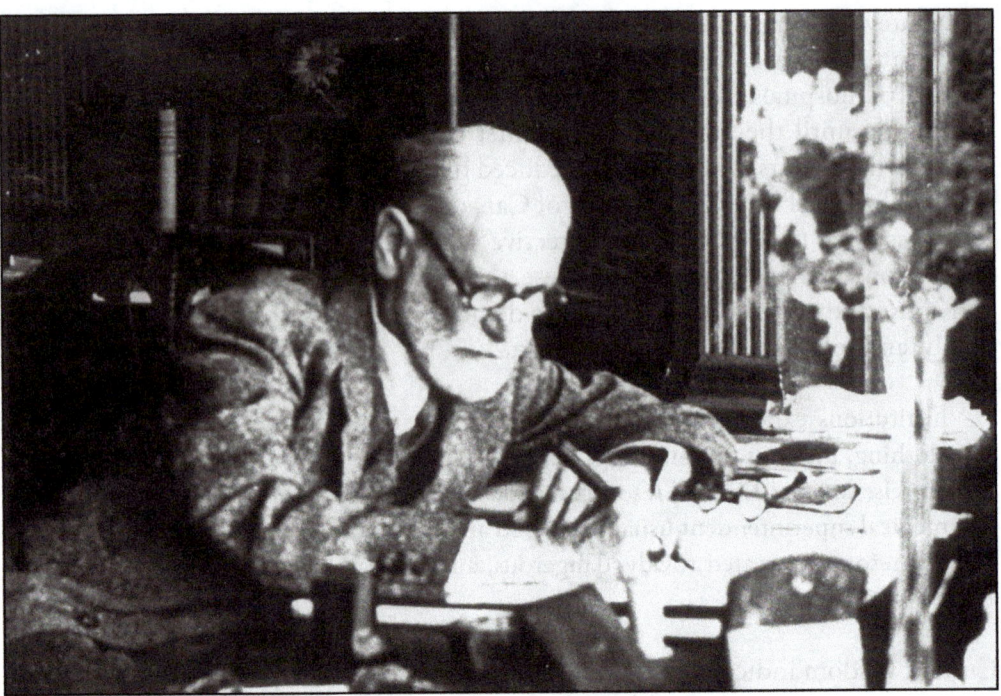

Figure 1.6: Sigmund Freud.

Source: GetStock/topham Picture Point

With the advent of psychoanalysis, a new era of psychotherapy (i.e., talk therapy) had begun. It became commonly accepted that the average person was likely to experience emotional challenges and might benefit from a course of psychotherapy. Previously, psychiatric or psychological treatment was thought to be something required only by individuals who had severe mental health challenges.

With the growing interest in psychotherapy in the mid-20th century, there was a large pendulum swing away from the biologically oriented ideas that had been dominant. Psychosocial theories became more prevalent, resulting in a generation of psychiatrists, psychologists, and other mental health practitioners who distanced themselves from the physical sciences. However, although this pendulum swing was extreme, it was brief. The dominance of psychosocial ideas was overthrown by a rapid succession of discoveries leading to the production of medications that could reduce symptoms of mental illnesses. The latter half of the 20th century was primarily an era of psychopharmacology, in which chemists, psychiatrists, and pharmaceutical companies worked in tandem to produce a panoply of medications to treat a variety of mental illnesses, including psychosis, depression, and anxiety.

Deinstitutionalization of People with Severe Mental Illnesses

The trend of institutionalizing people with severe mental illnesses had continued to increase until the 1960s, when the number of psychiatric beds peaked (see Figure 1.7, summarizing Quebec data, as an example). Concern regarding the dismal conditions of some psychiatric hospitals buoyed a large patient- and family-led movement in support for the policy of **deinstitutionalization, that is, plans by the government to decrease the use of psychiatric hospitals and replace them with community-based treatment.** This push from patients and families, coupled with the optimism that accompanied the introduction of antipsychotic medication, led Canada to begin the process of closing its institutions. Figure 1.7 also illustrates the profound downsizing of psychiatric hospitals over the years. It shows that, despite an increase in the number of general hospital beds available for psychiatric treatment, the total number of psychiatric beds has plummeted.

Deinstitutionalization resulted in the need to develop adequate services for people with severe mental illnesses in community settings through resources for family caregivers, placements in group homes and home shares, supports for independent living, and other services to assist individuals with mental illnesses in being included in their communities. Yet the creation of community-based services has proven to be a difficult and largely unmet challenge as a result of fiscal restraints, competing

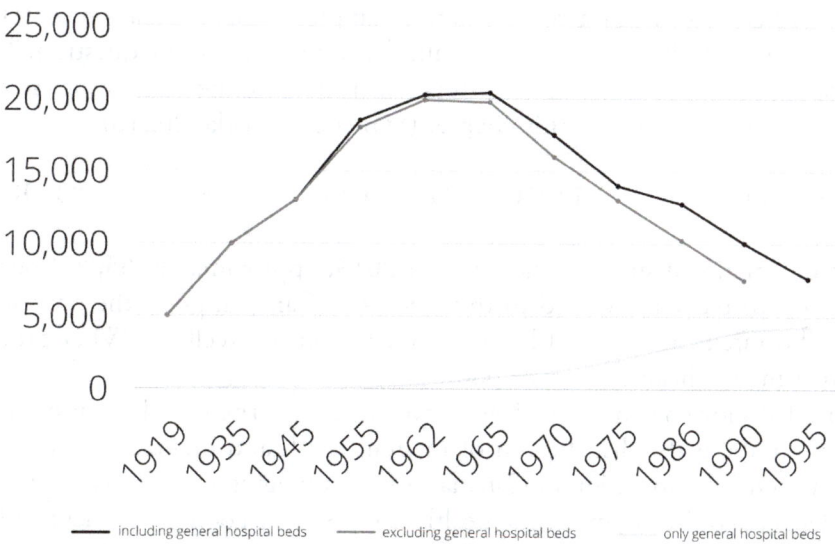

Figure 1.7: Psychiatric beds in Quebec, 1919–1995.

Source: Adapted from Lesage, A.D., Morissette, R., Fortier, L., Reinharz, D., & Contandriopoulos, A.-P. (2000). Downsizing psychiatric hospitals: Needs for care and services of current and discharged long-stay inpatients. *Canadian Journal of Psychiatry, 45*(6), 526–531.

demands for health budget dollars, and broad social factors. Despite intentions to replace institutional care with community supports, funds were often "poached" and diverted to other domains of health care. A system of community-based services that could replace institutional care for people with mental illnesses in Canada has not been adequately developed (Sealy, 2012).

In recent years, there has been profound concern regarding the abysmal health status of people living with severe mental illnesses and the high proportion of mental illnesses among the growing homeless populations in Canada (Krausz et al., 2013; Piat et al., 2015; Zhang et al., 2018). Such concern has been intensified by evidence of an influx of people experiencing mental illnesses to jails and the justice system in general, and high rates of violent criminal victimization of people affected by mental illnesses (Dupuis et al., 2013; Kouyoumdjian et al., 2016; Smith et al., 2019). This movement of individuals with mental illnesses into jails and other institutions, such as hospital emergency departments, is described as **transinstitutionalization** and is considered to be the consequence of inadequate community-based services and supports for individuals who require them (Paradis-Gagné & Jacob, 2020; Primeau et al., 2013; Testa, 2015).

Mental Health of Canadians

In an effort to monitor the mental health of people living in Canada, Statistics Canada gathers data from a representative sample of the population and asks respondents to assess their own mental health by responding to the question, "In general, would you say your mental health is …," providing the same response options as appear at the beginning of this chapter (Statistics Canada, 2021b):

EXCELLENT   VERY GOOD   GOOD   FAIR   POOR

As part of a national survey conducted in 2019, approximately 65,000 people 12 years of age or older responded to this question. Can you guess the proportion of people who rated their mental health as very good or excellent? What proportion rated their mental health as fair or poor?

Figure 1.8 shows a summary of the survey findings. These findings provide useful information about the distribution of mental health and mental health challenges across the general population in Canada. It is encouraging to find that 65 percent of respondents rated their own mental health as either very good or excellent. It is notable, however, that nearly 10 percent of the general population rated their own mental health as fair or poor, an increase over the previous version of this survey. Return to the exercise at the beginning of this chapter in which you and your friend were rating each other's mental health. How do your ratings compare with the general population in Canada?

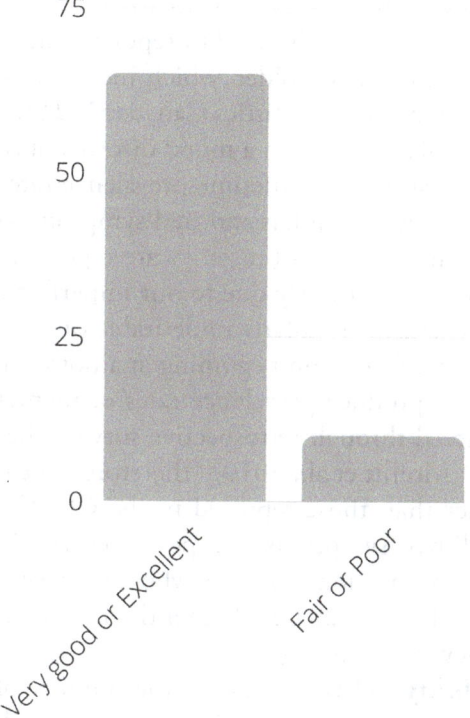

Figure 1.8: Self-rated mental health (percentage of population), Canada, 2019.

Source: Adapted from Statistics Canada. (2021b). *Perceived mental health, by age group* (Table 13-10-0096-03). https://www150.statcan.gc.ca/t1/tbl1/en/tv.action?pid=1310009603

Epidemiology and Mental Health

The type of survey described above is an example of the studies done in the field of **epidemiology**, defined as the study of the distribution of health and illness within populations. Epidemiological studies provide essential information about factors contributing to health and disease, including causation and risk factors, and lead to the development of clinical treatments and public health interventions.

There are a few important terms in epidemiology that you should know in order to understand the findings of epidemiological studies. **Prevalence** is one such term. It is defined as the proportion of individuals in a population who have a particular health condition. Prevalence may be measured at any one point in time (point prevalence) or over a period of time, often one year (12-month prevalence) or lifetime prevalence. For example, the 2019 Canadian Community Health Survey (CCHS), undertaken by Statistics Canada, reported the 12-month prevalence of heavy drinking (5 drinks or more at least once a month in the past year for males;

4 drinks or more for females) to be 18.3 percent (Statistics Canada, 2021a). Using a different type of prevalence measure, the CCHS reported the lifetime prevalence of mood disorders in Canadians 12 and older, which includes forms of depression and bipolar disorder, to be 9.0 percent (Statistics Canada, 2021a). This means that 9 in 100 Canadians have been diagnosed with a mood disorder at some point in their lives. However, it is generally agreed that lifetime prevalence rates, which are based on self-reports of whether an individual has *ever* had symptoms of specific illnesses in their lifetime, are gross underestimates (i.e., they are reported to be much lower than they are in reality). This is most likely due to our imperfect memories and our tendency to forget various events, particularly undesirable ones. In fact, prospective surveys (i.e., ones that gather information beginning at a point in time and looking forward) have been found to produce prevalence rates of mental illnesses that are twice as high as those gathered through retrospective surveys (i.e., ones that gather information about the past; Moffitt et al., 2010). Therefore, true lifetime prevalence rates are likely much higher than those reported in the CCHS and other surveys that require people to recall past symptoms or experiences. A related concept is **incidence**, which refers to the proportion of people who have a *new* case of the condition being studied. The prevalence estimate is higher than the incidence rate because prevalence includes both new and existing cases.

Years Lived with Disability (YLD) represents the number of years of life that have been accompanied by disability due to a disease or injury. YLD is estimated by multiplying the number of incident (new) cases of an illness in a population by the average duration of the condition and a weight factor that reflects the average degree of disability caused by the particular condition. Of the many different injuries and illnesses that exist, the illness that is estimated to be responsible for the greatest number of YLD worldwide is depression (WHO, 2017). This is because depression affects a very large proportion of the population, tends to begin relatively early in life, often recurs or persists, and frequently interferes with an individual's capacity to function across various aspects of their lives.

Years of Life Lost (YLL) is a measure of the number of years of life lost due to premature mortality (death) in the population. It is calculated by multiplying the number of deaths by the estimated number of years of life lost (determined by subtracting the age of death from the average life expectancy). In Nunavut, one of Canada's northern territories, suicide is responsible for more YLL than any other cause of death (Statistics Canada, 2018). Once again, one of the reasons for this high rate is that these suicides often occur relatively early in life and are thus responsible for the loss of many years of expected longevity. A critical question that needs to be addressed is how to best reduce high rates of suicide in Nunavut and other northern and rural communities in Canada.

Another important population health measure is **Disability Adjusted Life Years (DALY)**. It is created by combining the years lived with disability (YLD) and the years of life lost (YLL) and, consequently, provides a pooled measure of disability and premature mortality. DALYs have been used extensively by the WHO and by other public health scientists to estimate the **burden of disease** caused by various illnesses and injuries (Vos et al., 2012). According to recent data, mental illnesses are amongst the top two contributors to the global burden of disease (as measured by DALYs; Vigo et al., 2016). Further, in high income-countries, including Canada, depression is estimated to be *the* leading contributor to the burden of disease (WHO, 2010). As well as depression, other mental health challenges contribute significantly to the burden of disease. Both alcohol use disorders and self-inflicted injuries are among the top 20 contributors to burden of disease worldwide (Institute for Health Metrics and Evaluation, 2018).

Mental Health Epidemiology in Canada

A research project undertaken for the Mental Health Commission of Canada estimated the prevalence rates of mental illnesses in Canada in 2011 and projected forward in time to estimate expected rates in the year 2041. The project utilized data that had been collected by Statistics Canada and through other surveys to create the best possible epidemiological estimates (Mental Health Commission of Canada, 2013b). Figure 1.9 shows that, in the year 2011, the

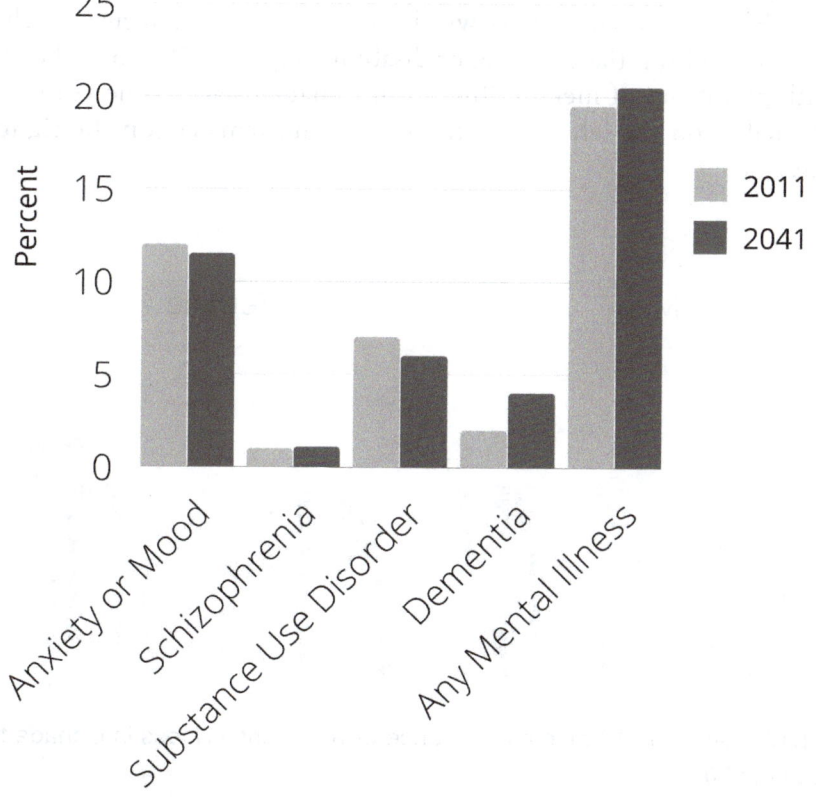

Figure 1.9: Estimated 12-month prevalence of specific mental illnesses in Canada.

Source: Adapted from Mental Health Commission of Canada. (2013a). *Making the case for investing in mental health in Canada*. https://www.mentalhealthcommission.ca/sites/default/files/2016-06/Investing_in_Mental_Health_FINAL_Version_ENG.pdf

12-month prevalence of mental illnesses was estimated to be about 20 percent. This means that, at that time, approximately one in five people had some form of mental illness, such as depression, an anxiety disorder, schizophrenia, substance use disorder, or dementia, in the past year. By modelling the expected growth of the population and anticipated demographic changes (such as the proportion of young and elderly people), the project was also able to estimate the 12-month prevalence of these mental health challenges in the year 2041. The projected increases are due to a predicted growth in the size of the population of older adults and, consequently, an increased prevalence of dementia expected to occur by 2041.

The project also estimated that, by the time Canadians reach the age of 40, approximately 50 percent will have or will have had a mental illness. If people reach the age of 90, approximately 65 percent of men and 70 percent of women will have had a mental illness. The high rate of mental illnesses in the population may surprise you. Indeed, these estimates indicate that most Canadians will experience a mental illness during their life. Of course, in many instances, individuals will have relatively short-lasting periods of illness that are mild to moderate in nature. However, many others will have long-lasting or recurring challenges that may cause substantial suffering or disability. Figure 1.10 shows the estimated 12-month prevalence of mental illnesses in Canadians aged nine years and older for both males (on the left side of the figure) and females (on the right side of the figure).

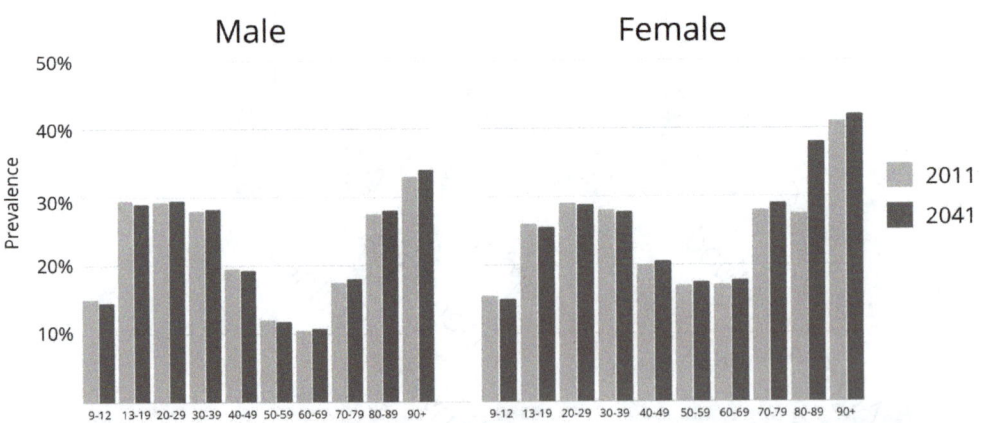

Figure 1.10: Estimated 12-month prevalence of any mental illness in Canada for select years, 2011 to 2041.

Source: Adapted from Mental Health Commission of Canada. (2013a). *Making the case for investing in mental health in Canada*. https://www.mentalhealthcommission.ca/sites/default/files/2016-06/Investing_in_Mental_Health_FINAL_Version_ENG.pdf

Males and females show a similar pattern, with the prevalence of mental illnesses rising relatively high in the teenage years and in early adulthood. The prevalence then drops in people in their forties, fifties, and sixties and then rises again among individuals living into their seventies, eighties, nineties, and beyond. The high rate of mental illnesses among people in the older age groups is due primarily to the incidence of dementia, a mental illness that most often begins later in life, becoming increasingly common as people age.

Overall, the prevalence of mental illnesses in males and females were found to be similar, with estimates among females somewhat higher than males (20.9 percent among females and 18.7 percent among males) in the year 2011. In Chapter 7, we discuss potential reasons for this disparity.

Figure 1.11 shows that, when we look across the lifespan at the absolute numbers of people with mental illnesses in any one year, the largest number of people are in their twenties. Unlike many other health challenges and illnesses, mental illnesses commonly emerge early in people's lives. As discussed above, this is one of the main factors contributing to the high YLD and the high burden of disease attributed to mental illnesses.

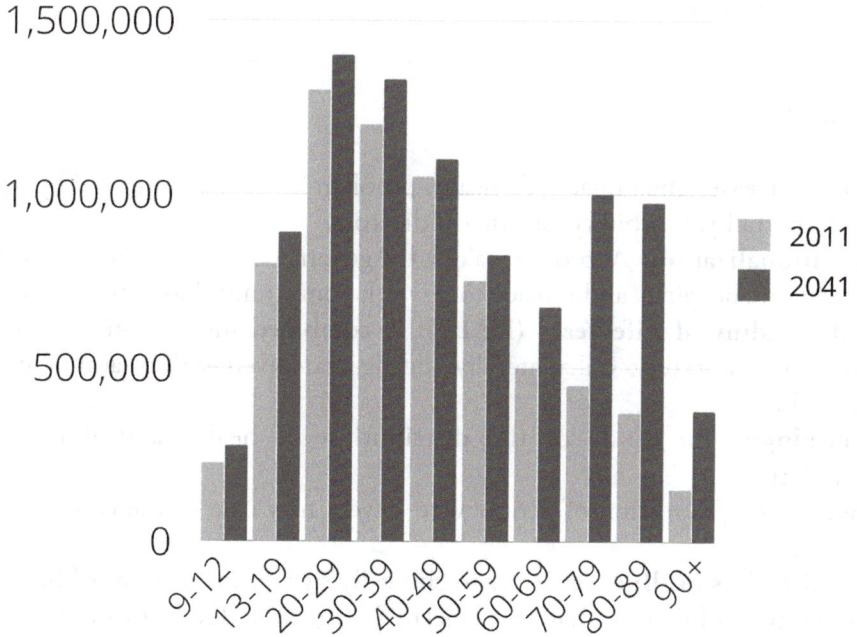

Figure 1.11: Number of people in Canada with mental illnesses by age group.

Source: Adapted from Mental Health Commission of Canada. (2013a). *Making the case for investing in mental health in Canada*. https://www.mentalhealthcommission.ca/sites/default/files/2016-06/Investing_in_Mental_Health_FINAL_Version_ENG.pdf

Conclusion

We started the chapter by asking the question "What is mental health?" It turns out that the answer is not straightforward. However, there is general agreement that mental health is not only the absence of mental illnesses but also the ability to enjoy and participate meaningfully in daily life. Mental health refers to the health of the "mind," a construct that includes the brain as well as the environment in which the brain functions.

There is a rich history in Canada of approaches taken to support mental health and respond to mental ill health. A prominent change over the past century has been a movement away from the institutionalization of people with severe mental illnesses to approaches that emphasize community-based services and supports. This change has been spurred by advancements in treatment, which have led to improvements in the trajectories of mental illnesses, particularly those that are considered severe and persistent. Epidemiological methods have provided useful measures to understand the distribution of mental health and illness within the population as well as changes over time.

Next, in Chapters 2 and 3, we will explore various factors that contribute to the mental health of people in Canada by applying, first, a physical sciences perspective and, second, a social sciences perspective.

Glossary

burden of disease: The impact of a health problem in an area measured by financial cost, mortality, morbidity, or other indicators.

deinstitutionalization: A process taken by governments to decrease the use of psychiatric hospitals and replace them with community-based treatment.

Disability Adjusted Life Years (DALY): A combined measure of disability and premature mortality. Calculated by adding years lived with disability and years of life lost.

epidemiology: The study of the distribution of health and illness within populations.

incidence: The proportion of people who have a new case of the condition being studied.

mental disorders or illnesses: Refer to clinically significant patterns of behavioural or emotional function that are associated with some level of distress, suffering (even to the point of pain and death), or impairment in one or more areas of functioning (e.g., school, work, social and family interactions).

mental health: A state of well-being in which an individual realizes their potential, can cope with the normal stresses of life, can work productively and fruitfully, and is able to make a contribution to their community.

mental health problems (or challenges): Refer to reduced capacities—whether cognitive, emotional, attentional, interpersonal, motivational, or behavioural—that impact an individual's enjoyment of life or negatively affect interactions with society and the environment.

mental status examination: A series of observations, structured questions, and tests undertaken by a health care professional to evaluate a person's mental health.

prevalence: The proportion of individuals in a population who have a particular health condition.

socioecological perspective: A conceptual model for understanding health as a product of the interactions between an individual and their broader family, community, and societal contexts.

transinstitutionalization: The process by which individuals who historically would have been detained inside mental health institutions are instead being transferred into detention by other state institutions (criminal justice system, general hospitals).

Years of Life Lost (YLL): A measure of the number of years of life lost due to premature mortality (death) in the population.

Years Lived with Disability (YLD): The number of years of life accompanied by disability due to a disease or injury.

Critical Thinking Questions

1. Describe the ways that mental health been defined.
2. What is the difference between the brain and the mind?
3. Define deinstitutionalization and explain how it has impacted services for those with mental illnesses.
4. What are some of the key terms that are used to describe the epidemiology of mental health and illness within a population?

Recommended Readings

Cairney, J., & Streiner, D. L. (Eds.). (2010). *Mental disorder in Canada: An epidemiological perspective*. University of Toronto Press.

Goffman, E. (1961). *Asylums: Essays on the social situation of mental patients and other inmates*. Doubleday.

Jenkins, E. (2014). The politics of knowledge: Implications for understanding and addressing mental health and illness. *Nursing Inquiry, 21*(1), 3–10.

Paris, J. (2015). *The intelligent clinician's guide to the DSM-5*. Oxford University Press.

Pietikainen, P. (2015). *Madness: A history*. Routledge.

Purtle, J., Nelson, K. L., Counts, N. Z., & Yudell, M. (2020). Population-based approaches to mental health: History, strategies, and evidence. *Annual Review of Public Health, 41*(1), 201–221.

Recommended Websites

Madness Canada. www.madnesscanada.com
The Mental Health Commission of Canada. www.mentalhealthcommission.ca
Network for Aboriginal Mental Health Research. www.namhr.ca
The World Health Organization—Mental Health and Substance Use. www.who.int/mental-health-and-substance-use
The World Mental Health Survey Initiative. www.hcp.med.harvard.edu/wmh

References

Austin, W., & Boyd, M. A. (2010). *Psychiatric and mental health nursing for Canadian practice*. Lippincott Williams & Wilkins.
Blows, W. T. (2016). *The biological basis of mental health* (3rd ed.). Routledge.
Dupuis, T., MacKay, R., & Nichol, J. (2013). *Current issues in mental health in Canada: Mental health and the criminal justice system* (Publication No. 2013-88-E). Library of Parliament. https://publications.gc.ca/collections/collection_2014/bdp-lop/bp/2013-88-eng.pdf
Ernst, W. (2016). Therapy and empowerment, coercion and punishment: Historical and contemporary perspectives on work, psychiatry, and society. In W. Ernst (Ed.), *Work, psychiatry, and society, c. 1750–2015* (pp. 1–30). Manchester University Press.
Howell, T., Auger, M., Gomes, T., Brown, F. L., & Leon, A. Y. (2016). Sharing our wisdom: A holistic Aboriginal health initiative. *International Journal of Indigenous Health, 11*(1), 111–132. https://doi.org/10.18357/ijih111201616015
Institute for Health Metrics and Evaluation. (2018). *Findings from the Global Burden of Disease study 2017*. IHME. http://www.healthdata.org/sites/default/files/files/policy_report/2019/GBD_2017_Booklet.pdf
Kilian, R., Becker, T., & Frasch, K. (2016). Effectiveness and cost-effectiveness of home treatment compared with inpatient care for patients with acute mental disorders in a rural catchment area in Germany. *Neurology, Psychiatry and Brain Research, 22*(2), 81–86. https://doi.org/10.1016/j.npbr.2016.01.005
Kirby, M. J. L., & Keon, W. J. (2004). *Mental health, mental illness and addiction: Overview of policies and programs in Canada*. The Standing Senate Committee on Social Affairs, Science and Technology. https://sencanada.ca/content/sen/Committee/381/soci/rep/report1/repintnov04vol1-e.pdf
Kohlberg, L., Levine, C., & Hewer, A. (1983). *Moral stages: A current formulation and a response to critics*. Karger.

Kouyoumdjian, F., Schuler, A., Matheson, F. I., & Hwang, S. W. (2016). Health status of prisoners in Canada: Narrative review. *Canadian Family Physician, 62*(3), 215–222.

Krausz, R. M., Clarkson, A. F., Strehlau, V., Torchalla, I., Li, K., & Schuetz, C. G. (2013). Mental disorder, service use, and barriers to care among 500 homeless people in 3 different urban settings. *Social Psychiatry and Psychiatric Epidemiology, 48*(8), 1235–1243. https://doi.org/10.1007/s00127-012-0649-8

Lesage, A. D., Morissette, R., Fortier, L., Reinharz, D., & Contandriopoulos, A.-P. (2000). Downsizing psychiatric hospitals: Needs for care and services of current and discharged long-stay inpatients. *Canadian Journal of Psychiatry, 45*(6), 526–531. https://doi.org/10.1177/070674370004500602

Mental Health Commission of Canada. (2013a). *Making the case for investing in mental health in Canada*. https://www.mentalhealthcommission.ca/wp-content/uploads/drupal/2016-06/Investing_in_Mental_Health_FINAL_Version_ENG.pdf

Mental Health Commission of Canada. (2013b). *Why investing in mental health will contribute to Canada's economic prosperity and to the sustainability of our health care system*. https://www.mentalhealthcommission.ca/sites/default/files/mhstrategy_case_for_investment_backgrounder_eng_0_0.pdf

Moffitt, T. E., Caspi, A., Taylor, A., Kokaua, J., Milne, B. J., Polanczyk, G., & Poulton, R. (2010). How common are common mental disorders? Evidence that lifetime prevalence rates are doubled by prospective versus retrospective ascertainment. *Psychological Medicine, 40*(6), 899–909. https://doi.org/10.1017/S0033291709991036

Paradis-Gagné, E., & Jacob, J. D. (2020). Judiciarization of people suffering from mental illness: A critical analysis of the psychiatric-judicial interface. *Journal of Psychiatric and Mental Health Nursing, 28*(2), 291–298. https://doi.org/10.1111/jpm.12667

Piat, M., Polvere, L., Kirst, M., Voronka, J., Zabkiewicz, D., Plante., M.-C., Isaak, C., Nolin, D., Nelson, G., & Goering, P. (2015). Pathways into homelessness: Understanding how both individual and structural factors contribute to and sustain homelessness in Canada. *Urban Studies, 52*(13), 2366–2382. https://doi.org/10.1177/0042098014548138

Primeau, A., Bowers, T. G., Harrison, M. A., & XuXu. (2013). Deinstitutionalization of the mentally ill: Evidence for transinstitutionalization from psychiatric hospitals to penal institutions. *Comprehensive Psychology, 2*, Article 2. https://doi.org/10.2466/16.02.13.CP.2.2

Sasakamoose, J., Scerbe, A., Wenaus, I., & Scandrett, A. (2016). First Nations and Métis youth perspectives of health: An Indigenous qualitative inquiry. *Qualitative Inquiry, 22*(8), 636–650. https://doi.org/10.1177/1077800416629695

Scull, A. (2018). Creating a new psychiatry: On the origins of non-institutional psychiatry in the USA, 1900–50. *History of Psychiatry, 29*(4), 389–408. https://doi.org/10.1177/0957154X18793596

Sealy, P. A. (2012). The impact of the process of deinstitutionalization of mental health services in Canada: An increase in accessing of health professionals for mental health concerns. *Social Work in Public Health, 27*(3), 229–237. https://doi.org/10.1080/19371911003748786

Smith, H. P., Sitren, A. H., & King, S. (2019). "A call to action": Mental illness and self-injurious behavior occuring in jails & prisons. *Journal of Health and Human Services Administration, 41*(4), 16–44.

Statistics Canada. (2018). *Mortality and potential years of life lost, by selected causes of death and sex, five-year period, Canada and Inuit regions* (Table 13-10-0157-01). https://www150.statcan.gc.ca/t1/tbl1/en/cv.action?pid=1310015701

Statistics Canada. (2021a). *Health characteristics, annual estimates* (Table 13-10-0096-01). https://www150.statcan.gc.ca/t1/tbl1/en/tv.action?pid=1310009601

Statistics Canada. (2021b). *Perceived mental health, by age group* (Table 13-10-0096-03). https://www150.statcan.gc.ca/t1/tbl1/en/tv.action?pid=1310009603

Testa, M. (2015). Imprisonment of the mentally ill: A call for diversion to the community mental health system. *Albany Government Law Review, 8*, 405–438.

Vigo, D., Thornicroft, G., & Atun, R. (2016). Estimating the true global burden of mental illness. *The Lancet Psychiatry, 3*(2), 171–178. https://doi.org/10.1016/S2215-0366(15)00505-2

Vos, T., Allen, C., Arora, M., Barber, R. M., Bhutta, Z. A., Brown, A., Carter, A., Casey, D. C., Charlson, F. J., Chen, A. Z., Coggeshall, M., Cornaby, L., Dandona, L., Dicker, D. J., Dilegge, T., Erskine, H. E., Ferrari, A. J., Fitzmaurice, C., Fleming, T., … Murray, C. J. L. (2012). Global, regional, and national incidence, prevalence, and years lived with disability for 310 diseases and injuries, 1990–2015: A systematic analysis for the Global Burden of Disease Study 2015. *The Lancet, 388*(10053), 1545–1602. https://doi.org/10.1016/S0140-6736(16)31678-6

Westerhof, G. J., & Keyes, C. L. M. (2010). Mental illness and mental health: The two continua model across the lifespan. *Journal of Adult Development, 17*, 110–119. https://doi.org/10.1007/s10804-009-9082-y

World Health Organization. (2004). *Promoting mental health: Concepts, emerging evidence, practice: A summary report*. https://www.who.int/mental_health/evidence/en/promoting_mhh.pdf

World Health Organization. (2010). *Mental health: Depression*. www.who.int/mental_health/management/depression/en/

World Health Organization. (2014). *Mental health: A state of well-being*. www.who.int/features/factfiles/mental_health/en/

World Health Organization. (2017). *Depression and other common mental disorders: Global health estimates*. https://apps.who.int/iris/bitstream/handle/10665/254610/WHO-MSD-MER-2017.2-eng.pdf

Zhang, L., Norena, M., Gadermann, A., Hubley, A., Russell, L., Aubry, T., To, M. J., Farrell, S., Hwang, S., & Papelu, A. (2018). Concurrent disorders and health care utilization among homeless and vulnerably housed persons in Canada. *Journal of Dual Diagnosis, 14*(1), 21–31. https://doi.org/10.1080/15504263.2017.1392055

Chapter 2

Understanding Mental Health through the Physical Sciences

> The hypothalamus is one of the most important parts of the brain, involved in many kinds of motivation, among other functions. The hypothalamus controls the "Four F's": fighting, fleeing, feeding, and mating.
> —Karl Pribram (neuroscientist and neurosurgeon)

Introduction

In this chapter, we present knowledge about mental health and illness generated through the physical sciences, which include biology, chemistry, physics, and neuroscience. The physical sciences have focused our understandings of mental health and illness heavily on the brain and associated activities. Healthy functioning of the brain is, of course, an important component of good mental health. The structural and electrochemical function of the brain is so highly sophisticated and advanced that the world's most impressive human-made technological achievements cannot begin to compare to its astounding features. The average brain consists of about 100 billion (100,000,000,000) **neurons** or cells (von Bartheld et al., 2016). Even more difficult to fathom is the number of interconnections among these neurons. Since each individual neuron may be connected to 10,000 others (Eysenck & Keane, 2015), the number of connections is so immense that it defies imagination and is thought to be similar to the number of elementary particles that exist in the entire universe.

To add to the astounding number of interconnections among neurons, the electrical impulses that fire rapidly through this enormous web of connections do so in parallel and they are modulated by the secretion of **neurotransmitters**—chemical messengers that alter electrical transmission by their release and uptake into the microscopic spaces, or synapses, present between the neurons. Neuroscience researchers have mapped the existence of a group of neurotransmitters with varying

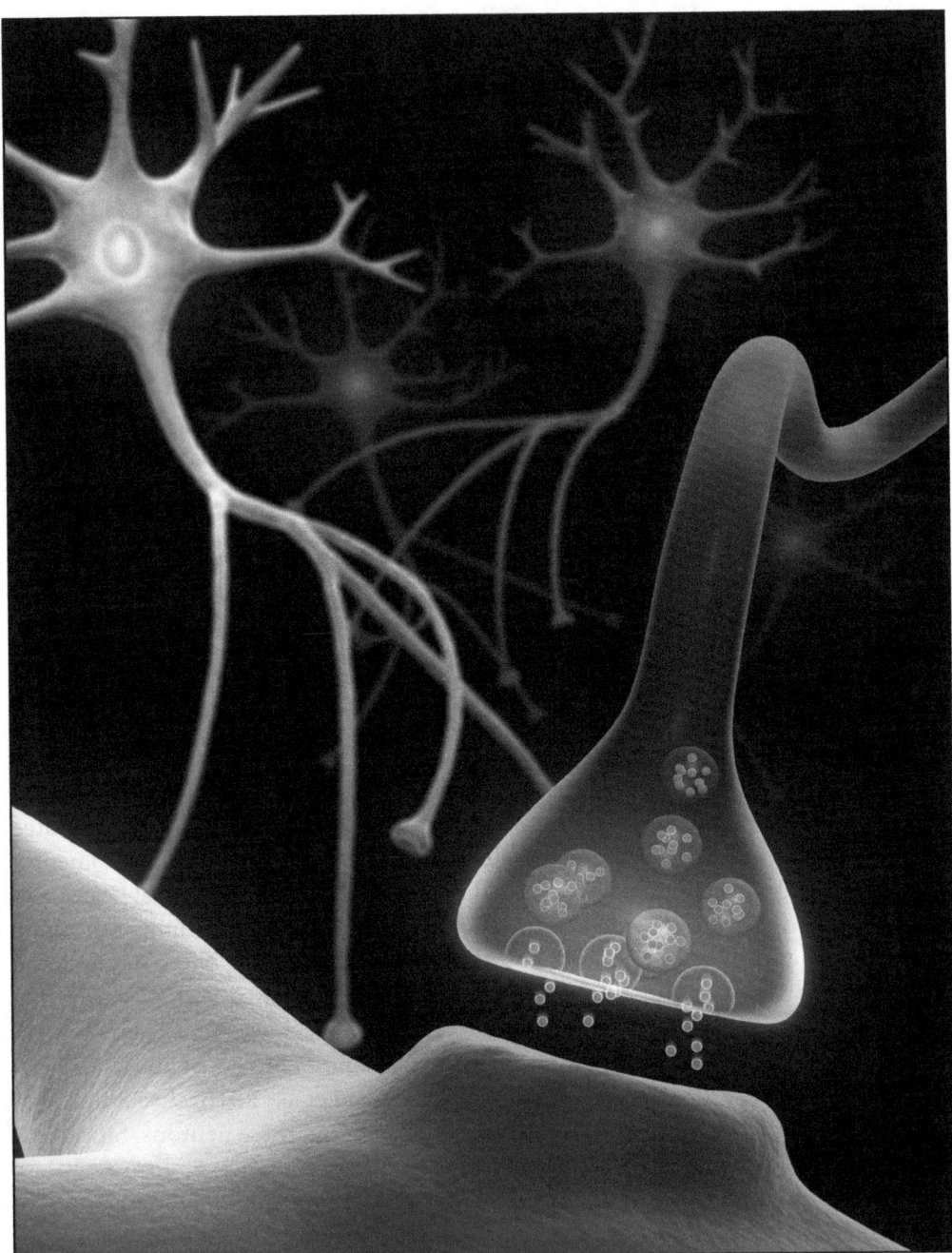

Figure 2.1: Neurotransmitters, the brain's "chemical messengers," are released into synapses and taken up by a receptor.

Source: iStockphoto/Xiaofeng Luo

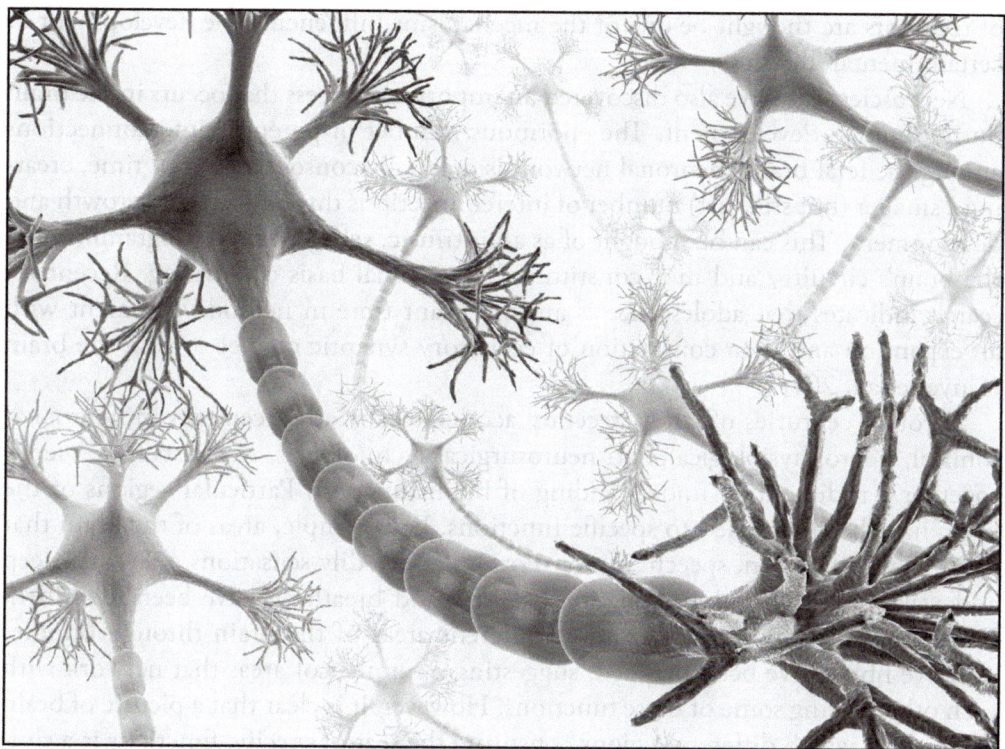

Figure 2.2: The average brain consists of 100 *billion* (100,000,000,000) neurons.

Source: iStockphoto/ktsimage

chemical composition, some of which tend to promote the transmission of electrical impulses across the synapse, whereas others may inhibit neurotransmission. The most abundant neurotransmitter in the brain is glutamate, which is excitatory, whereas the chief inhibitory neurotransmitter is GABA (gamma-amino-butyric acid). Other neurotransmitters include monoamines, such as norepinephrine, dopamine, and serotonin, and these appear to play important roles in regulation of mood and emotion. Various types of receptors have been identified that are responsive to the neurotransmitter molecules released into the synapses and it has been found that certain drugs have an influence on these and can modulate neurotransmission in particular areas of the brain. Psychoactive substances such as caffeine, cocaine, opioids, and cannabis appear to exert their effects in this way. Similarly, antidepressant and antipsychotic medications are thought to exert their therapeutic effects through the modulation of neurotransmitters at these receptor sites. Some receptors have been found to become less responsive (i.e., "downregulated") when they are repeatedly exposed to high levels of neurotransmitters. Such changes in the responsiveness of receptors are thought be one of the mechanisms influencing the development of certain mental illnesses.

Neuroscientists have also discovered an important process that occurs in the brain during human development. The enormous number of potential interconnections among the fetal brain's neuronal network is gradually consolidated over time, creating a smaller (but still vast) number of interconnections through a child's growth and development. This can be thought of as an intrinsic, self-generated programming of the brain's circuitry and may constitute the neuronal basis of learning. Recent research indicates that adolescence is an important time in neurodevelopment with an expansion and then contraction of excitatory synaptic connections in the brain (Guyer et al., 2016).

Through centuries of study, recently accelerated by advancements in neuroanatomical, neurophysiological, and neurosurgical technologies, scientists have pieced together a rudimentary understanding of brain function. Particular regions of the brain have been matched to specific functions. For example, areas of the brain that are involved in vision, speech, motor movements, bodily sensations, memory, sleep and wakefulness, emotion, appetite, balance, and breathing have been identified. Furthermore, pathways that connect different areas of the brain through bundles of nerve fibres have been mapped, suggesting a number of areas that network with each other during some of these functions. However, it is clear that a picture of brain function in which different regions constitute the seat of specific functions is a simplistic one. Brain functions involve multiple regions working in synchrony (Bowyer, 2016). The mind relies on complex brain activity and interposes past experiences, imbued with cultural meaning, fuelled with knowledge gained through a lifetime and accumulated through human history.

Box 2.1: The BRAIN Initiative

The BRAIN (Brain Research through Advancing Innovative Neurotechnologies) Initiative is a large and ambitious research project that, since 2013, has received many millions of dollars in funding from the US government. It involves researchers from more than 125 institutions in the US as well as collaboration with researchers in other countries, including Canada. The goal is to make substantial strides in uncovering the mysteries of brain disorders such as schizophrenia, autism, Alzheimer's disease, depression, and traumatic brain injury. It is hoped that the BRAIN Initiative will develop and apply new technologies that will enable researchers to produce dynamic images of the brain, show how individual brain cells and complex neural circuits process thought, language, and emotion; shed light on the complex links between brain function and behaviour; and examine potential new treatment technologies and interventions. Current priority areas for research include mapping the brain at multiple levels of scale, from individual synapses to the entire brain, and developing tools to identify and manipulate specific neurons responsible for health and disease.

In this chapter, we discuss a number of the prominent functions of the brain and features of mental activity. We also point to some of the key structures and functions that are relevant to mental health and illness.

Brain Functions and Mental Activity

Wakefulness/Arousal

Our minds function in different states of arousal, ranging from deep stages of sleep to highly stimulated wakefulness and arousal. An area known as the reticular formation, located deep in the core of the brain in the brainstem and midbrain, plays an important role in the regulation of sleep, wakefulness, and arousal. However, many brain areas appear to work in complex interaction to regulate these states. The healthy mind has a regular pattern of sleep and wakefulness, whereas injury or disease can result in disturbances in these states, including a prolonged loss of consciousness, known as a coma. We commonly alter our state of arousal through the use of substances that cause either stimulation or sedation. The use of coffee, tea, or other caffeine-containing drinks to stimulate arousal is common in many societies and cultures.

Box 2.2: Caffeine Drinks

Drinks containing caffeine, such as coffee, tea, and types of soda, stimulate areas of the brain, such as the reticular formation, involved in arousal and wakefulness (Cortés et al., 2016). The resulting feelings of alertness and heightened energy are responsible for the popularity and widespread use of these beverages. It is estimated that more than 75 percent of adults in Canada ingest caffeine on any given day (Statistics Canada, 2008), and it is likely that the majority would have great difficulty stopping. Does this mean that the vast majority of Canadians are physically dependent on caffeine? We will examine this question in more depth in Chapter 5, where we address substance use.

Other substances, such as alcohol, opiates, and various sedatives, commonly diminish alertness and arousal and may induce sleep. Mental activity during sleep remains largely mysterious, and although a number of theories about the language and meaning of dreams have been proposed, they remain unconfirmed.

Regulation of Physiological Activity

Another set of functions that involve brain areas in the brainstem and midbrain regulate rhythmic physiological activities such as breathing and heart rate. These functions occur mostly without our awareness. Yet changes in our overall state of mind may have a profound impact on these rhythms. For example, an intense state of fear will generally result in a marked increase in one's heart rate and breathing pattern, whereas feelings of deep relaxation and comfort may decrease heart rate and slow the pace of respiration. Numerous experimental studies have demonstrated that individuals who are accomplished at meditative and yogic practices are able to reliably induce such changes in physiological activity (Carter & Carter, 2016).

Sensation/Perception

A central function of the mind is integrating the extensive information collected through the body's many sources of sensory reception. Sensory input includes information about touch, pressure, pain, and temperature collected from nerve endings throughout the body. Areas of the cerebral cortex correspond to specific parts of the body. When these areas are activated by electrical stimulation, the result is a sensation in the corresponding body part. Figure 2.3 shows a strip of the cerebral cortex,

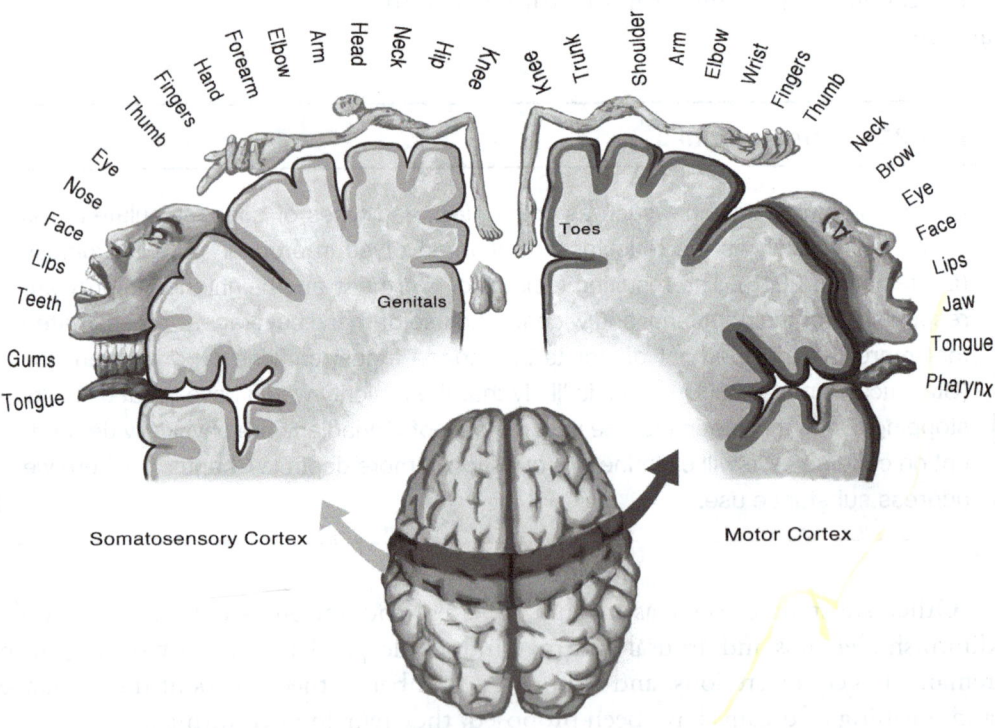

Figure 2.3: Somatosensory homunculus.

Source: Alamy Stock Photo/Science History Images

located on the postcentral gyri, which contains areas that correspond to different parts of the body. These are illustrated in a drawing of a *homunculus* (Latin for "little person") in which the size of various body parts on the drawing are representative of the area of cerebral cortex devoted to them. For example, the face and lips of the somatosensory homunculus are large because a relatively large area of cortex is connected to them and, correspondingly, they have more sensory receptivity than many other parts of the body. That is why being kissed on the face or lips can be so pleasurable.

Another type of sensory input is proprioceptive, coming from movement receptors in joints and muscles throughout the body. The mind also integrates sensory input from special visual, auditory (hearing), olfactory (smell), and gustatory (taste) receptors.

Many parts of the brain are involved with the processing of sensory input, and specific areas of the cerebral cortex have a role in processing special sensory information, such as visual and auditory input. The mind appears to make sense of the large amount of incoming information through the web of interconnections that are established in the brain. Instantaneously, meaning is assigned on the basis of recognized patterns and combinations. In this way, the mind accomplishes a complex perception of events through signals received from multiple sources. For example, a bright flash of light across the sky followed by a thunderous boom will immediately be identified as an electrical storm. The perception may also invoke a flood of emotions and memories.

When the mind is healthy, the analysis and perception of sensory input will be relatively accurate. Under the influence of various psychoactive substances or when mental health is impaired, the mind may create distorted perception. Thus, the rustling of wind might be misperceived to be a human voice or the touch of bedsheets on one's skin to be crawling insects.

Movement

Both simple and complex movements of the body are generated through mental activity involving multiple areas of the brain working together in synchrony. Areas of the **cerebral hemispheres**, called the motor cortex, play a key role in sending signals to the many muscles of the body. Movement is often modulated through the integration of sensory information received in rapid sequence and appears to be adjusted by information about balance and coordination through activity in the cerebellum, the lobe of the brain located at the back and bottom of the skull. Complex physical actions, such as running on uneven ground, require rapid coordination of muscle groups and immediate integration of proprioceptive and visual sensory information.

An individual's motor activity may reflect their mental state. Good mental health is generally associated with a good balance of motor activity, characterized by the ability to assume a comfortable resting state as well as the capacity to shift into motion easily. Someone who is in a state of hyperarousal and agitation may demonstrate hyperactive movements, with an inability to assume a resting state. This can result from the use of stimulant drugs such as cocaine, methamphetamine, or high doses of caffeine and may occur as a feature of certain mental illnesses. Conversely, some mental states will result in the profound slowing of psychomotor activity. This may occur in individuals with severe forms of depressive illness or accompany the use of drugs with sedative properties, for example, opioids and alcohol.

Thought, Emotion, and Memory

These complex mental functions form the foundation of humankind's accomplishments in science, art, literature, architecture, philosophy, and other endeavours. The capacity of the human mind to generate ideas, apply reasoning, attach emotional significance, and build banks of knowledge has distinguished humans from other animals and has permitted the creation of human civilizations.

We have barely scratched the surface in our attempts to understand the brain mechanisms that are involved with thought, emotion, and memory. These functions are interrelated and they involve simultaneous activity in many areas of the brain.

Thought and reasoning appear to draw on the immense interconnectivity of neurons in the cerebral hemispheres as well as those in other regions of the brain. The relative size and architectural complexity of the human cerebral hemispheres exceed parallel structures in other animals and facilitate the advanced capacity of the human mind for thinking and reasoning. With good mental health, an individual is able to think and reason clearly, make use of stored knowledge, and draw logical inferences. Once again, under the influence of certain psychoactive substances or with the presence of some mental illnesses, thinking and reasoning can become markedly distorted. In these circumstances, illogical or unlikely inferences can be drawn, resulting in delusions (i.e., fixed false beliefs).

Emotions frequently occur in connection with thoughts or ideas and are often initiated by sensory input and memories. The **limbic system** is a series of interconnected structures in different regions of the brain that are important in producing mood and emotions. Areas of the brain that are part of the limbic system include the cingulate gyrus, thalamus, hypothalamus, amygdala, and hippocampus. Some of these structures also appear to play an important role in long-term memory. Another structure with a central role in emotion is the nucleus accumbens, an area that becomes active with pleasurable behaviours, such as eating food or having sex. This area is also thought to be involved in the pleasurable feelings induced by various psychoactive substances.

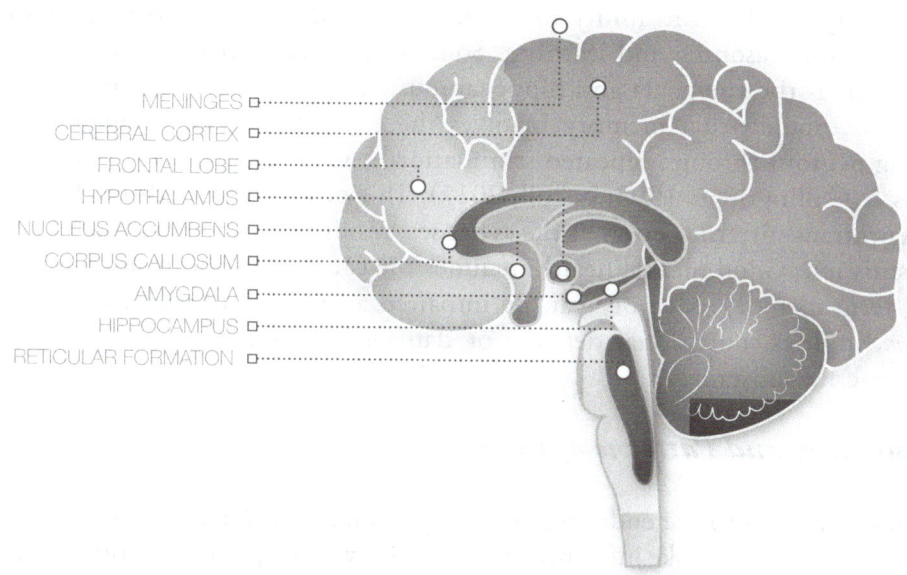

Figure 2.4: Brain structures. See Table 2.1 for description of the functions associated with each of these brain structures.

Source: Daniel Wierzbicki, Designer

Mood refers to the predominant background emotional state that persists in an individual over an extended period of time. A common mental health challenge is depressed mood, in which feelings of sadness, lack of pleasure, and decreased interest persist. Mood can also be elevated excessively as in manic or hypomanic states. Good mental health involves the capacity to be emotionally responsive without experiencing extreme or labile (i.e., rapidly shifting and unstable) mood swings.

Box 2.3: Anosognosia

Anosognosia is a symptom in which an individual does not have the ability to recognize that they have a specific health condition. It has been found to be the result of damage to areas in the cerebral hemispheres, that is, within the parietal and frontal lobes, and often occurs following a stroke (sudden damage to brain cells caused either by the rupture of blood vessels supplying the brain or by a blockage of blood vessels to the brain). An example of anosognosia would be a person with a paralyzed arm, who is completely unable to recognize this condition. Even if a physician tries to bring the paralyzed arm to the person's attention, they would not recognize or acknowledge the paralysis. More recently, the symptom of anosognosia has been considered to be operating among individuals with certain mental illnesses. For example, it is thought that individuals with schizophrenia may have anosognosia and are thus unable to recognize that they are experiencing hallucinations and delusions. Whether this symptom may be the result of some neurological impairment is not yet known and requires further research.

Memory involves the ability to store, retain, and retrieve information and is necessary for reasoning and learning. Some of the brain areas in the limbic system, such as the amygdala and hippocampus, appear to play an important role, and it is thought that memory involves the enhancement of interconnections among neurons through repeated stimulation, known as long-term potentiation (Bliss & Collingridge, 1993; Nicoll, 2017). This process occurs through changes in neurotransmitter function at the synapses, resulting in the potentiated neurotransmission. Good mental health includes the capacity for both short-term and long-term memory. Memory can be impaired as a result of various mental illnesses, injuries, nutritional deficits, or damage incurred through use of some psychoactive substances.

Personality and Patterns of Behaviour

Personality refers to the enduring behavioural traits and characteristics of an individual. We generally make inferences about an individual's personality on the basis of the characteristic behaviour patterns that are observed. For example, one personality dimension is introversion-extroversion, referring to the degree to which individuals tend to be shy, reserved, and inward-oriented (i.e., introverted) or outgoing and oriented towards interaction with others (i.e., extroverted). An individual's personality features are considered to exist along a continuum and, although some people will fall at extreme ends of the spectrum, the majority will be found closer to the middle. Research indicates that personality is both genetically determined and influenced by environmental factors (Sanchez-Roige et al., 2018). Although we each inherit a proclivity towards particular personality features, these features are shaped by interpersonal experiences and by repeated exposure to circumstances that either reinforce or inhibit particular traits.

Good mental health does not imply a particular set of personality characteristics; a wide variety of personality configurations and behaviour patterns are found in people with good mental health. Moreover, norms for personality and behaviour often vary across cultures and subcultures (LeVine, 2017). For instance, some cultures tend to consider extroverted, emotionally expressive behaviour to be normal, whereas other cultures favour more reserved and restricted emotional expression. We discuss this in more depth in Chapter 8.

If an individual's personality or pattern of behaviour deviates markedly from cultural expectations, and is inflexible and pervasive across many circumstances, then the person may be considered to have a personality disorder. Generally, an individual living with a personality disorder will experience distress or impairment in their capacity to function and relate to others. Individuals with certain forms of personality disorder may be likely to invoke distress in the people around them.

Table 2.1: Brain structures and associated functions

Brain Structure	Function
Cerebral Cortex	This outer layer of the cerebral hemispheres consists of grey matter (comprised primarily of neuronal cell bodies and unmyelinated axons) and has sensory, motor, and association areas. The association areas enable perception of the world and produce thought and language.
Frontal Lobe	This area at the front of the brain plays a large role in emotional expression, reasoning, judgment, memory, problem solving, planning, decision making, and language.
Hypothalamus	Controls appetite, sleep, aggression, and sex drive. Regulates body temperature, blood pressure, emotions, and hormone secretion.
Nucleus Accumbens	Often referred to as the pleasure centre of the brain; controls motivations.
Amygdala	Involved in emotional reactions (i.e., anger, fear, etc.).
Hippocampus	A structure involved in functions of memory.
Reticular Formation	Plays a key role in states of arousal and consciousness.
Corpus Callosum	Delivers messages between the two brain hemispheres.
Meninges	These structures wrap the brain in protective layers filled with cerebrospinal fluid and thus act as a "shock absorber" to help protect the brain from injury.

Brain Function and Mental Health

In the above section, we described many different mental functions. It is important to note that good mental health does not require perfect function in every sphere of mental life. The definition of mental health provided in Chapter 1 describes a state of emotional and psychological well-being in which an individual is able to use their cognitive and emotional capabilities, function in society, and meet the ordinary demands of everyday life. Thus, just as we might have a problem with high blood pressure yet be able to control this and enjoy good overall physical health, we may also have a particular challenge with one or more mental functions, yet still achieve overall good mental health.

Genetics and Epigenetics of Mental Health and Illness

While we inherit physical characteristics from our biological parents, we also appear to inherit mental characteristics. If both of your biological parents are tall and have green eyes, then you are much more likely than average to be tall and have green eyes. However, despite your tall, green-eyed parents, you could be short and have brown eyes. Similarly, if both of your biological parents are very shy and introverted, you are more likely to be shy and introverted, but you might be socially confident and outgoing instead. Although the likelihood of sharing traits with your ancestors is heightened as a result of genetic transmission, it remains very possible that you will demonstrate a different combination of traits.

Genes are segments of DNA that are contained in the nuclei of all cells in our bodies. The coding of the segments provides "instructions" that guide the development and function of our bodies. Thus, just as there are certain genes (DNA sequence segments) that determine the colour of our eyes, there are genes that determine our mental characteristics, such as whether we are likely to be shy and introverted or confident and extroverted. However, genetic transmission of mental characteristics appears to be highly complex, involving multiple gene loci (Hoskin et al., 2019).

Even if we inherit the genes for a certain trait or illness, we may not develop the condition. This is partly due to **epigenetics**, which can be defined as functions at the molecular level affecting gene expression that operate in addition to DNA sequencing transmission. Thus, the "epi" in epigenetics can be thought of as meaning "in addition to" genetics. This explains why "identical" (monozygotic) twins

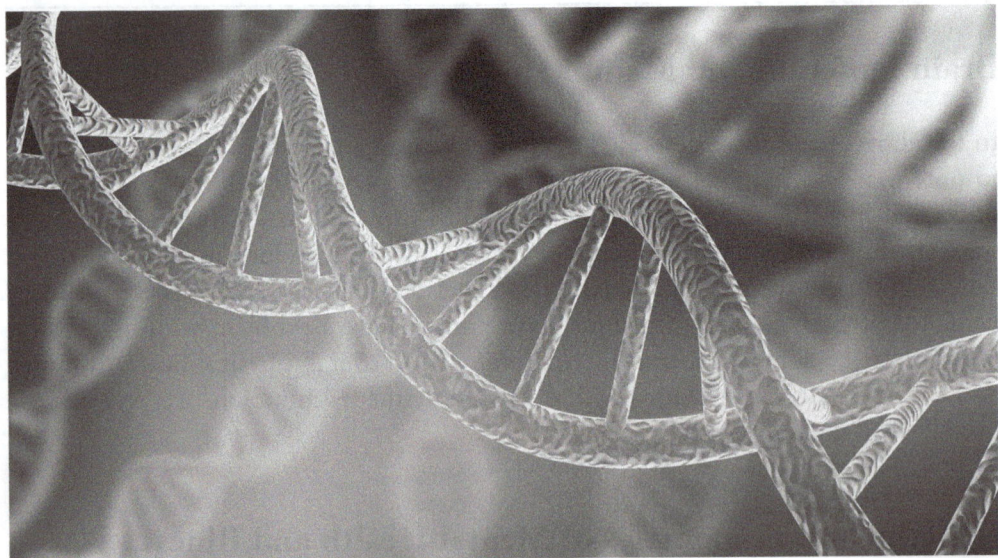

Figure 2.5: Pictured here is a strand of DNA, which is contained within the nuclei of all cells in our bodies. The coding of the segments provides "instructions" that guide the development and function of our bodies.

Source: iStockphoto/artisteer

are not really identical, physically or mentally. Although they have nearly identical DNA, monozygotic twins are exposed to different environmental influences both in the womb and throughout the rest of their lives, during which genes are switched on or off. These epigenetic variations and other environmental influences alter the phenotype (i.e., the observable characteristics that result from the interaction of the genotype—or genetic makeup of a cell or organism—and environmental factors). For example, monozygotic twins do not have the same fingerprints because environmental factors in the womb result in different whorls and patterns developing at the fingertips. If one monozygotic twin experiences a mental illness such as schizophrenia, the chance that the other twin will also have schizophrenia is only about 33 percent (Hilker et al., 2017). Although this is much higher than the risk among the general population of having schizophrenia (less than 1 percent), a monozygotic twin of someone with schizophrenia does not have a 100 percent chance of having the illness, which would be the case if genetic transmission were completely deterministic. Once again, this shows that genetic factors have significant influence but play only a partial role in determining mental health and illness.

Cellular Activity in the Brain

As discussed earlier in this chapter, the brain contains approximately 100 billion brain cells or neurons that comprise an intricate web of electrochemical connections sending multiple electrical signals shooting at a rapid pace throughout the brain and along nerves leading to all other parts of the body. How is the electrical energy supplied to fuel the brain cells? What serves as the "battery" to keep the brain going strong? The answer is adenosine triphosphate (ATP), a macromolecule that, along with DNA (another macromolecule), constitutes the most important building block of all living organisms. ATP powers virtually every activity of the cell and organism, including generating electrical energy in neurons. ATP is a complex molecule that contains the nucleoside adenosine and a tail consisting of three phosphates, which have high-energy bonds. Energy is released from the ATP molecule by a reaction that breaks off one of the phosphates, leaving ADP, or adenosine diphosphate. Immediately, the cell mitochondria reattach a phosphate group, thus producing ATP and "recharging" the battery: "hooking and unhooking that last phosphate [on ATP] is what keeps the whole world operating" (Trefil, 1992).

At any one instant, there are about a billion ATP molecules in each cell of the human body. As they release energy (by the breaking of the high-energy phosphate bonds), they are being replenished continually. Food and oxygen are required to provide the necessary molecular ingredients to rebuild the ATP molecules. In neurons, ATP supplies the energy needed for electrical activity, for transport of chemical messengers across synapses, and for other cellular functions. Neurons require approximately twice the energy supply of other cells, and the brain uses about

10 percent of the entire supply of energy in the human body due to the high demands of neural electrical transmission.

Brain Nutrients and the Blood-Brain Barrier

Unlike other cells in the human body, which use various nutrients derived from food as fuel, brain cells or neurons use only glucose. Other nutrients do not fuel the brain because of the **blood-brain barrier.** This structure surrounds the blood capillaries that supply the brain and spinal cord and allows only small molecules to pass through its membranes. The blood-brain barrier allows essential metabolites, such as oxygen and glucose, to pass from the blood to the brain but blocks most larger molecules, including most drugs, hormones, viruses, and bacteria. Despite the protection of the blood-brain barrier, it is possible for some harmful toxins to reach the brain. Molecules that are small and those that are lipid-soluble can pass through the barrier. Some viruses and certain toxins, such as lead and mercury, can enter and have damaging effects on brain function; children, whose brains are developing, are particularly susceptible.

Neurons cannot store glucose and, consequently, a constant supply must be delivered for the brain to be adequately fuelled. Glucose is supplied from carbohydrates, which are found primarily in grains (such as rice, pasta, bread), legumes, fruits and vegetables, and refined sugar, that we eat. Glucose levels are usually maintained at adequate levels by various homeostatic mechanisms. However, in unusual circumstances that cause blood glucose levels to drop to low levels, such as prolonged starvation (including that which occurs in people with the eating disorder anorexia nervosa) or when someone with diabetes receives too high a dose of insulin (a hormone that facilitates the uptake of glucose by cells), brain function is adversely affected. Without adequate levels of glucose, brain cells cannot function properly and one quickly becomes unable to think clearly. Very low blood glucose will disable brain function, cause loss of consciousness, and possibly lead to death.

The brain also requires a constant supply of oxygen to be delivered via the bloodstream and utilizes much more oxygen than other parts of the body. The brain uses about 20 percent of the body's oxygen yet constitutes about 2 percent of the body's weight. Consequently, the brain is particularly sensitive to a lack of oxygen (hypoxia) and large numbers of brain cells will begin to die after about five minutes without oxygen.

In addition to glucose and oxygen, the brain requires an adequate supply of certain vitamins for healthy function. A number of the B vitamins, particularly B1 (thiamine), B3 (niacin), and B12 (cyanocobalanin), are necessary for healthy neuronal activity. The body generally maintains adequate stores of these vitamins, but in unusual circumstances these vitamins can become depleted. Prolonged starvation or malnutrition can lead to deficiencies in B vitamins, as can chronic use of alcohol and certain forms of cancer and other diseases. Deficiencies in these B vitamins can cause serious brain deficits, including disturbances of memory and thinking.

The Brain's Shock Absorbers: The Meninges and Cerebrospinal Fluid

Since the precious supercomputer that we carry around on top of our necks is so essential to human life, it is not surprising that the body has a series of protective envelopes and shock absorbers to diminish the likelihood of damage or trauma to the brain. Inside the hard casing of the skull, there are three separate protective membranes surrounding the brain, called the **meninges**. The brain is bathed in cerebrospinal fluid, a fluid shock absorber held tightly in place by the meninges.

When we sustain a blow to the head, the brain is protected by the meninges and cerebrospinal fluid. However, if the trauma is too great for the protective shock absorption they provide, bleeding or damage to brain tissue may occur. Repeated studies now confirm that even minor repeated trauma to the head (without loss of consciousness) can cause substantial damage to the human brain (Bieniek et al., 2019). These findings have led to increased public health efforts, for example, encouraging or mandating the use of helmets and protective headgear in various sports activities and enhancing safety features (such as seatbelts and airbags) in motor vehicles.

Hormones and Mental Health

In addition to the complex and sophisticated electrochemical network of neurons, the human body produces various **hormones** (i.e., chemical messengers released by cells that affect other cells elsewhere in the body). Hormones provide an additional mechanism for regulating and changing mental function and behaviour. They are located in many different sites in the body, usually stored in glands that secrete them into the bloodstream under certain conditions. For example, hormones are stored in the pituitary gland (a small structure located at the base of the brain), the thyroid gland (a gland wrapped around the trachea in the front of the neck), the adrenal glands (triangular glands that sit on top of each kidney), the pancreas (located in the abdomen), and in the ovaries and testes.

The different hormones secreted by these and other glands each have specific effects on the body's function, and many of these hormones can affect the brain and nervous system. For example, adrenaline, the hormone secreted by the adrenal glands, stimulates the brain and snaps it into an emergency, high-alert mode. Adrenaline is secreted when we are under threat or experience fear, pain, and other danger signals. It can also be secreted when we are in a competitive situation and need to push our bodies to operate at peak physical performance.

Hormones can be thought of as controls on a music sound system, like those controlling volume or tone. Although changing these parameters will not change the piece of music that is being played, shifts in volume or tone will create profound changes in the character of the sound. Similarly, the release of hormones can create changes in general characteristics of mental activity, such as speeding up or slowing down thought and intensifying or diminishing memory and emotional responsiveness.

Females may experience changes in mood in association with hormonal changes that occur during menstrual cycles, during and following pregnancy, and through menopause. Estrogen and progesterone, the ovarian hormones that regulate menstruation, appear to have significant impact on mood and other mental functions. However, the mechanism of action is not yet understood. Testosterone, a hormone released by the testes in males (and released in smaller amounts by the ovaries) also appears to have a significant effect on mental function and behaviour, including regulation of one's libido (i.e., sexual drive) and levels of mental energy. Testosterone levels decline with aging, and some individuals, regardless of sex, may experience an associated loss of libido and a decrease in mental energy associated with this drop. We will discuss some of the unique interactions between sex, gender, and mental health in Chapter 7.

The "master control" for the release of the many hormones is the hypothalamus, a complex region of the brain containing a number of nuclei involved in the regulation of emotion, appetite, body temperature, and other functions. The hypothalamus is directly connected to the pituitary gland, which is located directly below the area of the brain where the hypothalamus is situated. The hypothalamus signals the pituitary gland to release particular hormones (i.e., releasing factors) into the bloodstream, which in turn signal glands in other parts of the body, such as the thyroid gland, adrenal glands, and ovaries, to release their hormones.

Usually, levels of hormones are well regulated by the body. However, certain illnesses can cause hormone levels to be too high or low; this can lead to mental changes, such as increased anxiety or decreased mental energy. Research studies indicate that children who are exposed to repeated stress may develop changes in their hormonal regulatory systems that are associated with major depressive disorder. This appears to occur as a result of changes that cause the adrenal glands to attenuate the release of cortisol (Staufenbiel et al., 2013; Steudte-Schmiedgen et al., 2017).

Light, Darkness, and Mental Health

Similar to other mammals, human biology appears to be affected by changes in the seasons and cycles of light and darkness. Changes in exposure to daylight that occur throughout the seasons, and which may occur more abruptly when we travel to very different time zones or different latitudes, alter the synchronization of our internal biological rhythms. We each have a type of internal biological clock that can be reset by changes in exposure to bright light. If we travel to a very different time zone, we are likely to experience jet lag, in which our internal biological clock becomes confused and our internal biological rhythms go out of sync. That is why we can feel so crummy and can have difficulty sleeping. People who travel frequently across time zones, such as pilots and other airline crew, are trained to maintain their patterns according to a fixed time zone in order to minimize the de-synchronization of their biological clocks.

During the winter months in Canada, daylight hours shorten and many people experience an unpleasant response known as Seasonal Affective Disorder (SAD), which is characterized by difficulty sleeping and other symptoms of depression. People who live at high latitudes, that is, either in the far northern or southern hemisphere, will go through long periods in the winter during which there is very little daylight. Research studies have shown that people who live in areas with long periods of darkness are more prone to developing SAD (Meesters & Gordijn, 2016). There may be biological reasons why people tend to feel happy and energetic in sunny climates and more moody when there is little light.

Researchers have found that people with SAD often experience relief from depressive symptoms when exposed to bright light each morning (Nussbaumer et al., 2015). Special light boxes that generate enough bright light (10,000 LUX for 30 minutes) have been created and are sometimes prescribed for use by people with SAD.

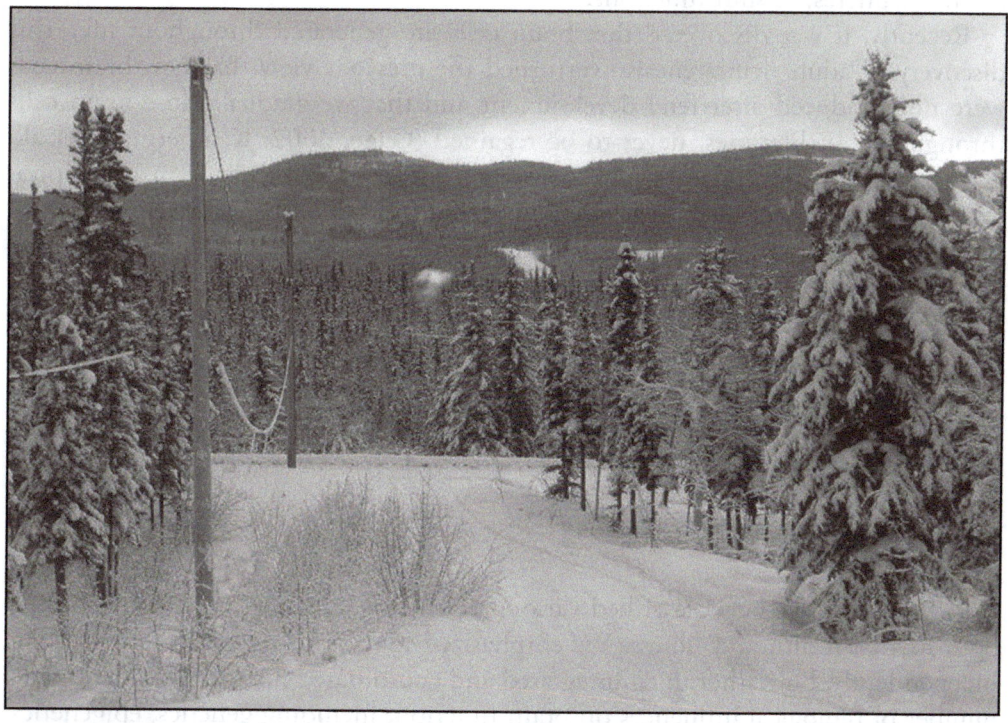

Figure 2.6: Some individuals will experience Seasonal Affective Disorder (SAD) in response to the longer dark hours during winter months. This photo was taken in the small northern community of Carmacks in the Little Salmon/Carmacks First Nation, Yukon Territory, where there is as little as five hours of daylight in the winter months.

Source: Brenden Westman, Photographer

Plasticity and Regenerativity of the Brain

As described earlier in this chapter, the brain is more than a collection of independent centres, each responsible for particular functions; these centres work together in a coordinated, integrated manner. Furthermore, the brain has a high degree of plasticity so that functions of the brain may be taken over by different areas if there is damage or loss of brain tissue. For example, such plasticity can occur between the two sides of the brain. If a line is drawn, dividing the brain equally into left and right halves, it can then be seen that the brain is similar to many other parts of the body, with symmetry in structure between its left and right sides. A large band of fibres called the corpus callosum connects the two sides of the brain.

Scientists have found differentiation of function between the right and left sides of the brain. You may have heard that the left side of the brain is more focused on functions such as mathematics and logic, whereas the right side of the brain is more involved in artistic and intuitive functions and abilities; however, the reality is more complex. The plasticity of the brain allows different regions, including the right and left hemispheres, to shift functions.

Recently, it was discovered that brain cells are generated throughout life. This discovery of adult neurogenesis overturned the previous view that new brain cells were not produced after fetal development and that we gradually lose brain cells throughout our lifetimes, never to be regained (Gage, 2002; Kempermann et al., 2018). Many neuroscientists now consider generation of neurons in the hippocampus to be important for learning and memory. As disturbances of hippocampal function are thought to be present in various mental illnesses, including mood, anxiety, and certain psychotic disorders, scientists hope that discoveries regarding adult hippocampal neurogenesis may help to develop new treatments and interventions (Schoenfeld & Cameron, 2015). The important discovery of adult neurogenesis reversed a long-standing scientific belief and is a good reminder to us that some of our current scientific ideas will be revised in the future as we acquire new information.

Conclusion

In this chapter, we have described various structures and functions of the brain in both mental health and illness. We emphasized that brain regions do not operate independently, but rather in an integrated and coordinated manner. We identified a number of biological influences on brain function, including genetics, epigenetics, psychoactive substances, nutrition, hormones, and exposure to cycles of light and darkness. We also discussed the capacity of the brain to shift functions from one region to another (i.e., plasticity) and its ability to regenerate its own cells.

Brain function is fascinating and complex; it is no wonder that so many students and scientists are captivated by the study of the brain. However, do not fall into the trap of reductionism and convince yourself that all mental processes and human behaviour can be explained by brain function. In the next chapter, we hope to convince you that a full understanding of mental health and illness also requires knowledge provided by the social sciences.

Glossary

blood-brain barrier: The structure that surrounds the blood capillaries that supply the brain and spinal cord, allowing only small molecules to pass through its membranes.
cerebral hemisphere: One of two regions of the brain; the left and right cerebral hemispheres.
epigenetics: Functions at the molecular level affecting gene expression that operate in addition to DNA sequencing transmission.
hormones: Chemical messengers released by cells that affect other cells elsewhere in the body.
limbic system: A series of interconnected structures in different regions of the brain that are important in producing mood and emotions.
meninges: Three separate protective membranes surrounding the brain.
mood: The predominant background emotional state that persists in an individual over an extended period of time.
neurons: Cells of the brain.
neurotransmitters: Chemical messengers that allow the transmission of signals from one neuron to another.
personality: The enduring behavioural traits and characteristics of an individual.

Critical Thinking Questions

1. How do neurons transmit messages?
2. Select a region of the brain and describe how it can affect a person's mental health.
3. What role do genetics play in determining mental health and illness?
4. Name two hormones that can affect a person's mental health.
5. What role does biology play in understanding human behaviour and mental health?

Recommended Readings

Eagleman, D. (2017). *The brain: The story of you*. Vintage.
Kendler, K. S., & Prescott, C. A. (2006). *Genes, environment, and psychopathology: Understanding the causes of psychiatric and substance use disorders*. Guildford Press.
O'Keane, V. (2021). *A sense of self: Memory, the brain, and who we are*. W.W. Norton.

Stetka, B. (2021). *A history of the human brain: From the sea sponge to CRISPR, how our brain evolved*. Timber Press.

Tost, H., Champagne, F. A., & Meyer-Lindenberg, A. (2015). Environmental influence in the brain, human welfare and mental health. *Nature Neuroscience, 18*(10), 4121–4131. https://doi.org/10.1038/nn.4108

Recommended Websites

The Brain from Top to Bottom. www.thebrain.mcgill.ca
The Franklin Institute—The Human Brain. www.fi.edu/exhibit/your-brain
The Hormones of the Human—Kimball's Biology Pages. http://biology-pages.info/H/Hormones.html
The Medical Biochemistry Page—Michael W. King. Biochemistry of Nerve Transmission. www.themedicalbiochemistrypage.org/nerves.html

---

References

Bieniek, K. F., Blessing, M. M., Heckman, M. G., Diehl, N. N., Serie, A. M., Paolini II, M. A., Boeve, B. F., Savica, R., Reichard, R. R., & Dickson, D.W. (2019). Association between contact sports participation and chronic traumatic encephalopathy: A retrospective cohort study. *Brain Pathology, 30*(1), 63–74. https://doi.org/10.1111/bpa.12757

Bliss, T. V. P., & Collingridge, G. L. (1993). A synaptic model of memory: Long-term potentiation in the hippocampus. *Nature, 361*(6407), 31–39.

Bowyer, S. M. (2016). Coherence a measure of the brain networks: Past and present. *Neuropsychiatric Electrophysiology, 2*, Article 1. https://doi.org/10.1186/s40810-015-0015-7

Carter, K. S., & Carter III, R. (2016). Breath-based meditation: A mechanism to restore the physiological and cognitive reserves for optimal human performance. *World Journal of Clinical Cases, 4*(4), 99–102. https://doi.org/10.12998/wjcc.v4.i4.99

Cortés, A., Casadó-Anguera, V., Moreno, E., & Casadó, V. (2016). Caffeine, adenosine A_1 receptors, and brain cortex: Molecular aspects. In V. R. Preedy (Ed.), *Neuropathology of drug addictions and substance misuse—Volume 3: General processes and mechanisms, prescription medications, caffeine and areca, polydrug misuse, emerging addictions and non-drug addictions* (pp. 741–752). Elsevier.

Eysenck, M. W., & Keane, M. T. (2015). *Cognitive psychology: A student's handbook* (7th ed.). Psychology Press.

Gage, F. H. (2002). Neurogenesis in the adult brain. *Journal of Neuroscience, 22*(3), 212–213. https://doi.org/10.1523/JNEUROSCI.22-03-00612.2002

Guyer, A. E., Silk, J. S., & Nelson, E. E. (2016). The neurobiology of the emotional adolescent: From inside out. *Neuroscience & Biobehavioral Reviews, 70*, 74–85. https://doi.org/10.1016/j.neubiorev.2016.07.037

Hilker, R., Helenius, D., Fagerlund, B., Skytthe, A., Christensen, K., Werge, T. M., Nordentoft, M., & Glenthøj, B. (2017). Heritability of schizophrenia and schizophrenia spectrum based on nationwide Danish twin register. *Biological Psychiatry, 83*(6), 492–498. https://doi.org/10.1016/j.biopsych.2017.08.017

Hoskin, D. J., Hunt, J., & Wedell, N. (Eds.). (2019). *Genes and behaviour: Beyond nature–nurture.* John Wiley & Sons.

Kempermann, G., Gage, F. H., Aigner, L., Song, H., Curtis, M. A., Thuret, S., Kuhn, H. G., Jessberger, S., Frankland, P. W., Cameron, H. A., Gould, E., Hen, R., Abrous, D. N., Schinder, A. F., Zhao, X., Lucassen, P. J., & Frisén, J. (2018). Human adult neurogenesis: Evidence and remaining questions. *Cell Stem Cell, 23*(1), 25–30. https://doi.org/10.1016/j.stem.2018.04.004

LeVine, R. A. (2017). *Culture, behavior and personality: An introduction to the comparative study of psychosocial adaptation* (2nd ed.). Routledge.

Meesters, Y., & Gordijn, M. C. M. (2016). Seasonal affective disorder, winter type: Current insights and treatment options. *Psychology Research and Behavior Management, 9*, 317–327. https://doi.org/10.2147/PRBM.S114906

Nicoll, R. A. (2017). A brief history of long-term potentiation. *Neuron, 93*(2), 281–290. https://doi.org/10.1016/j.neuron.2016.12.015

Nussbaumer, B., Kaminski-Hartenthaler, A., Forneris, C. A., Morgan, L. C., Sonis, J. H., Gaynes, B. N., Greenblatt, A., Wipplinger, J., Lux, L. J., Winkler, D., Van Noord, M. G., Hofmann, J., & Gartlehner, G. (2015). Light therapy for preventing seasonal affective disorder. *Cochrane Database of Systematic Reviews, 11*, Article CD011269. https://doi.org/10.1002/14651858.CD011269.pub2

Sanchez-Roige, S., Gray, J. C., MacKillop, J., Chen, C.-H., & Palmer, A. A. (2018). The genetics of human personality. *Genes, Brain and Behaviour, 17*(3), e12439. https://doi.org/10.1111/gbb.12439

Schoenfeld, T. J., & Cameron, H. A. (2015). Adult neurogenesis and mental illness. *Neuropsychopharmacology, 40*(1), 113–128. https://doi.org/10.1038/npp.2014.230

Statistics Canada. (2008). Beverage consumption of Canadian adults (Catalogue no. 82-003-X). *Health Reports, 19*(4). www.statcan.gc.ca/pub/82-003-x/2008004/article/6500240-eng.htm

Staufenbiel, S. M., Penninx, B. W. J. H., Spijker, A. T., Elzinga, B. M., & van Rossum, E. F. C. (2013). Hair cortisol, stress exposure, and mental health in humans: A systematic review. *Psychoneuroendocrinology, 38*(8), 1220–1235. https://doi.org/10.1016/j.psyneuen.2012.11.015

Steudte-Schmiedgen, S., Wichman, S., Stalder, T., Hilbert, K., Muehlhan, M., Lueken, U., & Beesdo-Baum, K. (2017). Hair cortisol concentrations and cortisol stress reactivity in generalized anxiety disorder, major depression and their comorbidity. *Journal of Psychiatric Research, 84*, 184–190. https://doi.org/10.1016/j.jpsychires.2016.09.024

Tortora, G., & Grabowski, S. R. (2002). *Principles of anatomy and physiology* (10th ed.). John Wiley & Sons.

Trefil, J. (1992). *1001 things everyone should know about science.* Doubleday.

von Bartheld, C. S., Bahney, J., & Herculano-Houzel, S. (2016). The search for true numbers of neurons and glial cells in the human brain: A review of 150 years of cell counting. *Journal of Comparative Neurology, 524*(18), 3865–3895. https://doi.org/10.1002/cne.24040

Chapter 3

Mental Health Examined through the Social Sciences

> For the past century, people have looked to the physical and biological sciences to solve important problems. The social sciences offer equal promise for improving human welfare; our lives can be greatly improved through a deeper understanding of individual and collective behavior.
> —Nicholas A. Christakis (sociologist and physician)

Introduction

In this chapter, we draw on knowledge about mental health and illness accumulated by the social sciences. The social sciences use the methods of scientific inquiry: careful and systematic data collection, analysis, and interpretation. Examples of social sciences include the disciplines of anthropology, criminology, economics, geography, history, political science, psychology, and sociology. A contrast is often drawn between these sciences and physical sciences such as biology, chemistry, and neuroscience. In this chapter, we examine some of the more important factors associated with mental health identified within the realm of social sciences, both at the level of the individual and the level of populations. Since a vast body of knowledge relevant to mental health and illness has been explored by social scientists, we will only be able to touch on a small sample of important ideas and discoveries. This chapter will highlight some topics we find intriguing, and we recommend additional readings at the end of the chapter for those who would like to explore social sciences in more depth.

Theories of Individual and Group Behaviour

As we mentioned in the first chapter, psychoanalysis has had a substantial influence on ideas about mental health and illness. Developed in the beginning of the 20th century by Sigmund Freud, a Viennese psychiatrist, psychoanalysis included many ideas; some of these continue to receive attention, whereas others have been dismissed. Freud believed that the human behaviour we observe may be understood only by looking into deeper forces and conflicts operating below the level of awareness, that is, in the **unconscious mind** (Freud, 1901).

Freud asserted that humans are embroiled in a constant conflict between two aspects of the mind: the id, which is the source of instinctual drives (aggression and sexual desire), and the superego, an inner representation of societal norms and cultural conventions (Freud, 1901). Instinctual drives are passed on as part of our evolutionary heritage, whereas societal norms are shaped by our family and social environment. For example, an ordinary college student experiences the sudden wish to embrace a fellow student passionately while in the middle of a class; this represents a conflict between an instinctual drive and a societal norm and would cause stress for this student. Freud theorized that such conflicts are typically resolved by repressing the unacceptable drive, that is, by pushing it below awareness. When this mechanism of repression is unsuccessful, a person may develop mental health challenges such as depression or anxiety. Freud daringly proposed that, during childhood, we all have sexual desires towards our parents that are in direct conflict with our societal norms, and, as a result, we end up with emotional conflicts and problems (Freud, 1910). According to psychoanalytic theory, we are unaware of this conflict and repression, because it occurs in the unconscious mind. Psychoanalytic ideas are considered a part of "depth psychology," which plumbs the depths of the human psyche (Gay, 1995). In recent decades, the fields of psychiatry, psychology, nursing, and social work have mostly distanced themselves from psychoanalytic ideas (Bornstein, 2001). However, the appeal of these ideas remains strong in various creative disciplines such as literature, dance, and the visual arts.

Whether we embrace or dismiss his ideas and theories, Freud is considered to have had a great impact on Western thought—in part, because he initiated an awakening of interest in the human psyche and sparked exploration and analysis of human behaviour. In the first half of the 20th century, psychoanalytic theories were the subject of intense intellectual debate in Europe, soon spreading to other continents. Many creative thinkers devoted themselves to extending psychoanalytic theory and practice. Two of the most famous individuals who emerged from Freud's immediate circle were Alfred Adler and Carl Jung. Adler was concerned with the ways in which social structures may cause humans to feel helpless or powerless—he labelled this the **inferiority complex** (Adler, 1956). Adler asserted that much of human striving can be understood as an attempt to overcome the inferiority complex and increase one's sense of personal power and self-esteem. Meanwhile, Carl Jung took a radically different approach and asserted that we all share a very deep level of our mind in the form of the **collective unconscious** (Jung, 1981). Jung understood human personality in terms of archetypes, mythic figures contained in the collective unconscious that show us different ways we might be in the world. For example, the archetype of the *puer aeternus* is like a perpetual child who never settles down or accepts commitment. Jung's ideas appeal to those who favour a more spiritual and non-materialistic approach to understanding mental health.

However, many theorists and practitioners became skeptical of these "depth psychology" approaches and sought frameworks that would be less complicated and esoteric. From the field of psychology emerged a straightforward theoretical framework called **behaviourism** that explains how behaviour is shaped by the application of various stimuli, that of rewards and punishments (Skinner, 1938; Watson, 1924). In its early phases, behaviourism used animal research (often studying laboratory mice and rats) to examine the effects of various patterns of reward and punishment on behaviour. The Russian physiologist Ivan Pavlov was one of the first to examine behaviour in relation to environmental stimuli through his research on dogs (Pavlov, 1927). Such research on behaviour proved to be accurate in describing how humans learn behaviour, too. For example, if you reward a behaviour intermittently and unpredictably, the resulting behaviour change will last longer than if the reward is given every time the behaviour is carried out (think about how stubbornly people will continue gambling, where the rewards are intermittent and unpredictable).

Behaviour therapy applies behaviourist principles to help individuals with mental health challenges. It aims to identify the ways that people with mental health challenges have learned maladaptive responses to their environments. One type of behavioural learning involves **classical conditioning**. An example of this would be to pair a stimulus that elicits a strong negative response (e.g., an electric shock) with a neutral stimulus (e.g., a soft light). As these two stimuli are repeatedly paired, the light begins to elicit a strong negative response as well. At a more complex level, imagine someone who has been harshly disciplined by several teachers. This person might develop a conditioned fear response to all authority figures, resulting in a marked tendency to avoid contact with such figures. This would amount to a phobia that could severely limit this person's ability to complete education or function successfully in a job. Another way in which a maladaptive response might be learned is through **instrumental conditioning**, in which a person has been rewarded or punished for a particular kind of behaviour, increasing or decreasing the frequency of the behaviour (Skinner, 1953). Most of our learning occurs through instrumental conditioning. For example, when you receive a high mark for demonstrating your knowledge of course material, you have been rewarded for working hard to reach that level of achievement and this is likely to increase your tendency to work hard in other courses and jobs. When you receive a very low mark for a course you have not been giving much attention, this is a punishment that will likely discourage future inattentive behaviour. This can be considered a form of adaptive learning. In contrast, a child who cannot obtain the interest or attention of their parents or siblings other than when they exhibit disruptive, bothersome behaviour may experience maladaptive learning. By conceptualizing mental health challenges as expressions of maladaptive learning, whether through classical or instrumental conditioning, we gain a powerful tool to understand behaviours shown by individuals with mental illnesses that would otherwise be difficult to understand. Over recent decades, behaviour therapy has largely been supplanted by a more wide-ranging approach called cognitive behavioural therapy (CBT; Rachman, 1997). This approach adds a focus on our thoughts or cognitions and how they relate to our behaviours. We'll learn more about CBT when we review treatments for mental health challenges in Chapter 14.

Social scientists have also been intrigued by the way behaviour changes when people are in large groups or crowds. Sociologists have noted many examples of people acting differently when in large groups than they would normally as individuals, and this is sometimes referred to as **herd behaviour** (Kameda et al., 2015). For example, people in a large group are more likely to help an individual in distress when they see others extending help, but more likely to do nothing if others are ignoring the individual's distress.

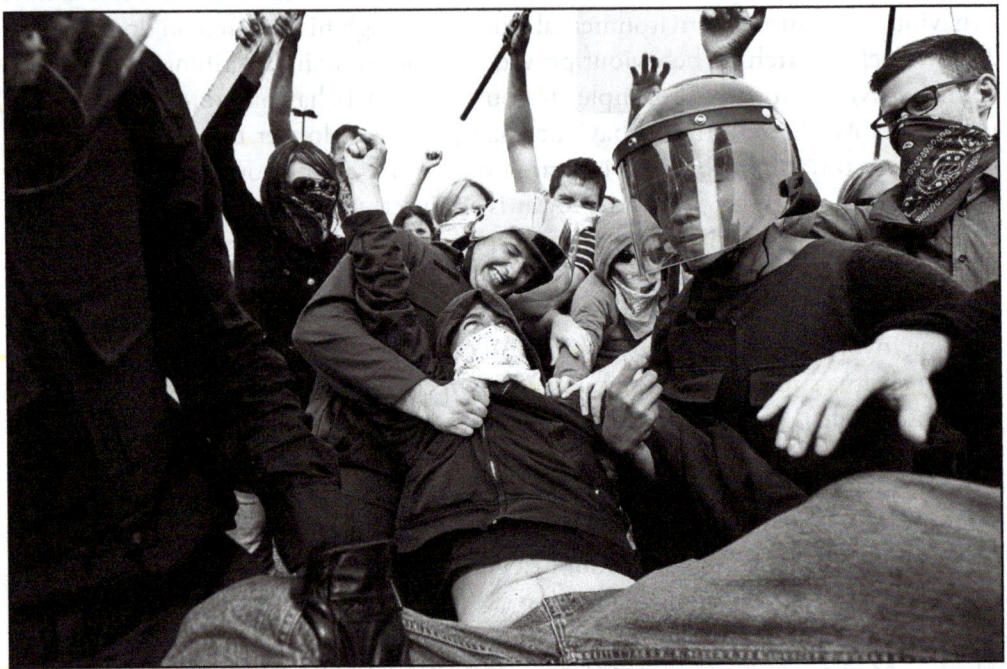

Figure 3.1: Riots provide an example of how crowd behaviour can quickly become out of control. This picture shows a young man being arrested by police during a riot.

Source: iStockphoto/Nicole S. Young

Box 3.1: The Mental Health of Social Groups

In sociology, it has been questioned whether social groups themselves can be viewed as having good or poor mental health. Consider the surprising behaviour of crowds: excited mobs have been known to act more violently and irrationally than any one individual member would. This phenomenon has been referred to as "the madness of crowds" (Mackay, 1841). Crowd members may lose their individuality and be subsumed by the group's emotions. Each person is subject to contagion and suggestion, virtually hypnotized into doing things that might otherwise be repugnant. When viewed in this way, one can think of the crowd as exhibiting poor mental health when it engages in actions that are irrational, impulsive, and destructive.

Developmental Trajectories and Mental Health

Some social scientists have focused attention on childhood development because it is a time when individuals learn extensive amounts of information at a very rapid pace. Childhood is a critical period that establishes lifelong patterns of personality and behaviour, echoing the famous dictum of the Jesuit priesthood: "Give me a child up until he is seven and I will give you the man." Although it is true that childhood is a particularly important period for mental development, our minds continue to develop and change throughout our lives (Kail & Cavanaugh, 2016).

Among the best-known theories of development are those of Erik Erikson, who presented a view of identity development as proceeding through a series of stages across the lifespan (Erikson, 1950; Erikson & Erikson, 1987). Through infancy and childhood, our identities are defined by our parents and immediate social environment. In adolescence, we begin to question the identity we have been "given" and think about our *own* values and goals. By adulthood, we have preferably worked out our own identity and are striving to reach goals that have personal meaning (see Table 3.1). According to Erikson's theory, failure to navigate each of the stages of identity development can result in mental health challenges, whose form will reflect the particular transition that was unsuccessfully completed. For example, the late adolescence/early adult stage of identity formation involves the establishment

Table 3.1: Summary of Erik Erikson's developmental stages

Stage	Ages	Basic Conflict	Summary
1. Oral-Sensory	Birth to 18 months	Trust vs. Mistrust	The infant must form a first loving, trusting relationship with the caregiver or develop a sense of mistrust.
2. Muscular-Anal	18 months to 3 years	Autonomy vs. Shame/Doubt	The child's energies are directed toward the development of physical skills, including walking, grasping, and rectal sphincter control. The child learns control but may develop shame and doubt if not handled well.
3. Locomotor	3 to 6 years	Initiative vs. Guilt	The child continues to become more assertive and to take more initiative, but may be too forceful, leading to guilt feelings.

(continued)

Table 3.1: Summary of Erik Erikson's developmental stages

Stage	Ages	Basic Conflict	Summary
4. Latency	6 to 12 years	Industry vs. Inferiority	The child must deal with demands to learn new skills or risk a sense of inferiority, failure, and incompetence.
5. Adolescence	12 to 18 years	Identity vs. Role Confusion	The teenager must achieve a sense of identity in occupation, sex roles, politics, and religion.
6. Young Adulthood	19 to 40 years	Intimacy vs. Isolation	The young adult must develop intimate relationships or suffer feelings of isolation.
7. Middle Adulthood	40 to 65 years	Generativity vs. Stagnation	Each adult must find some way to satisfy and support the next generation.
8. Maturity	65 to death	Ego Integrity vs. Despair	The culmination is a sense of oneself as one is and of feeling fulfilled.

Source: Cramer, C., Flynn, B., & LaFave, A. (1997). *Erik Erikson's 8 stages of psychosocial development: Summary chart*. https://web.cortland.edu/andersmd/ERIK/sum.HTML

of occupational and relationship choices—individuals who have difficulty completing this stage may remain in a state of identity diffusion, in which they feel lost, directionless, and anxious (Becht et al., 2016). In recent years, the developmental transitions during adolescence and adulthood have become notably delayed—taking longer to complete for many. Young people are living longer with their parents, they are taking more time to complete their education, and they are getting married and having children later. Social scientists have hypothesized that this delay is a result of complex social and economic factors, including shifts in educational requirements for entry-level jobs as well as higher costs of living (Barroso et al., 2019; Statistics Canada, 2014). Another stage, associated with the elderly, is that of *ego integrity*, in which individuals must find meaningful ways to look back on their lives; individuals who have difficulty with this stage may experience despair, feeling that their lives have been empty or meaningless.

Erikson's theory is only one of a number of sophisticated theories of psychological development. We won't be able to discuss most of these, but it is worth noting Kohlberg's theory of moral development. This theory explains the stages by which individuals develop the ability to reason out the moral aspects of situations in order to make appropriate ethical decisions (see Table 3.2). Although Kohlberg described six stages of moral development, he proposed that most adults do not progress beyond the third or fourth stage and many operate at more primitive levels throughout their lives (Kohlberg, 1976). At the most advanced stage, individuals choose their actions by viewing situations from various perspectives and trying to achieve the best balance of benefits for the most people, according to universal principles of justice.

How does Kohlberg's theory help us to understand mental health? It can help to explain how certain people become anti-social, that is, willing to ignore others' rights and act in violent or destructive ways. Even violent criminals will typically express some kind of moral justification for their actions, though their moral reasoning is crude and maladaptive (e.g., built on a primitive notion of personal vengeance) and corresponds to the lower stages of Kohlberg's developmental framework.

Table 3.2: Kohlberg's stages of moral development

Level	Stage	Summary
Level One: Pre-Conventional Morality	Stage 1: Punishment-Obedience Orientation	An action is perceived to be morally wrong if punishment is received. Young children use this form of reasoning.
	Stage 2: Instrumental Relativist Orientation	Actions are determined by "What's in it for me?" Others' needs are considered only on the basis of self-interest.
Level Two: Conventional Morality	Stage 3: Good Boy-Nice Girl Orientation	Individuals are receptive to approval or disapproval by others and moral decisions are influenced by a desire to be liked and accepted.
	Stage 4: Law and Order Orientation	Actions are based on social conventions and what is right and wrong, and obligations to uphold laws and societal rules.
Level Three: Post-Conventional Morality	Stage 5: Social Contract Orientation	Individuals are understood to hold different positions and decisions are made based on wishes of the majority and through compromise.
	Stage 6: Universal Ethical Principle Orientation	Decisions are made through abstract reasoning about what is right according to universal ethical principles.

Since our behaviour and development is strongly influenced by our families, various theories have been advanced to explain family interactions and create family therapy approaches. For example, a family systems theory model, developed by Olson and colleagues (1989), describes families in terms of three dimensions: family cohesion, flexibility, and communication. "Family cohesion" is defined by the degree of emotional bonding among family members and is viewed as connected, separated, disengaged, or enmeshed. "Family flexibility" refers to the amount of change that is tolerated in the family's leadership and relationship rules and is flexible, structured, rigid, or chaotic. "Family communication" describes the listening skills, self-disclosure, clarity, and respect in communications among family members.

In recent years, family theorists have questioned traditional theories and have criticized the contention that there is a "normal" set of behaviours that characterizes families. It has been proposed that certain kinds of families and family members have been dominated and oppressed by those in more powerful positions in society (including scientists and therapists), and therefore we should be wary of theories that prescribe what is "normal." Some family theorists have embraced **social constructionism**, which posits that there is no objective truth, only a variety of subjective views developed through dialogue with others (Burr, 2015). We discuss this perspective in the following section.

Society and Mental Health

It has long been recognized that there is a relationship between an individual's mental health and the sense of connection and cohesion within their society. This relationship was articulated by Emile Durkheim, a sociologist who argued that people living in societies undergoing a high degree of turbulence or fragmentation would experience a state of **anomie**, that is, a condition where social and/or moral norms are confused, unclear, or simply absent. Durkheim felt that this lack of connectedness would result in feelings of alienation and isolation (Durkheim, 1897). Durkheim also believed that individuals experiencing anomie would be at an increased risk of suicide. Recent sociological and psychological research has built upon Durkheim's foundation to show that individuals with low levels of connections to social networks, that is, lacking family connections, friendships, or membership in religious or voluntary groups, have relatively poor mental health and higher rates of mortality (Holt-Lunstad & Smith, 2015). Conversely, connectedness to social networks is positively correlated with mental health.

Social scientists have concluded that each of us must feel that we are meeting the expectations of our social group, yet some experience this as a painful struggle. Those who perceive large discrepancies between their self-image and the person they feel they ought to be, may feel considerable anxiety and distress. To escape these painful feelings, these individuals may use coping strategies, some of which may be unhealthy, such as alcohol and drug use, overeating, self-harm, and even suicide.

> **Box 3.2: Generations and Birth Cohorts**
>
> You have likely heard of generational groups such as the "Baby Boomers" (born approximately 1946–1960), "Generation X" (born approximately 1960–1980), "Millennials" (born 1980–1994), "Generation Z" (born 1995–2010), and "Generation Alpha" (born 2011–present). Epidemiologists and social scientists often refer to such generational groupings as **birth cohorts** (i.e., groups of people born at the same time who then grow up together) and have found that various facets of our behaviour seem to be strongly predicted by membership in a specific birth cohort. People in the same birth cohort are generally exposed to the same social events and these often have powerful impacts on key beliefs, values, worries, and behaviour patterns. Baby Boomers came of age during a time of rapid social change, increased freedom, and relative affluence. Experimentation with psychoactive substances was common and socially accepted during their teenage and young adult years. Even as they age, they continue to have high rates of substance use. Members of the Generation X birth cohort, when compared to previous generations, have been found to be more heterogeneous and socially diverse in regard to characteristics such as ethnicity, culture, sexual orientation, gender identity, and religious affiliation. Millennials are unique in their facility and comfort with technology in everyday life since they grew up at a time when computer, internet, and mobile device technology advanced at a rapid pace. Members of Generation Z are characterized as being extremely dependent on technology—including for their social interactions. As a result of this reliance on social media and other aspects of the rapidly changing digital world, they are said to be particularly good at multitasking; however, their attention spans have been said to have taken a hit. Finally, Generation Alpha are the latest birth cohort and have been described as "Millennials on steroids." However, it is difficult to predict the key characteristics of this cohort so early in their development. Rates of depression, anxiety, substance use, and other mental health characteristics have been shown to be strongly associated with birth cohorts.

A provocative theory that emerged in the social sciences is social constructionism, which is grounded in the notion that "scientific concepts" and "facts" are based upon social norms, rather than a bedrock of absolute reality (Burr, 2015). According to this view, scientific concepts or laws are constructed within the context of science itself as a type of social organization. The social constructionist view holds that conceptions of mental health are socially constructed, and thus, they vary across societies. From this perspective, there are many equally valid ways to define mental health and construe mental ill health.

> **Box 3.3: Social Constructionism**
>
> Imagine a man who states that he is inhabited by a god and has been chosen as a sacred spokesman. This man would be viewed by conventional mental health practitioners in Western society as suffering from a delusional belief, a symptom of psychosis. However, in another society, that same person's experience might be understood differently. In the science magazine *Nautilus*, Susie Neilson (2016) tells the story of Frank, a man who was first diagnosed as experiencing psychosis as a teenager and subsequently underwent various pharmaceutical treatments for 15 years. His life changed when he met a *titiyulo*, or shaman, from the Dagara tribe in Burkina Faso, who immediately recognized Frank as a fellow shaman. While psychosis is considered to be a symptom of mental illness in North America, Neilson observes that "had Frank been born into the Dagara tribe ... the community would have immediately rallied around him" and afforded him a prominent position within the tribe. The social constructionist would not be surprised to find such different views of this man's mental health and, further, would insist that each is "correct" for its respective society. Needless to say, social constructionism has engendered a great deal of controversy within the social sciences and beyond. You might want to explore this fascinating controversy, but don't assume that social constructionism is easily disproven. Consider the experiences of Frank, who we described above. Some would argue that he must be experiencing schizophrenia and that schizophrenia is caused by a dysfunctional brain. However, there isn't a laboratory test to prove that schizophrenia is a result of brain pathology. And if we can't prove that this person has a mental illness, would we acknowledge that he *might* be a shaman?

Politics, Economics, and Mental Health

Stable political and economic conditions foster good mental health, whereas periods of political or economic instability have detrimental impacts on populations. For example, suicide rates increased dramatically in Asia during the economic crisis of 1997–98, during which many people lost their jobs (Chang et al., 2009). Similarly, suicide in Greece increased during the economic crisis that hit the nation in 2011–12 (Rachiotis et al., 2015). During the COVID-19 pandemic, populations globally have experienced mental health consequences related to job loss and economic uncertainty, as well as political unrest (Galea et al., 2020; Jenkins et al., 2021). The atrocities of war, which may include substantial loss of life and property, displacement from communities, and even extrajudicial execution and torture, can also have far-reaching effects on population mental health (Miller & Rasmussen, 2016).

Canadians have enjoyed relative political and economic stability and peace for many decades. However, there are groups within Canadian society who have experienced political and economic hardships similar to those living in poor and

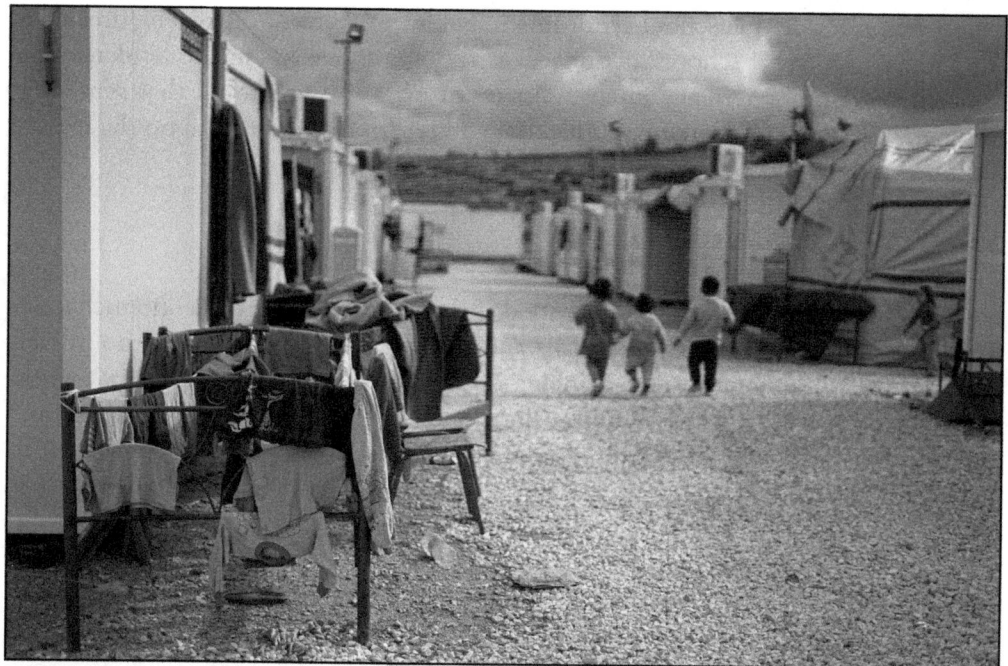

Figure 3.2: A Syrian refugee camp in Greece.
During years of civil war, millions of Syrians have been forced to flee their homes as refugees and asylum seekers. Experiences of war and life as a refugee can contribute to a multitude of mental health challenges, including post-traumatic stress, despair and hopelessness, and severe depression and anxiety.

Source: Unsplash/Julie Ricard

war-ravaged countries. For example, refugees who have fled or been forced out of countries in which they were subjected to human rights abuses frequently experience substantial mental health challenges. Members of Canada's armed forces who have served in combat zones or have witnessed traumatic events are also at high risk of mental health challenges. Studies of Canadian military personnel returning from deployment have found that 38 percent suffered from at least one moderate to severe mental health challenge (Thompson et al., 2016).

Many members of Canada's Indigenous communities have experienced terrible losses as a result of colonization. Over a period of more than 100 years, Indigenous children were forcibly placed in residential schools where they were separated from their families and forced to abandon their cultural and linguistic heritages. Many people who went through the residential school system describe psychological, physical, and sexual abuse while they were residents in the schools. The detrimental effects of residential schools on Indigenous peoples are considered by some to a condition similar to post-traumatic stress disorder (PTSD) termed **residential school syndrome**. According to Canadian psychiatrist Charles Brasfield, people experiencing residential school syndrome may have "recurrent distressing dreams of the Indian residential schools, act or feel as though the events in the residences are re-occurring, and experience intense distress at exposure to stimuli that symbolize residential schools" (Robertson, 2006). We will return to a discussion on the mental health of Indigenous populations in Canada in Chapter 8.

Social Determinants of Health

Social determinants of health are defined as the sociopolitical and economic factors that influence the health of individuals and broad populations. There is no universally accepted list of social determinants of health; however, public policy experts Juha Mikkonen and Dennis Raphael have undertaken a detailed exploration and identified the following 14 social determinants of health as particularly relevant to Canadians (Mikkonen & Raphael, 2010):

- Income and its distribution
- Housing
- Education
- Early childhood development
- Gender
- Employment and working conditions
- Unemployment and employment security
- Indigenous status
- Social exclusion
- Social safety net
- Food security
- Health services
- Race/racism
- Disability

Social determinants have a profound influence on health; in fact, they have a greater impact on health than behavioural risk factors such as diet, physical activity, smoking, and use of alcohol (Donkin et al., 2018). Researchers continue to explore which social determinants have the strongest influence on the health of individuals and populations. It is important to recognize that social determinants of health do not operate in isolation. Rather, they are often experienced simultaneously, interacting at multiple levels—a concept that is detailed in the theory of "intersectionality" (Hankivsky & Jordan-Zachery, 2019). Emerging from Black feminist theory, sociologists such as Patricia Hill Collins, argue that patterns of oppression are often tied together and influenced by the intersectional systems of society (Hill Collins, 2000). As an example, it has been identified that the experiences of white, middle-class women were often very different from those of immigrant, poor, or disabled women. When considering how gender affects health, it became evident that women are not a homogeneous group and that consideration of the relationships between various social determinants are critical to understanding and promoting health outcomes.

The World Health Organization (WHO) has described poverty as the greatest cause of suffering on Earth (WHO, 2013). It will not surprise you that poverty is strongly correlated with poor health; the relationship between individual income and health is well established. This holds true for mental health conditions such as mood disorders, anxiety disorders, developmental problems, hyperactivity, and suicidal behaviour, each of which has been found to be much more prevalent among people living in poverty (Burns, 2015; Pickett & Wilkinson, 2015). Table 3.3 presents findings from a study by Sareen and colleagues (2011), which examined the relationship between income and mental illness in a large population-based sample. Individuals in the lowest income bracket (i.e., income less than $20,000 per year) were far more likely to have had mood disorders or have made suicide attempts than those in higher income groups. This relationship was also identified in recent research carried out by members of our team, when examining the mental health impacts of the COVID-19 pandemic. Indeed, our national survey findings showed that individuals in with the lowest household income (i.e., less than $25,000 per year) were much more likely to report a deterioration in mental health, challenges with coping, and experiences of suicidal thoughts (Jenkins et al., 2021).

Poverty is thought to have an impact on mental health through various mechanisms. These mechanisms include the stress of obtaining material necessities and sustaining oneself or one's family. Poverty also increases the likelihood that one will live in an unsafe environment and be exposed to criminal activity, violence, and problematic or harmful substance use. Exposure to each of these will, in turn, increase the likelihood of developing significant mental health challenges. People who are living in poverty will also have greater limitations in their abilities to access treatment or get time away from work.

Table 3.3: Rates of mood disorders, suicide attempts, and other mental health conditions by income

Lifetime Outcome	Annual Household Income			
	≤ $19,999	$20,000 – $39,999	$40,000 – $69,999	≥ $70,000
Mood Disorder Adjusted Odds Ratio (Confidence Interval)	1.80 (1.50–2.16)	1.36 (1.18–1.37)	1.05 (0.95–1.24)	1.00 (Reference)
Suicide Attempt Adjusted Odds Ratio (Confidence Interval)	3.66 (2.56–5.24)	2.33 (1.44–2.87)	1.52 (1.09–2.13)	1.00 (Reference)

Source: Sareen, J., Afifi, T. O., McMillan, K. A., & Asmundson, G. J. G. (2011). Relationship between household income and mental disorders: Findings from a population-based longitudinal study. *Archives of General Psychiatry, 68*(4), 419–426. https://doi.org/10.1001/archgenpsychiatry.2011.15

Although the mental health of populations increases as income levels rise, the relationship between individual income and emotional well-being is not linear. Moreover, there is a point at which the relationship between mental health and income level plateaus, a finding that has been described as the "law of diminishing marginal utility" (Marx, 1949). According to this theory, lower incomes are correlated with poorer mental health; however, at a certain level there is little added benefit to one's emotional well-being through having a greater income (Jantsch & Veenhoven, 2019; Kahneman & Deaton, 2010). This relationship is depicted in Figure 3.3.

The relationship between mental health or emotional well-being and income levels is complex. In countries such as Canada and the US, which have experienced increasing affluence over recent decades, people are less happy and experience poorer emotional well-being than during preceding decades when people had less material wealth (Oishi & Kesebir, 2015). This has been explained by relative deprivation theory, which posits that individuals assess their satisfaction with their material wealth by comparing themselves with others. When people perceive themselves to be deprived relative to those around them, it can lead to considerable psychosocial stress (Smith & Pettigrew, 2015). Citizens of countries with large gaps between those who are rich and those who are poor (i.e., income inequality) tend to have poorer health overall than citizens of countries in which there is a smaller disparity between the wealthiest and poorest (WHO, 2016).

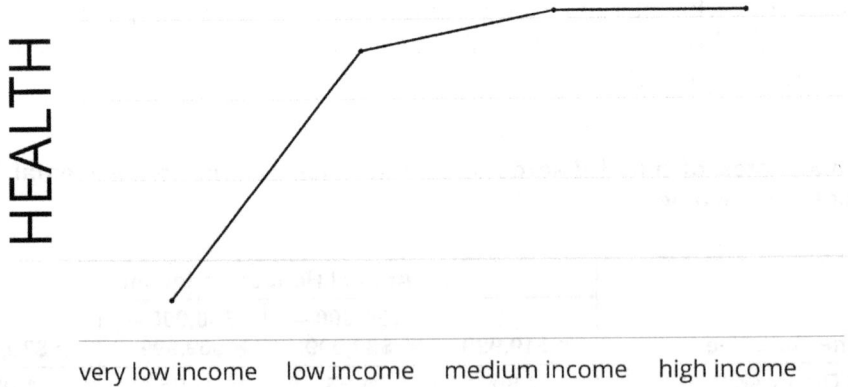

Figure 3.3: Relationship of individual income and emotional well-being. Kahneman and Deaton (2010) found that although emotional well-being rises with income, there is a marginal increase, and an increase in income above median income levels does not lead to further increases in emotional well-being.

Source: Adapted from Kahneman, D., & Deaton, A. (2010). High income improves evaluation of life but not emotional well-being. *Proceedings of the National Academy of Sciences of the United States of America, 107*(38), 16489–16493. https://doi.org/10.1073/pnas.1011492107

> **Box 3.4: Gross National Happiness**
>
>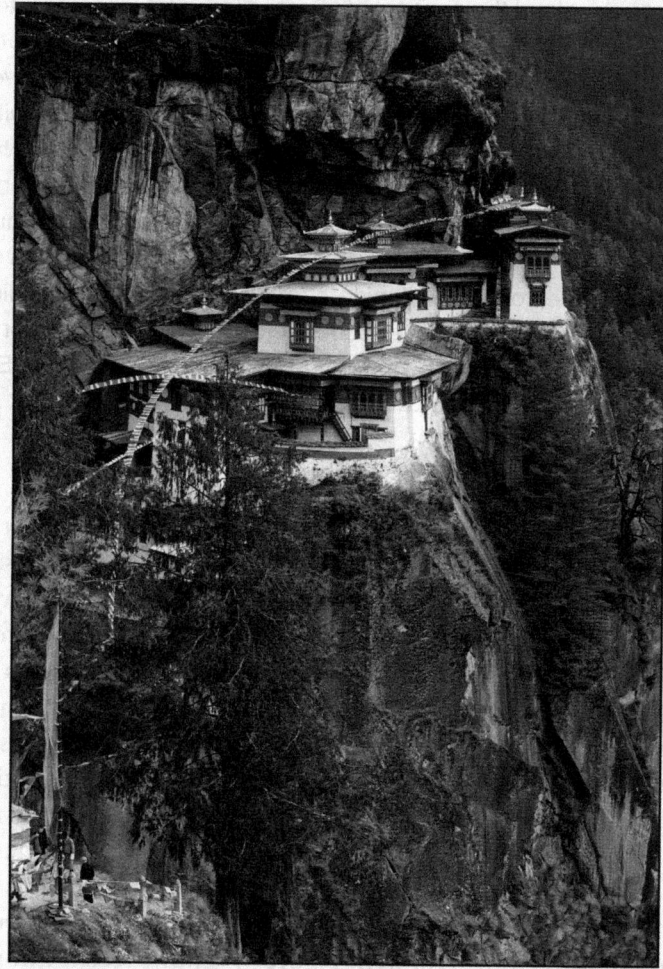
>
> **Figure 3.4:** A cliffside monastery in Bhutan, where former King Jigme Singye Wangchuck began measuring Gross National Happiness as opposed to Gross Domestic Product.
>
> *Source*: iStockphoto/Steve Geer
>
> At the population level, good mental health is associated with life satisfaction, as well as subjective happiness. The Kingdom of Bhutan is a nation in Asia that has made a commitment to promoting these factors through a strong sense of spirituality and a resistance of modern materialism. Despite being a relatively poor country, Bhutan's population has been found to have high levels of subjective happiness, though in

> recent years, the country's relative happiness ranking has fallen considerably to 95/156 countries (Canada ranks 9th; Helliwell et al., 2019). Former King Jigme Singye Wangchuck coined the concept of "Gross National Happiness" to emphasize the importance of well-being as opposed to the widespread drive for material wealth, which is reflected in the measure of Gross Domestic Product. However, while the idea of Gross National Happiness may sound nice in theory, it is not without its critics. Dr. David Luechauer at Purdue University suggests that a Gross National Happiness measure may serve as a distraction from tackling real social and economic problems: "I questioned why Bhutanese leaders were out promoting Bhutan's Gross National Happiness as an economic development model to follow when conditions in the country were so deplorable—dilapidated housing, unsanitary medical facilities, inability to procure healthcare …" (Luechauer, 2013). These conditions may offer insights into the recent deterioration in reported happiness among the Bhutanese.

Housing and Mental Health

Housing is one of the social determinants of health, and certainly, the absence of adequate housing has a huge impact on mental health. Stable and secure housing provides the safety that people need to be able to function in their day-to-day lives. Those without such security are often subject to substantial levels of fear and stress.

The term "homelessness" refers to situations in which people lack a regular, fixed, or adequate nighttime address. It includes those who live in temporary shelters or in public or private spaces that are not intended for human habitation, such as streets, parks, cars, bus stations, or abandoned buildings. In Canada, it is estimated that at least 235,000 people are homeless in a given year, not accounting for those living in precarious housing (e.g., couch surfing, staying temporarily with friends or family) or individuals living in housing that does not meet basic standards (Gaetz et al., 2016). The homeless population includes adults, youth who have run away from home, and families with young children. Figure 3.5 shows recent information about the homeless population in Vancouver as an example. Many people may be homeless for a brief period, but there is a group of people who are chronically homeless. A large proportion of homeless individuals have mental health challenges, including difficulties with substance use that predated their homelessness (To et al., 2016). Moreover, if one's mental health was okay before becoming homeless, living without stable shelter would certainly create mental health challenges.

For those of us who have never had to contemplate surviving without stable housing, it may be difficult to imagine why someone would consider living on the street or sleeping in a doorway or under a bridge. In particular, it might be hard to understand why someone would choose to sleep on the street even when a temporary shelter is offered as an alternative. Yet many people who experience homelessness prefer life on the street because they consider shelters or low-quality housing to hold greater dangers, including bedbugs, rodents, fires, or encounters with people who

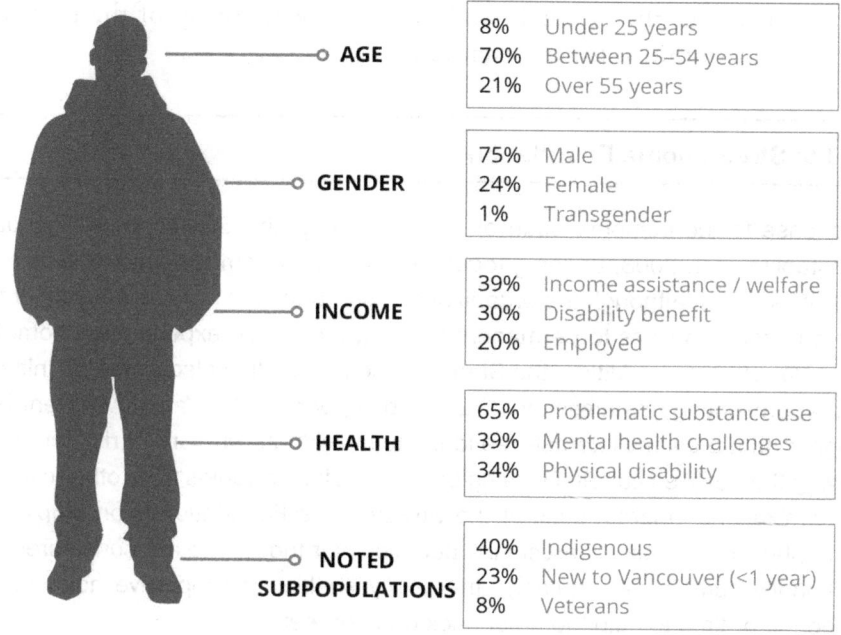

Figure 3.5: Who is experiencing homelessness?

Source: Adapted from Urban Matters CCC & BC Non-Profit Housing Association. (2018). *Vancouver homeless count 2018.* https://vancouver.ca/files/cov/vancouver-homeless-count-2018-final-report.pdf

are threatening or aggressive. You might also question why safe and secure housing is not provided to all citizens in Canada. To answer this question, you may consider that people who are poor, who experience mental health challenges, and who are stigmatized are often without much political influence. A prominent research study, known as the "At Home/Chez Soi" trial, was undertaken by the Mental Health Commission of Canada and improved understandings about the relationship between mental illness and homelessness. Specifically, the study, which was conducted in five Canadian Cities (Vancouver, Winnipeg, Toronto, Montreal, and Moncton), examined the outcomes associated with employing a "Housing First" approach to those experiencing homelessness. Unlike traditional strategies, which require that people accept treatment for mental illnesses or stop using drugs or alcohol before they are provided with housing, the Housing First model removes these barriers. Instead, people who experience homelessness are moved immediately into their own apartments. Findings showed the Housing First model to be effective in enabling people experiencing mental illnesses and homelessness to find and maintain stable housing for extended periods of time. Individuals who received Housing First spent 73 percent of their time in stable housing, whereas a comparison group spent 32 percent of their time in stable housing (Aubry et al., 2015). Housing First also led to improvements in functioning and quality of life. Unfortunately, despite the positive results, once this research study was complete, many of the participating jurisdictions discontinued the intervention.

Box 3.5: Streetohome Foundation

In response to the complex issue of homelessness, the Streetohome Foundation was established in 2008, bringing together individuals from the private, public, and non-profit sectors. Although the organization itself does not provide housing, it functions to increase access to permanent housing for people experiencing homelessness in Vancouver. In addition, the Streetohome Foundation also works on initiatives aimed at preventing homelessness, including supporting the Vancouver Rent Bank, a program that provides interest-free loans to individuals who are at risk for eviction or having their utilities cut off. Drawing on successful strategies from other cities and like-organizations, a large focus of the Streetohome Foundation is on employment and job placement. This is particularly beneficial for those who are considered to be transitionally homeless—requiring emergency shelter or supportive housing for a brief period of time to help them get back on their feet.

Conclusion

In this chapter, we have examined mental health through the social sciences. Some prominent theories developed to understand and explain individual and group behaviour are psychoanalysis, behaviourism, family systems theory, and social constructionism. Theories have also been formulated to describe the development of identity and moral reasoning throughout the life course. The social determinants play a key role in influencing mental health and illness for individuals and populations.

Glossary

anomie: A condition where social and/or moral norms are confused, unclear, or simply absent.
behaviourism: Understanding how behaviour is shaped by the application of various stimuli, such as rewards and punishments.
birth cohorts: Groups of people who were born around the same time and therefore often have had the same exposure to various social and temporal events that may shape their behaviour.

classical conditioning: A learning response that involves associations between environmental stimulus and a naturally occurring stimulus.
collective unconscious: The very deep level of our minds, shared by all humans.
herd behaviour: Describes how people act differently when in large groups than they would normally as individuals.
inferiority complex: The ways in which social structures may cause humans to feel helpless or powerless.
instrumental conditioning: A learning response in which reward or punishment for a particular behaviour increases or decreases the frequency of the behaviour.
residential school syndrome: A form of post-traumatic stress disorder resulting from the detrimental effects of residential schools on Indigenous peoples.
social constructionism: A theory that states that there is no objective truth, only a variety of subjective views developed through dialogue with others.
social determinants of health: The sociopolitical and economic factors that influence the health of individuals and populations.
unconscious mind: The part of the mind that holds feelings, thoughts, desires, and conflicts that the person is unaware of.

Critical Thinking Questions

1. Describe one social science theory related to mental health that is of interest to you.
2. Compare and contrast classical conditioning and instrumental conditioning.
3. How does Erikson's theory of psychosocial development help us to understand mental health?
4. Explain how an individual's mental health is related to their sense of connection to the society in which they live.
5. Choose one of the social determinants of health and explain how that determinant can affect the mental health of an individual and population.

Recommended Readings

Alegría, M., NeMoyer, A., Falgas, I., Wang, Y., & Alvarez, K. (2018). Social determinants of mental health: Where we are and where we need to go. *Current Psychiatry Reports, 20*(11), Article 95. https://doi.org/10.1007/s11920-018-0969-9

Goering, P., Veldhuizen, S., Watson, A., Adair, C., Kopp, B., Latimer, E., Nelson, G., MacNaughton, E., Streiner, D., & Aubry, T. (2014). *National At Home/Chez Soi final report.* https://mentalhealthcommission.ca/resource/national-at-home-chez-soi-final-report/

Green, L. D., & Ubozoh, K. (2019). *We've been too patient: Voices from radical mental health—Stories and research challenging the biomedical model.* North Atlantic Books.

Greenwood, M., de Leeuw, S., & Lindsay, N. M. (2018). *Determinants of Indigenous peoples' health: Beyond the social*. Canadian Scholars.

Kirmayer, L. J., Lemelson, R., and Cummings, C. A. (2017). *Re-visioning psychiatry: Cultural phenomenology, critical neuroscience, and global mental health*. Cambridge University Press.

Morrow, M., & Halinka Malcoe, L. (2017). *Critical inquiries for social justice in mental health*. University of Toronto Press.

Raphael, D. (2016). *Social determinants of health: Canadian perspectives* (3rd ed.). Canadian Scholars.

Rogers, A., & Pilgrim, D. (2020). *A sociology of mental health and illness* (6th ed.). Open University Press.

Recommended Websites

Canadian Housing First Toolkit. https://housingfirsttoolkit.ca

Government of Canada—Social Determinants of Health and Health Inequalities. https://www.canada.ca/en/public-health/services/health-promotion/population-health/what-determines-health.html

Homeless Hub. www.homelesshub.ca

Streetohome. www.streetohome.org

The World Health Organization—Social Determinants of Mental Health. https://apps.who.int/iris/bitstream/handle/10665/112828/9789?sequence=1

References

Adler, A. (1956). *The individual psychology of Alfred Adler*. (H. L. Ansbacher & R. R. Ansbacher, Eds.). Basic Books.

Aubry, T., Nelson, G., & Tsemberis, S. (2015). Housing first for people with severe mental illness who are homeless: A review of the research and findings from the At Home–Chez Soi demonstration project. *Canadian Journal of Psychiatry, 60*(11), 467–474. https://doi.org/10.1177/070674371506001102

Barroso, A., Parker, K., & Fry, R. (2019, October 23). Majority of Americans say parents are doing too much for their young adult children. *Pew Research Centre*. https://www.pewsocialtrends.org/2019/10/23/majority-of-americans-say-parents-are-doing-too-much-for-their-young-adult-children/

Becht, A. I., Nelemans, S. A., Branje, S. J., Vollebergh, W. A., Koot, H. M., Denissen, J. J., & Meeus, W. H. (2016). The quest for identity in adolescence: Heterogeneity in daily identity formation and psychosocial adjustment across 5 years. *Developmental Psychology, 52*(12), 2010–2021. https://doi.org/10.1037/dev0000245

Bornstein, R. F. (2001). The impending death of psychoanalysis. *Psychoanalytical Psychology, 18*, 3–20. https://doi.org/10.1037/0736-9735.18.1.2

Brasfield, C. R. (2001). Residential school syndrome. *British Columbia Medical Journal, 43*(2), 78–81.

Burns, J. K. (2015). Poverty, inequality and a political economy of mental health. *Epidemiology and Psychiatric Sciences, 24*(2), 107–113. https://doi.org/10.1017/S2045796015000086

Burr, V. (2015). *Social constructionism* (3rd ed.). Routledge.

Chang, S. S., Gunnell, D., Sterne, J. A. C., Lu, T. H., & Cheng, A. T. A. (2009). Was the economic crisis 1997–1998 responsible for rising suicide rates in East/Southeast Asia? A time-trend analysis for Japan, Hong Kong, South Korea, Taiwan, Singapore and Thailand. *Social Science & Medicine, 68*(7), 1322–1331. https://doi.org/10.1016/j.socscimed.2009.01.010

Cramer, C., Flynn, B., & LaFave, A. (1997). *Erik Erikson's 8 Stages of psychosocial development: Summary chart.* https://web.cortland.edu/andersmd/ERIK/sum.HTML

Donkin, A., Goldblatt, P., Allen, J., Nathanson, V., & Marmot, M. (2018). Global action on the social determinants of health. *BMJ Global Health, 3*(Suppl 1), e000603. http://dx.doi.org/10.1136/bmjgh-2017-000603

Durkheim, E. (1897). *Suicide.* The Free Press.

Erikson, E. (1950). *Childhood and society.* W.W. Norton & Company.

Erikson, E., & Erikson, J. M. (1987). *The life cycle completed.* W.W. Norton & Company.

Freud, S. (1901). *The psychopathology of everyday life.* T. Fisher Unwin.

Freud, S. (1910). The origin and development of psychoanalysis. *American Journal of Psychology, 21*(2), 181–218.

Gaetz, S., Dej, E., Richter, T., & Redman, M. (2016). *The state of homelessness in Canada, 2016.* https://homelesshub.ca/sites/default/files/SOHC16_final_20Oct2016.pdf

Galea, S., & Abdalla, S. M. (2020). COVID-19 pandemic, unemployment, and civil unrest: Underlying deep racial and socioeconomic divides. *JAMA, 324*(3), 227–228. https://doi.org/10.1001/jama.2020.11132

Gay, P. (1995). *The Freud reader.* Norton.

Hankivsky, O., & Jordan-Zachery, J. S. (Eds.). (2019). *The Palgrave handbook of intersectionality in public policy.* Palgrave MacMillan.

Helliwell, J. F., Layard, R., & Sachs, J. D. (2019). *World happiness report 2019.* https://s3.amazonaws.com/happiness-report/2019/WHR19.pdf

Hill Collins, P. (2000). Gender, Black feminism, and Black political economy. *Annals of the American Academy of Political and Social Science, 568*, 41–53. https://doi.org/10.1177/000271620056800105

Holt-Lunstad, J., & Smith, T. B. (2015). Loneliness and social isolation as risk factors for mortality: A meta-analytic review. *Perspectives on Psychological Science, 10*, 227–237. https://doi.org/10.1177/1745691614568352

Jantsch, A., & Veenhoven, R. (2019). Private wealth and happiness: A research synthesis using an online findings-archive. In G. Brulé & C. Suter (Eds.), *Wealth(s)*

and subjective well-being: Social indicators research series, volume 76 (pp. 17–50). Springer.

Jenkins, E. K., McAuliffe, C., Hirani, S., Richardson, C., Thomson, K. C., McGuinness, L., Morris, J., Kousoulis, A., & Gadermann, A. (2021). A portrait of the early and differential mental health impacts of the COVID-19 pandemic in Canada: Findings from the first wave of a nationally representative cross-sectional survey. *Preventive Medicine, 145*, 106333. https://doi.org/10.1016/j.ypmed.2020.106333

Jung, C. (1981). *The archetypes and the collective unconscious.* Princeton University Press.

Kahneman, D., & Deaton, A. (2010). High income improves evaluation of life but not emotional well-being. *Proceedings of the National Academy of Sciences of the United States of America, 107*(38), 16489–16493. https://doi.org/10.1073/pnas.1011492107

Kail, R. V., & Cavanaugh, J. C. (2016). *Human development: A life-span view* (7th ed.). Cengage Learning.

Kameda, T., Inukai, K., Wisdom, T., & Toyokawa, W. (2015). The concept of herd behaviour: Its psychological and neurological underpinnings. In S. Grundmann, F. Möslein, & K. Riesenhuber (Eds.), *Contract governance: Dimensions in law and interdisciplinary research* (pp. 61–71). Oxford University Press.

Kohlberg, L. (1976). Moral stages and moralization: The cognitive-developmental approach. In T. Lickona (Ed.), *Moral development and behavior: Theory, research, and social issues* (pp. 31–53). Holt, Rinehard, and Winston.

Luechauer, D. L. (2013). Gross National Happiness of Bhutan and its false promises. *Global South Development Magazine.* www.gsdmagazine.org/the-false-promises-of-bhutans-gross-national-happiness/

Mackay, C. (1841). *Extraordinary popular delusions and the madness of crowds.* Harmony Books.

Marx, W. (1949). The law of diminishing marginal utility of income: An investigation of its utility. *Kyklos, 3*(3), 254–272.

Mikkonen, J., & Raphael, D. (2010). *Social determinants of health: The Canadian facts.* York University School of Health Policy and Management.

Miller, K. E., & Rasmussen, A. (2016). The mental health of civilians displaced by armed conflict: An ecological model of refugee distress. *Epidemiology and Psychiatric Services, 26*(2), 129–138. https://doi.org/10.1017/S2045796016000172

Neilson, S. (2016, September 15). A mental disease by any other name. *Nautilus.* https://nautil.us/issue/40/learning/a-mental-disease-by-any-other-name

Oishi, S., & Kesebir, S. (2015). Income inequality explains why economic growth does not always translate to an increase in happiness. *Psychological Science, 26*(10), 1630–1638. https://doi.org/10.1177/0956797615596713

Olson, D. H., Russell, C. S., & Sprenkle, D. H. (1989). *Circumplex model: Systemic assessment and treatment of families.* Haworth Press.

Pavlov, I. P. (1927). *Conditioned reflexes: An investigation of the physiological activity of the cerebral cortex* (G. V. Anrep, Ed. and Trans.). Oxford University Press.

Pickett, K. E., & Wilkinson, R. G. (2015). Income inequality and health: A causal review. *Social Science & Medicine, 128*, 316–326. https://doi.org/10.1016/j.socscimed.2014.12.031

Rachiotis, G., Stuckler, D., McKee, M., & Hadjichristodoulou, C. (2015). What has happened to suicides during the Greek economic crisis? Findings from an ecological study of suicides and their determinants (2003–2012). *British Medical Journal Open, 5*(3), e007295–e007295. https://doi.org/10.1136/bmjopen-2014-007295

Rachman, S. (1997). The evolution of cognitive behaviour therapy. In D. Clark, C. G. Fairburn, & M. G. Gelder (Eds.), *Science and practice of cognitive behaviour therapy* (pp. 1–26). Oxford University Press.

Robertson, L. H. (2006). The residential school experience: Syndrome or historic trauma. *Pimatisiwin: A Journal of Aboriginal and Indigenous Community Health, 4*(1). https://www.pimatisiwin.com/uploads/291994116.pdf

Sareen, J., Afifi, T. O., McMillan, K. A., & Asmundson, G. J. G. (2011). Relationship between household income and mental disorders: Findings from a population-based longitudinal study. *Archives of General Psychiatry, 68*(4), 419–426. https://doi.org/10.1001/archgenpsychiatry.2011.15

Skinner, B. F. (1938). *The behavior of organisms.* Appleton-Century-Crofts.

Skinner, B. F. (1953). *Science and human behavior.* Macmillan.

Smith, H. J., & Pettigrew, T. F. (2015). Advances in relative deprivation theory and research. *Social Justice Research, 28*(1), 1–6. https://doi.org/10.1007/s11211-014-0231-5

Statistics Canada. (2014). *Delayed transitions of young adults.* https://www150.statcan.gc.ca/n1/pub/11-008-x/2007004/10311-eng.htm

Thompson, J., Sweet, J., VanTil, L., Poirier, A., & MacKinnon, K. (2016). *Correlates of mental health problems in Canadian Armed Forces veterans—2013 Life After Service survey.* Veterans Affairs Canada. https://cimvhr.ca/vac-reports/data/reports/Thompson%202016_Correlates%20of%20Mental%20Health%20Problems%20in%20CAF%20Veterans%20LASS%202013.pdf

To, M. J., Palepu, A. Aubry, T., Nisenbaum, R., Gogosis, E., Gadermann, A., Cherner, R., Farrell, S., Misir, V., & Hwang, S. W. (2016). Predictors of homelessness among vulnerably housed adults in 3 Canadian cities: A prospective cohort study. *BMC Public Health, 16*, 1041. https://doi.org/10.1186/s12889-016-3711-8

Urban Matters CCC & BC Non-Profit Housing Association. (2018). *Vancouver homeless count 2018.* City of Vancouver. https://vancouver.ca/files/cov/vancouver-homeless-count-2018-final-report.pdf

Watson, J. B. (1924). *Behaviorism.* Norton.

World Health Organization. (2013). *The economics of social determinants of health and health inequalities: A resource book.* https://apps.who.int/iris/bitstream/handle/10665/84213/9789241548625_eng.pdf?sequence=1

World Health Organization. (2016). *World health statistics 2016: Monitoring health for the SDGs, sustainable development goals.* https://reliefweb.int/sites/reliefweb.int/files/resources/9789241565264_eng.pdf

Chapter 4

◆

The Spectrum of Mental Health Challenges

They called me mad, and I called them mad, and damn them, they outvoted me.
—Nathaniel Porter (playwright)

Introduction

Now that you are familiar with the paradigms used to inform understandings of mental health and illness, in this chapter, we will turn to explore the spectrum of mental health challenges. We will begin with an orientation to the ways that mental disorders are organized and classified. In doing so, we will touch on some of the limitations and problems associated with these approaches. We will then provide an overview of the main categories of mental disorders. This will set the stage for further, more nuanced discussion of these various mental health challenges in subsequent chapters.

Systems of Diagnostic Classification

There are many different forms of mental health challenges, and they vary widely in terms of the course and pattern of illness, the type and severity of symptoms, and the degree of disability or functional impairment experienced. An individual may have only one episode of illness or may have repeated occurrences. Some mental illnesses are episodic or cyclical in nature, whereas others are more persistent, with lengthy or frequently recurring episodes.

In Canada, two systems are used in the diagnostic classification of mental illnesses: the *International Classification of Diseases* (ICD), Mental Health Section, published by the World Health Organization (WHO), and the *Diagnostic and*

Statistical Manual of Mental Disorders (DSM) published by the American Psychiatric Association. The ICD system is used internationally and addresses all types of illness, whereas the DSM classification system solely addresses psychiatric disorders and is used exclusively in North America. Expert panels refine these classification systems regularly in an effort to enhance diagnostic accuracy and incorporate new research evidence. These two classification systems provide the official definitions of the various mental illnesses that may be diagnosed; each classification system includes more than 300 separate mental illnesses. Although Canadian psychiatrists tend to use the DSM system, we have chosen to summarize the ICD system here because it is international in scope. Further, despite the pervasive influence of the DSM in North America, Canada's official classification system is the ICD. Updated in 2018, the ICD is in its 11th version and its sixth chapter addresses mental, behavioural, and neurodevelopmental disorders. In this current edition, attempts have been made to move from what has been termed a "categorical" system of diagnosis—where a person either meets the criteria for diagnosis or not—to a "dimensional" system, in which symptoms are viewed along a continuum. This new approach is considered to be more flexible and patient-centred than previous versions (Gaebel & Kerst, 2019). The ICD-11 groups together classes of mental illnesses considered to share etiological or causal factors. Table 4.1 lists the main ICD-11 Chapter VI groupings. Later in this chapter, we will provide a brief description of a selection of these main blocks and summarize prominent diagnostic categories. Individuals who develop mental illnesses often meet criteria for more than one mental illness at the same time, and many will experience a number of different mental illnesses at various points across their lives (Fried et al., 2017).

The introduction of the latest version of the DSM classification system, the DSM-5, has raised considerable controversy and triggered discussion of fundamental issues concerning the act of diagnosing mental illnesses. As we indicated in Chapter 1, a basic problem of psychiatric diagnosis is that laboratory tests are not available to help establish the presence of mental illnesses. Consequently, there is a great reliance upon clinician experts for diagnosis and considerable room for disagreement. Notably, the DSM-5 is much less cautious about labelling individuals as "mentally ill" than were previous DSM versions; it loosens the criteria in such a way that many more individuals may now receive psychiatric diagnoses. The developers of the DSM-5 insist that their approach is one that will extend the benefits of psychiatric treatment to a larger proportion of individuals, and that this advantage outweighs the risk of labelling large numbers of people as "mentally ill." However, concerns persist. For example, Allen Frances (2013), a psychiatrist who led the development of the previous DSM version, states: "DSM-5 pushes psychiatric diagnosis in the wrong direction, will create new false epidemics, and promotes even more medication misuse. The right goal for DSM-5 would have been diagnostic restraint and deflation, not a further unwarranted expansion of diagnosis and treatment."

Table 4.1: List of blocks of diagnoses in Chapter VI of the ICD-11 covering mental, behavioural, and neurodevelopmental disorders

ICD-11 Mental, Behavioural, or Neurodevelopmental Disorders
Neurodevelopmental disorders
Schizophrenia or other primary psychotic disorders
Catatonia
Mood disorders
Anxiety or fear-related disorders
Obsessive-compulsive or related disorders
Disorders specifically associated with stress
Dissociative disorders
Feeding or eating disorders
Elimination disorders
Disorders of bodily distress or bodily experience
Disorders due to substance use or addictive behaviours
Impulse control disorders
Disruptive behaviour or dissocial disorders
Personality disorders and related traits
Paraphilic disorders
Factitious disorders
Neurocognitive disorders
Mental or behavioural disorders associated with pregnancy, childbirth, or the puerperium
Psychological or behavioural factors affecting disorders or diseases classified elsewhere
Secondary mental or behavioural syndromes associated with disorders or diseases classified elsewhere
Other specified mental, behavioural, or neurodevelopmental disorders
Mental, behavioural, or neurodevelopmental disorders, unspecified

Source: Adapted from World Health Organization. (2018). *ICD-11 for mortality and morbidity statistics (ICD-11 MMS): 2018 version*. https://icd.who.int/browse11/l-m/en

Concerns about Diagnostic Classification

Unfortunately, receipt of a psychiatric diagnosis can cause an individual to experience various challenges. People who are designated as "mentally ill" are often subject to serious discrimination within Canadian society because of widespread fear and misunderstanding. A person who carries a diagnosis of mental illness may suffer loss of relationships, ostracism at work, or exclusion from employment and housing opportunities (Sickel et al., 2014). Some people who have been given diagnoses of

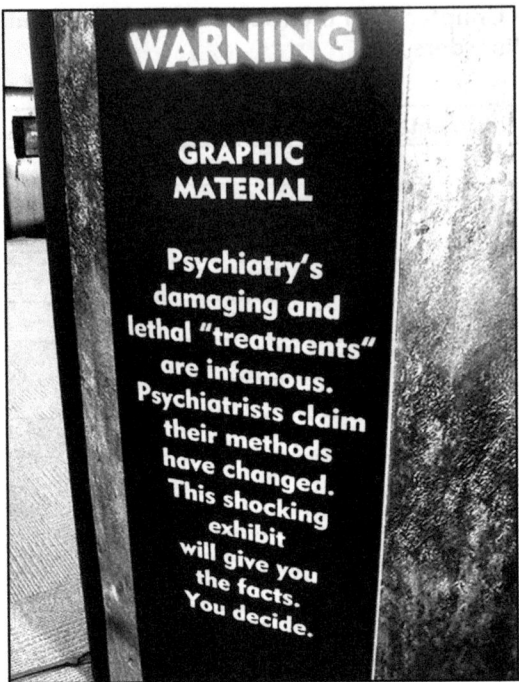

Figure 4.1: Display panel from Psychiatry: An Industry of Death Museum, Los Angeles, CA.

Source: Wikimedia Commons/gruntzooki

mental illness feel that their lives have been damaged as a result (Stolzenburg et al., 2017), and it is not uncommon to find anti-psychiatry protests organized to bring attention to such concerns (see Figure 4.1).

Criticisms regarding the diagnosis of mental illnesses include problems with reliability and validity, adverse effects of labelling, cultural relativity of symptoms, and political and economic misuses of diagnoses. We will discuss each of these in turn.

Problems with Reliability and Validity

Reliability refers to the *consistency* of results when a measurement (including a diagnostic test) is repeated. For example, if someone is examined and diagnosed with schizophrenia at one point in time, will that person receive the same diagnosis if examined at a different point in time? Will different examiners produce the same diagnosis? As is the case with other medical diagnoses, the reliability of mental illness diagnoses is far below 100 percent. **Validity** refers to whether a measurement (including a diagnostic test) really captures what it purports to measure. Thus, when a diagnostician describes someone as having schizophrenia, does this truly indicate that the person has schizophrenia? Perhaps this person presents with similar symptoms as a result of substance use or some other mental health challenge. Even if a diagnosis has high reliability (consistency), its validity may be poor. Thus, in our example, a diagnostician might consistently give a diagnosis of schizophrenia (i.e., high reliability) to a person who has similar symptoms but doesn't really have schizophrenia (i.e., poor validity).

Diagnostic descriptions of mental illnesses are criticized as being vague, arbitrary, and unscientific (Cooper, 2014). These criticisms reflect the fact that most mental illness diagnoses are simply descriptive of patterns of observed symptoms. Very few are clearly linked to specific causes or mechanisms of action, that is, specific biochemical or psychological processes that explain how the illness occurs. For example, the diagnosis of depressive disorder describes a core set of symptoms often found together (e.g., sadness, loss of interest, lack of energy), but there may be many mechanisms that lead to the same symptom complex; there may be any variety of different underlying problems. Imagine that we have used the term "abdominal

> **Box 4.1: Validity of Psychiatric Diagnoses**
>
> A famous experiment conducted by David Rosenhan in the 1970s highlighted the questionable validity of psychiatric diagnoses. Rosenhan assembled a group of students and others who pretended to have mental illnesses and sought admission to 1 of 12 different psychiatric hospitals. When they were assessed, the "fake patients" (who gave false names and employment information but provided other biographical information accurately) pretended to be hearing voices, but claimed no other symptoms or problems. All were admitted and received diagnoses of schizophrenia or bipolar disorder. Once they were admitted, they acted "normally" and no longer reported any symptoms. None were identified as imposters by the hospital staff. Only after they agreed to accept the diagnosis that they were given and take antipsychotic medications were they allowed to leave; their hospital stays ranged from 7 to 52 days. In a second part of the study, staff members at one psychiatric hospital were asked to detect fake patients over a three-month period, yet none had actually been admitted to that hospital. Nevertheless, the hospital staff members identified large numbers of patients they considered to be impostors. In his publication in the journal *Science*, Rosenhan (1973) concluded: "It is clear that we cannot distinguish the sane from the insane in psychiatric hospitals."

pain disorder" to describe a group of different conditions (e.g., peptic ulcer disease, stomach cancer, and appendicitis) without knowing the cause of these conditions. If we did this, each of these conditions would be considered an instance of abdominal pain disorder, and we would not understand the actual problem. Such a vague diagnosis would contribute little to our understanding of the illness, its appropriate treatment, or its likely outcome. Analogously, the diagnosis of depressive disorder may be far too broad to be of much benefit. Without understanding underlying causes and mechanisms, the current diagnostic classification of mental disorders may not provide a valid or meaningful reflection of the actual conditions.

Effects of Labelling

Labelling theory emerged from the disciplines of sociology and criminology and describes the tendency of dominant groups to negatively label minority groups (Murphy, 1976; Scheff, 1966). The theory states that when individuals internalize a label, they eventually take on the traits and behaviours that conform to that label (Roman & Trice, 1968). Psychiatric diagnoses are considered by some to constitute an example of labelling that carries negative consequences (Link & Phelan, 2012). However, some individuals who experience mental illnesses are working to "reclaim" labels that have historically been used as pejorative or discriminatory. For example, the Toronto Mad Pride (2021) organization advocates for the use of "labels" such as "mad" or "crazy" as a way to challenge discrimination and empower people with mental health challenges. Yet it is important to note that while some people who experience mental illnesses may choose to self-identify with these terms, it is considered inappropriate for people who do not experience mental health challenges to use these terms to describe others.

Cultural Relativity

The extent to which diagnoses of mental illnesses are valid across different cultures has been questioned (Murphy, 1976). Indeed, a classification of mental illness developed in one culture may not be applicable to other cultural groups

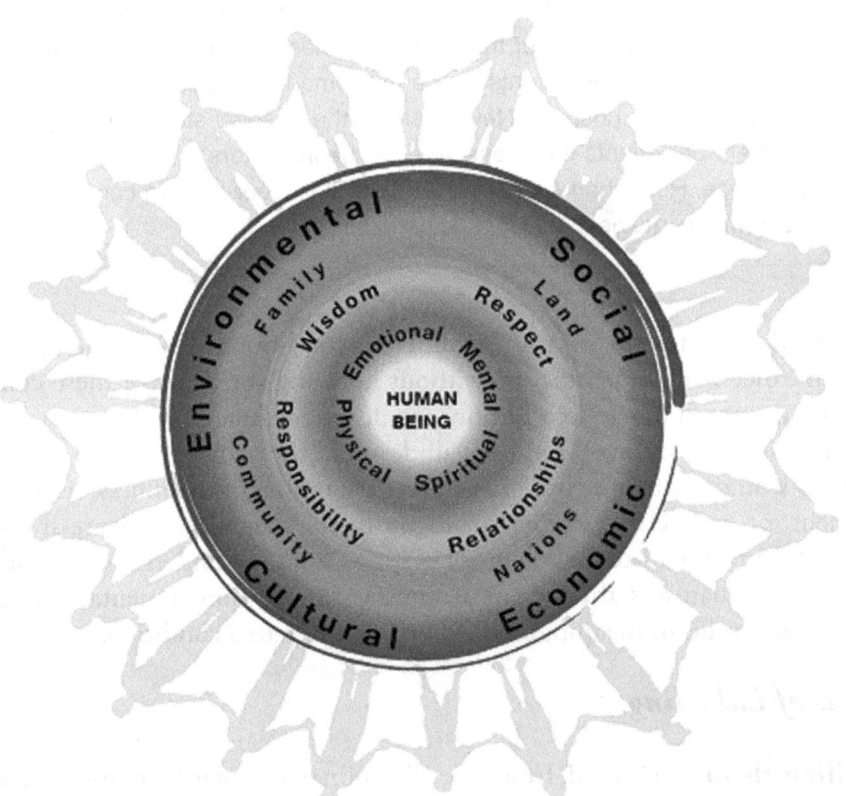

Figure 4.2: Mental health and mental illness are construed in different ways by people of various cultural backgrounds. In comparison to the dominant approach in psychiatric diagnostic systems, Indigenous peoples in Canada tend to think about mental health in more holistic and spiritual terms. Pictured here is a conceptualization of health and wellness, including mental health, endorsed by the First Nations Health Authority in British Columbia.

Source: First Nations Health Authority.

(Bredström, 2019). For example, many Indigenous peoples in Canada have declared that the descriptions of mental disorders listed in the DSM and the ICD may not be relevant or meaningful to members of their communities. Many feel that the unique historical and cultural events—including colonization—that have shaped the type of mental health challenges they encounter are not reflected in the existing diagnostic systems. The psychiatric diagnostic system utilized in Canadian health services may not fit with the spiritual and philosophical frameworks that are embraced by many Indigenous peoples (Smye & Mussell, 2001; Vukic et al., 2011).

Political and Economic Misuses of Diagnoses

The issue has been raised that psychiatric diagnosis may serve a number of covert agendas. One concern is that various governments have imprisoned individuals for political purposes by falsely applying diagnoses of mental illness (Buoli & Giannuli, 2017). This can be a nefarious means of circumventing legal and judicial procedures and has been used to detain minority groups and political prisoners for lengthy periods. Another concern is that diagnoses are promulgated and over-identified for the purpose of selling medications. The pharmaceutical industry and the psychiatric profession have been accused of colluding to manufacture illusory mental illnesses (Atrens, 2011; Cosgrove et al., 2017). For example, the diagnosis of attention deficit disorder is made when children have difficulty focusing their attention, are easily distracted, and have difficulty sitting or standing still. Standard treatment includes prescription of medications such as methylphenidate (also known by the brand name Ritalin). Critics contend that psychiatrists and pharmaceutical companies inflate the prevalence of attention deficit disorder for their own economic benefit, while needlessly medicating children who may simply be bored or overstimulated (Parikh et al., 2016).

Diagnostic Categories

Given the significant concerns we have identified regarding the diagnosis of mental disorders, you might ask: why not discard the whole enterprise? What is the purpose of diagnosing people with mental illnesses if it risks causing harm? The answer is that diagnosis is meant to provide a framework for understanding and responding to mental illnesses and for guiding the correct treatment to fit the condition. The assumption is that the benefits of applying a diagnosis outweigh potential risks.

In the following sections, we provide a short description of a selection of the ICD-11 Chapter VI diagnostic categories. As we can't adequately discuss all of the possible diagnoses here, we offer recommendations at the end of the chapter for additional reading with more comprehensive listings and explanations.

Mood Disorders

Mood disorders include depressive disorders, bipolar disorder, and a number of related diagnostic categories (WHO, 2018) and are among the most commonly occurring mental illnesses in Canada and globally (McRae et al., 2016). As is the case for almost all mental illness diagnoses, mood disorders cover a very wide spectrum of severity and disability. In some situations, a mood disorder can constitute a mild, brief episode that resolves spontaneously. At the other extreme, mood disorders can be tremendously debilitating, persistent, recurrent, and resistant to treatment. Depressive disorders are among the most common mental disorders and are characterized by one or more depressive episodes lasting at least two weeks. People with depressive disorders experience depressed mood (i.e., sadness, emptiness) alongside other symptoms such as fatigue or loss of energy, insomnia or sleeping too much, feelings of worthlessness or guilt, and/or hopelessness (WHO, 2018). Bipolar disorder, which used to be known as "manic depressive illness," is a condition that involves both substantial elevations of mood as well as depressed or low mood (WHO, 2018). These elevations in mood are referred to as mania or hypomania. **Mania** can involve feelings of euphoria, intense or agitated mood, hyperactivity and high energy, and diminished perceived need for sleep or food. Oftentimes, people experiencing a manic episode will engage in dangerous or unsafe behaviours, such as overspending or high-risk sexual activities. Symptoms of mania are extremely disruptive, to the point that they interfere with everyday life. **Hypomania** is a less intense form of elevated mood compared to mania. It typically lasts for a shorter period of time and does not lead to the same level of disruption to activities of daily living. Bipolar disorder most often begins in late adolescence or early adulthood but can also develop during childhood or later in adulthood.

While the differences in terminology between the ICD-11 and the DSM-5 make it challenging to communicate accurate estimates of prevalence, some research indicates that nearly 30 percent of people will experience what the DSM-5 calls major depressive disorder in their lifetime and 15.2 percent will experience persistent depressive disorders (Vandeleur et al., 2017). Bipolar I, the more severe of the bipolar types, has a lifetime prevalence of 0.9 percent (McDonald et al., 2015).

Anxiety or Fear-Related Disorders

This diagnostic category includes various anxiety disorders such as generalized anxiety disorder (GAD), specific phobias, panic disorder, agoraphobia, and social anxiety disorder (WHO, 2018). Like mood disorders, anxiety disorders are also relatively common, with a lifetime prevalence (averaging across anxiety disorder categories) of 14.5 to 33.7 percent (Bandelow & Michaelis, 2015). Generalized anxiety disorder is defined by an extended period of anxiety and worry accompanied by multiple symptoms such as muscle tension, fatigue, poor concentration, insomnia, and irritability. Specific phobias are anxiety disorders involving excessive fears in relation to certain objects or situations. For example, common specific phobias include a fear of certain animals or insects, heights, or elevators. Panic disorder is diagnosed when an individual has experienced multiple panic attacks. Panic attacks are episodes of intense and acute distress. They often include a sense of impending doom and are accompanied by characteristic physical symptoms (e.g., sweating, palpitations, difficulty breathing, dizziness) in addition to persistent concern about the likelihood of having more attacks. Social anxiety disorder involves significant fear of particular social situations (e.g., giving a presentation, having a conversation) due to concerns about being judged by others. As a result, people with social anxiety disorder tend to avoid these situations or else experience extreme fear or anxiety in persisting through them. Anxiety disorders tend to start early in life (during childhood or adolescence) and often persist for many years.

Obsessive-Compulsive and Related Disorders

While historically classified within the anxiety disorder block, in the ICD-11, obsessive-compulsive disorder is now contained in a separate group alongside a selection of disorders differentiated by cognitive experiences including obsessions, intrusive thoughts or ideas, and preoccupations. These experiences are often accompanied by repetitive or ritualistic behaviours intended to ease distress. With obsessive-compulsive disorder, the person experiences obsessions, consisting of intrusive and persistent thoughts, impulses, or images that are inappropriate or irrational and lead to significant anxiety or distress. In an effort to ease this distress, the person will often engage in compulsions, which are repetitive or ritualistic behaviours (such as handwashing) or mental acts (such as counting). Also included in this block are hoarding disorder and hypochondriasis. Hoarding disorder is associated with the excessive accumulation of and/or challenges in letting go of possessions, irrespective of their actual worth. This leads to unsafe or disorderly living spaces and related risks to health and safety. Hypochondriasis involves a preoccupation with the possibility of having a serious or life-threatening illness. Individuals who experience this disorder often seek out excessive medical intervention and are not reassured even by the receipt of encouraging test results.

Schizophrenia and Other Primary Psychotic Disorders

Schizophrenia and other psychotic disorders usually emerge in adolescence or early adulthood, but occasionally develop during childhood or later in adulthood (Miettunen et al., 2019). Schizophrenia is a relatively infrequent disorder, with a lifetime prevalence of approximately 0.48 percent (although there is considerable variation between geographic regions; Simeone et al., 2015). Schizophrenia affects the way the brain processes and interprets information and leads people to experience **psychosis**, or to "lose touch with reality" through the presence of delusions, (i.e., intensely held irrational beliefs), hallucinations, impaired cognition, and changes in behaviour (i.e., bizarre or unpredictable). Delusions come in a variety of forms. Paranoid delusions involve beliefs that there is some imminent danger or that someone is being followed or persecuted. These delusions can be extremely frightening and often create terrible distress and suffering. Grandiose delusions are also common. They comprise false beliefs about possessing superior abilities, powers, or influence over others or world events. Religious delusions can also occur, for example, believing oneself to be a spiritual saviour.

Hallucinations (i.e., false sensory experiences generated by an individual's mind) are also typical features of schizophrenia and related disorders. Most often, people with schizophrenia experience auditory hallucinations, convinced that they hear voices or sounds despite the absence of external stimuli. Hallucinations involving other senses can also occur. Delusions and hallucinations are categorized as *positive* symptoms of schizophrenia. This does not mean that they are beneficial or desirable, only that they are symptoms that occur in addition to usual cognitive and sensory experiences. Schizophrenia and related disorders are also characterized by *negative* symptoms, in which the person has reduced motivational drive or activity level and may experience cognitive impairment, such as poor attention span or memory. Schizophrenia and related disorders usually begin slowly with prodromal symptoms (i.e., early symptoms that indicate the start of illness) and often manifest in cycles of alternating remission and relapse. Many people who experience schizophrenia have **anosognosia**, which means that they lack insight into their illness and do not recognize or understand their symptoms or the need for treatment.

Box 4.2: "The Son Who Vanished..." by Erin Anderssen

On a September evening almost nine years ago, Susan and Jay Bigelow called 911, then sat down to dinner in their Toronto home, waiting for the police to come and take away the stranger at the dining-room table who was once their son.

For 19 years, they had raised a cheerful, outgoing boy named Jesse Bigelow, who had lots of friends, was chased by girls and sang in a rock band called, in an odd foreshadowing, Mental Distortion.

Then, slowly, helplessly, they watched Jesse Bigelow vanish, as surely as if he had been kidnapped. They didn't recognize the shaggy, bearded intruder who now lay like a zombie in the bedroom upstairs and ranted at them about God.

Jay: The first thing you notice is that, all of a sudden, he is not associating with his friends as regularly as he had been. He became very withdrawn. And he was not having as much social contact.

Jesse: I went from being very sociable to being weird and more reserved and very moody. I became paranoid. If there was a group of people in the schoolyard talking and laughing, I started to believe they were laughing at me.

Susan: Then one day, he came home and told me that he thought people on the subway had been talking about him.

For several months, Jesse's parents hoped that it really was just "a bad patch." But by the late spring of 1999, Jesse was clearly psychotic.

It was devastating: Jay had always been close to Jesse, but now his son refused to speak to him and began to refer to his father as the Devil. The family, who'd never attended church, couldn't make sense of this newly found religious fervour. "It was very scary," his mother says, as Jesse's delusions intensified.

Jesse: I started hearing voices. I would hear my own voice in my head as my regular thoughts, but then I had additional voices. On my left side, I heard a very disruptive commanding male voice that I thought was the Devil. On the right side, I would hear a very soothing, calming female voice that I thought was the Virgin Mary.

Jay: There'd be times when he'd go to his room and spend hours and hours on end lying in bed, doing nothing but basically staring at the ceiling. And every hour or so, you might hear maniacal laughter, or sometimes you'd hear talking. Of course, what he was really doing was interacting with the voices.

Jesse: ... But I really, really believed I was Jesus Christ at that time. Now I look back, no human being can be Jesus Christ. That's impossible....

In the elevator after the first meeting with Jesse's doctor at the Centre for Addiction and Mental Health in Toronto, his parents were reeling from the diagnosis. Susan looked at Jay: "This is a death sentence," she said. Only about one-third of people diagnosed with schizophrenia make a full recovery and, even then, the disease is a chronic condition....

For four months, his doctors experimented with medications... At last he showed progress on a new antipsychotic called Clozapine.

Even so, it was a year before they began to see signs of the old Jesse. He could follow a conversation. He showered. He spoke less often about the voices. He began to talk about getting a job....

If you met Jesse Bigelow today, more than eight years since his release from the hospital, it would never cross your mind that he had a mental illness....

Over the years, he has reclaimed his life, piece by piece, and in many ways started fresh. He falls within the lucky percentage of people with schizophrenia who are able, through medication, to control the disease.

Now 29, he attends a United Church faithfully (something he never would have done before his diagnosis) and sings with a band in a local pub on Sunday nights....

> Healthy as he is, Jesse is not cured. At times, he has experienced "breakthrough symptoms," times when his medication, which comes with a risk of serious side effects, must be increased....
>
> **Susan:** The thing that bothers me is that there were so many times we could have said, "Just get out." And he would have been living on the street—or dying on the street. I think that's the most frightening. There are so many people on the street with mental illness, and that's what happened. I understand. You just can't put up with them anymore. But you have to.
>
> **Jay:** Don't give up hope. When it looks really bleak, there is room to get better.
>
> *Source*: Anderssen, E. (2008, June 20). The son who vanished... *The Globe and Mail.* http://www.theglobeandmail.com/life/health-and-fitness/the-son-who-vanished/article560793/

Schizoaffective disorder is another psychotic illness in which an individual simultaneously meets the diagnostic criteria for both schizophrenia and a mood disorder (i.e., mania, depression, or a mixed state). Schizotypal disorders refer to conditions in which disturbances in thinking and eccentric behaviour occur that are similar to symptoms seen in schizophrenia and schizoaffective disorder, but generally milder in nature. A variety of other diagnoses are included in this group, and they are characterized by the existence of delusional symptoms that may be transient or persistent (WHO, 2018).

Disorders Due to Substance Use or Addictive Behaviour

While the use of psychoactive substances is common in Canadian society, their use can lead to challenges. A diagnosis within this block of mental disorders indicates that the cause is related to the use of psychoactive substances, which may or may not have been medically prescribed (WHO, 2018). The specific diagnosis given is based on the type of substance that is implicated, for example, alcohol use disorder or opioid use disorder. Other substances that may contribute to a substance use disorder include cannabinoids, sedatives, cocaine or other stimulants, psychedelics, nicotine, volatile inhalants, and others.

While substance use occurs across a spectrum, from beneficial through to problematic use, disorders are associated with what the ICD-11 describes as harmful patterns of use:

> [substance use] that has caused damage to a person's physical or mental health or has resulted in behaviour leading to harm to the health of others ... Harm to health of the individual occurs due to one or more of the following: (1) behaviour related to intoxication; (2) direct or secondary toxic effects on body organs

and systems; or (3) a harmful route of administration. Harm to health of others includes any form of physical harm, including trauma, or mental disorder that is directly attributable to behaviour related to [substance use] intoxication on the part of the person to whom the diagnosis of harmful pattern of [substance] use applies.

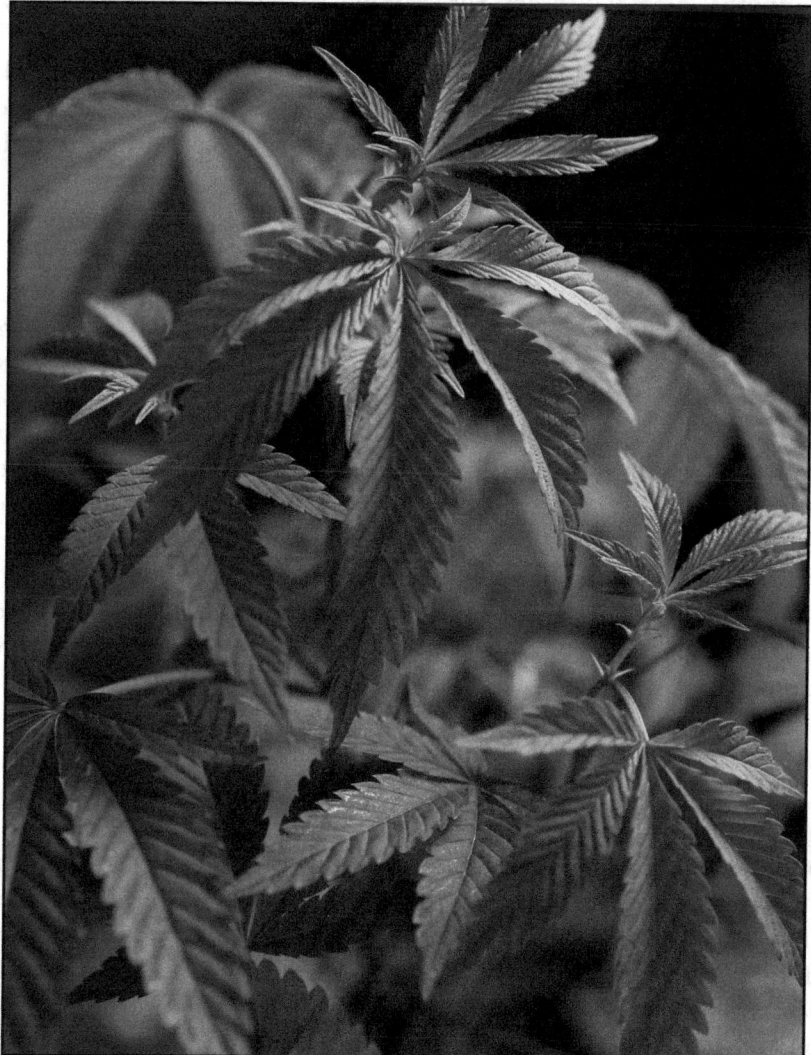

Figure 4.3: Shown here in plant form, cannabis was historically the most commonly used illicit substance in Canada, although its use is no longer considered a Criminal Code violation as of October 17, 2018 (Cox, 2018). Persistent, high-frequency use is associated with a number of mental health challenges.

Source: Pexels/Kindel Media

Other clinical conditions that may be designated within this block include syndromes involving dependence, withdrawal, and psychosis secondary to substance use. We consider the topic of substance use to be so important that we have devoted an entire chapter to its discussion (Chapter 5) and we define these syndromes there.

Concurrent disorders refer to the co-occurrence of a substance use disorder alongside another mental disorder. For example, someone who meets the diagnostic criteria for both alcohol dependence and major depressive disorder would be considered to have a concurrent disorder. Epidemiological studies have found that concurrent disorders are very common (Khan, 2017), and in our chapter on treatment (Chapter 14), we will discuss specialized approaches to concurrent disorders that have been developed in recent years.

Disorders Specifically Associated with Stress

A new category in the ICD-11 is disorders specifically associated with stress, which includes disorders directly resulting from an exposure to or ongoing experiences of stressful or traumatic events. Included in this category is post-traumatic stress disorder, or PTSD, which develops in response to profoundly threatening or horrifying incidents. PTSD involves flashbacks, disturbing dreams, persistent frightening thoughts and memories, anger, or irritability in response to a terrifying experience. Adjustment disorders also fall within this category and are conditions that are considered to be a response to some particular stressor, such as the loss of a job or a death in the family. The diagnosis of adjustment disorder indicates that the individual has developed symptoms in response to the event that are more intense or prolonged than expected.

Feeding or Eating Disorders

Feeding and eating disorders involve a serious disturbance in feeding or eating behaviour. Feeding disorders are characterized by behaviours such as eating non-edible materials and do not relate to concerns over body weight, size, or shape. In contrast, eating disorders involve atypical eating behaviours and perseveration on food. Individuals with eating disorders experience profound worry centring on body weight and shape (WHO, 2018). As a result of the nutritional and metabolic consequences of severe feeding and eating disorders, they can cause very serious medical problems that may be life-threatening (Fitcher & Quadflieg, 2016). Avoidant-restrictive food intake disorder, referred to in clinical circles as ARFID, is a recently classified, serious disorder involving extreme food "pickiness" or restrictiveness. The associated feeding and eating behaviours result in inadequate amounts or varieties of foods being consumed, leading to nutritional and functional deficiencies.

> **Box 4.3: "Why Picky Eating Could Be a Sign of an Eating Disorder" by Gabby Bess**
>
> For people with avoidant/restrictive food intake disorder (ARFID), tasting or even being around foods that they would rather avoid is, indeed, a huge deal. First defined in the 2013 update of the DSM-5, the recently classified eating disorder is marked by at least one of the following symptoms: "significant weight loss, significant nutritional deficiency, dependence on enteral feeding or oral nutritional supplements, or marked interference with psychosocial functioning."
>
> Though the condition goes far beyond your typical picky toddler, ARFID typically starts in early childhood and manifests most frequently in young boys, according to a study published in the *Journal of Eating Disorders*. Young people diagnosed with ARFID refuse to eat or eat very little. But what makes it different from other eating disorders is that ARFID is not rooted in body image issues.
>
> "Prior to the DSM-5 update, we were seeing a lot of kids who you would now say 'fit the diagnosis,' but they had to be lumped into the category of 'eating disorder not otherwise specified' or 'feeding disorders of early childhood' or they were just not diagnosed," says Dr. Debra K. Katzman, a leading researcher on the disorder and senior associate scientist at the SickKids hospital at the University of Toronto. "Classically we think of eating disorders as either anorexia nervosa or bulimia nervosa. In those eating disorders, young people have distortions about their body weight, shape, or size. In this particular eating disorder, they don't have those distortions, which is very interesting."
>
> Those with the condition often display a literal fear or suspicion of certain foods, sometimes following a traumatic event. However, there is no known cause. In the [journal] *Paediatrics and Child Health*, Dr. Katzman writes about a 10-year-old boy who had to go to the emergency room because he refused to eat solid foods for eight weeks; he feared choking after a previous incident involving steak, and his weight was rapidly declining. "He became progressively more restricted in the type of foods that he considered to be 'safe,'" Dr. Katzman writes. "Despite his parents' best attempt to feed him soft and pureed food, he failed to gain any weight."
>
> Like any eating disorder, ARFID can be dangerous, leading to malnutrition and fatal weight loss. And if not deadly, extreme picky eating habits can carry on into adulthood. (Some might think of 30-year-old Kelly, a subject on the TLC show *Freaky Eaters* who went viral for her diet consisting of only cheesy potatoes. On the show, she cried from anxiety when confronted with vegetables.) In *Scientific American*, Dr. Katzman underscores that early awareness—and awareness of the disorder in general—is key. "Once we identify and characterize these cases, we can begin to study different types of treatments, long-term outcomes and root causes of the illness," she tells the publication. There's still a lot of research to be done.
>
> *Source:* Bess, G. (2016, January 6). Why picky eating could be a sign of an eating disorder. *Vice*. https://www.vice.com/en_us/article/mgmzga/some-picky-eaters-eating-disorder-arfid

The most common eating disorders are binge eating disorder and bulimia nervosa. Binge eating disorder is a condition characterized by episodes in which an individual feels compelled to eat large amounts of food in an uncontrolled manner, experiencing profound distress and self-denigration. The episodes of binge eating are not followed by any compensatory activities (i.e., self-induced vomiting, intense exercise, or laxative use to avert weight gain). Bulimia nervosa, in contrast, is marked by both binge eating episodes and regular compensatory activities. Anorexia nervosa involves disturbed eating behaviour, low body weight, intense fear of weight gain, and an inaccurate perception of one's own body weight or shape. Eating disorders often arise in adolescence and affect girls and women disproportionately (National Eating Disorder Information Centre, 2019).

Personality Disorders and Related Traits

Personality disorders include a number of personality traits or patterns that vary considerably in their characteristics and related behaviours. However, they all share the following: an enduring pattern of inner experience and behaviour that deviates from the expectations of society; and behavioural patterns that are pervasive, inflexible, and stable over time, creating distress and/or impairment. The onset of personality disorders usually occurs in adolescence or early adulthood, though they can also become apparent in mid-adulthood.

In the ICD-11, the categorization of personality disorders was altered to focus on central personality dysfunction, while allowing flexibility in the classification of severity (i.e., mild, moderate, and severe). In addition, pronounced trait patterns can be specified, including negative affectivity, detachment, disinhibition, dissociality, and anankastia (i.e., a narrow focus on perfectionism or one's own sense of right and wrong). Borderline pattern (which replaces borderline personality disorder in the ICD-11) can also be denoted. This pattern of personality disruption is characterized by persistent volatility in interpersonal relationships and affect as well as significant impulsivity.

Some personality disorder traits result in suffering that primarily affects the individual, for example, detachment, which is characterized by feelings of extreme discomfort and intense self-criticism in social circumstances. This can lead to marked loneliness and isolation, despite intense longings for social contact. Other personality disorder traits tend to cause distress to those who are in proximity to the individual. For example, dissociality involves a pervasive pattern of disregard for and violation of the rights of others and often includes a lack of empathy, attention-seeking behaviours, and self-centredness.

Neurodevelopmental Disorders

In the ICD-11, neurodevelopmental disorders are a category of "behavioural and cognitive disorders that arise during the developmental period. These disorders involve significant difficulties in the acquisition and execution of specific intellectual, motor, or social functions" (WHO, 2018). Included in this category are disorders of intellectual development, autism spectrum disorder, and attention deficit hyperactivity disorder, among others. Disorders of intellectual development are comprised of a group of diverse conditions that are distinguished by below average cognitive or intellectual abilities and onset during the developmental period (WHO, 2018). In Canada, the terms "developmental disability" or "intellectual disability" are commonly used to describe these disorders. Disorders of intellectual development are further classified by level of severity or impairment, from mild through to profound.

Autism spectrum disorder is a condition that arises in the early years of life and involves challenges in social interactions, relationships, and communication. Further, those diagnosed with this disorder tend to have distinctive, intense, and inflexible patterns of behaviour or interests. For example, some young children diagnosed with autism spectrum disorder become consumed by their interests (such as elevators, particular animals, or even sensations) and their caregivers describe great difficulty in redirecting their child's attention or managing the behaviour if the focus needs to change. Attention deficit hyperactivity disorder—often referred to simply as ADHD—is a relatively common neurodevelopmental condition that tends to be diagnosed in early to mid-childhood. This disorder is characterized by an ongoing pattern of inattention, hyperactivity, and impulsivity that leads to impairment in school, work, or social functioning (WHO, 2018). In recent years, the number of children diagnosed with ADHD has skyrocketed in some jurisdictions (though remained stable in others), leading to concerns about over-diagnosis and over-treatment (Vasiliadis et al., 2017).

We will return to discussing some of these disorders further in Chapter 9, which is devoted to examining mental health and illness in children and adolescents.

Conclusion

A great deal of effort has gone into the diagnostic classification of mental illnesses. Although these efforts are limited by problems of reliability and validity, they remain a central means of organizing our understanding of mental and behavioural conditions and delineating treatment approaches. Care must be taken to avoid harms that may occur as a result of diagnostic labelling, including perpetuating stigma and discrimination towards people who live with mental illnesses. In forthcoming chapters, we will delve deeper into several of these disorder categories in relation to their impacts within various sub-groups of the population.

Glossary

anosognosia: Also referred to as a "lack of insight," anosognosia is a symptom of certain mental illnesses, including schizophrenia and other psychotic disorders, that interferes with a person's ability to recognize their illness.

hypomania: A less intense form of elevated mood than mania, it is most often experienced by people with bipolar disorder.

labelling theory: The theory that when individuals who are labelled internalize the label, they eventually take on the traits and behaviours that conform to that label.

mania: An intense, elevated mood that is often experienced as part of bipolar disorder and results in significant disruption to life activities and responsibilities.

psychosis: A condition that causes people to lose touch with reality. It is common among those who have schizophrenia.

reliability: The consistency of results when a measurement (including a diagnostic test) is repeated.

validity: Whether a measure (including a diagnostic test) really captures what it purports to measure.

Critical Thinking Questions

1. What are the differences between mental health challenges and mental illnesses?
2. What are some of the challenges with current diagnostic classification?
3. Provide examples of political and economic misuses of diagnosis.
4. What role does culture play in understanding mental health and illness?
5. Select and describe one of the ICD-11 Chapter VI blocks.

Recommended Readings

Conrad, P. (2007). *The medicalization of society: On the transformation of human conditions into treatable disorders.* Hopkins Fulfillment Service.

Kutchins, H., & Kirk, S. A. (2003). *Making us crazy: DSM: The psychiatric bible and the creation of mental disorders.* Free Press.

Lavallee, L. F., & Poole, J. M. (2010). Beyond recovery: Colonization, health and healing for Indigenous people in Canada. *International Journal of Mental Health and Addiction, 8,* 271–281. https://doi.org/10.1007/s11469-009-9239-8

Stein, D. J., Szatmari, P., Gaebel, W., Berk, M., Vieta, E., Maj, M., de Vries, Y. A., Roest, A. M., de Jonge, P., Maercker, A., Brewin, C. R., Pike, K. M., Grilo, C. M., Fineberg, N. A., Briken, P., Cohen-Kettenis, P. T., & Reed, G. M. (2020). Mental, behavioural and neurodevelopmental disorders in the ICD-11: An international perspective on key changes and controversies. *BMC Medicine, 18,* Article 21. https://doi.org/10.1186/s12916-020-1495-2

Recommended Websites

Anxiety Canada. www.anxietycanada.com
Canadian Mental Health Association. www.cmha.ca
eMentalHealth.ca—A-Z Mental Health Topics and Conditions. www.ementalhealth.ca/index.php?m=azConditions
National Eating Disorder Information Centre. www.nedic.ca
Public Health Agency of Canada—Mental Health. www.phac-aspc.gc.ca/mh-sm/index-eng.php
Schizophrenia Society of Canada. https://schizophrenia.ca
World Health Organization—ICD-11 for Mortality and Morbidity Statistics (ICD-11 MMS): 2018 version. https://icd.who.int/browse11/l-m/en
World Health Organization—Mental Health. www.who.int/topics/mental_health/en

References

Anderssen, E. (2008, June 20). The son who vanished … *The Globe and Mail.* http://www.theglobeandmail.com/life/health-and-fitness/the-son-who-vanished/article560793/

Atrens, D. M. (2011). Big pharma and the manufacture of madness. *Quadrant, 55*(1–2).

Bandelow, B., & Michaelis, S. (2015). Epidemiology of anxiety disorders in the 21st century. *Dialogues in Clinical Neuroscience, 17*(3), 327–355. https://doi.org/10.31887/DCNS.2015.17.3/bbandelow

Bess, G. (2016, January 6). Why picky eating could be a sign of an eating disorder. *Vice.* https://www.vice.com/en_us/article/mgmzga/some-picky-eaters-eating-disorder-arfid

Bredström, A. (2019). Culture and context in mental health diagnosing: Scrutinizing the DSM-5 revision. *Journal of Medical Humanities, 40*(3), 347–363. https://doi.org/10.1007/s10912-017-9501-1

Buoli, M., & Giannuli, A. S. (2017). The political use of psychiatry: A comparison between totalitarian regimes. *International Journal of Social Psychiatry, 63*(2), 169–174. https://doi.org/10.1177/0020764016688714

Cooper, R. (2014). *Diagnosing the Diagnostic and Statistical Manual of Mental Disorders*. Routledge.

Cosgrove, L., Krimsky, S., Wheeler, E. E., Peters, S. M., Brodt, M., & Shaughnessy, A. F. (2017). Conflict of interest policies and industry relationships of guideline development group members: A cross-sectional study of clinical practice guidelines for depression. *Accountability in Research, 24*(2), 99–115. https://doi.org/10.1080/08989621.2016.1251319

Cox, C. (2018). The Canadian Cannabis Act legalizes and regulates recreational cannabis use in 2018. *Health Policy, 122*(3), 205–209. https://doi.org/10.1016/j.healthpol.2018.01.009

Fitcher, M. M., & Quadflieg, N. (2016). Mortality in eating disorders: Results of a large prospective clinical longitudinal study. *International Journal of Eating Disorders, 49*(4), 391–401. https://doi.org/10.1002/eat.22501

Frances, A. (2013). *Saving normal: An insider's revolt against out-of-control psychiatric diagnosis, DSM-5, Big Pharma, and the medicalization of ordinary life.* HarperCollins Canada.

Fried, E. I., van Borkulo, C. D., Cramer, A. O. J., Boschloo, L., Schoevers, R. A., & Borsboom, D. (2017). Mental disorders as networks of problems: A review of recent insights. *Social Psychiatry and Psychiatric Epidemiology, 52*(1), 1–10. https://doi.org/10.1007/s00127-016-1319-z

Gaebel, W., & Kerst, A. (2019). ICD-11 Mental, behavioural and neurodevelopmental disorders: Innovations and managing implementation. *Archives of Psychiatry and Psychotherapy, 3*, 7–12. https://doi.org/10.12740/APP/111494

Khan, S. (2017). Concurrent mental and substance use disorders in Canada (Catalogue no. 82-003-X). *Health Reports, 28*(8), 3–8. https://iogt.org/wp-content/uploads/2017/08/54853-eng.pdf

Link, B. G., & Phelan, J. C. (2012). Labelling and stigma. In C. S. Aneshensel, J. C. Phelan, & A. Bierman (Eds.), *Handbook of the sociology of mental health* (pp. 525–543). Springer.

McDonald, K. C., Bulloch, A. G. M., Duffy, A., Bresee, L., Williams, J. V. A., Lavorato, D. H., & Patten, S. B. (2015). Prevalence of bipolar I and II disorder in Canada. *Canadian Journal of Psychiatry, 60*(3), 151–156. https://doi.org/10.1177/070674371506000310

McRae, L., O'Donnell, S., Loukine, L., Rancourt, N., & Pelletier, C. (2016). Report summary—Mood and anxiety disorders in Canada, 2016. *Health Promotion and Chronic Disease Prevention in Canada, 36*(12), 314–315.

Miettunen, J., Immonen, J., McGrath, J. J., Isohanni, M., & Jääskeläinen, E. (2019). The age of onset of schizophrenia spectrum disorders. In G. de Girolamo, P. McGorry, & N. Sartorius (Eds.), *Age of onset of mental disorders: Etiopathogenetic and treatment implications* (pp. 59–73). Springer.

Murphy, J. (1976). Psychiatric labeling in cross-cultural perspective: Similar kinds of disturbed behavior appear to be labeled abnormal in diverse cultures. *Science, 191*, 1019–1028.

National Eating Disorder Information Centre. (2019). *General information.* https://nedic.ca/general-information/

Parikh, K., Fleischman, W., & Agrawal, S. (2016). Industry relationships with pediatricians: Findings from the Open Payments Sunshine Act. *Pediatrics, 137*(6), e20154440. https://doi.org/10.1542/peds.2015-4440

Roman, P. M., & Trice, H. M. (1968). The sick role, labeling theory, and the deviant drinker. *International Journal of Social Psychiatry, 14*, 245–251. https://doi.org/10.1177/002076406801400401

Rosenhan, D. L. (1973). On being sane in insane places. *Science, 179*(70), 250–258. https://doi.org/10.1126/science.179.4070.250

Scheff, T. J. (1966). *Being mentally ill: A sociological theory*. Aldine.

Sickel, A. E., Seacat, J. D., & Nabors, N. A. (2014). Mental health stigma update: A review of consequences. *Advances in Mental Health, 12*(3), 202–215. https://doi.org/10.1080/18374905.2014.11081898

Simeone, J. C., Ward, A. J., Rotella, P., Collins, J., & Windisch, R. (2015). An evaluation of variation in published estimates of schizophrenia prevalence from 1990–2013: A systematic literature review. *BMC Psychiatry, 15*, Article 193. https://doi.org/10.1186/s12888-015-0578-7

Smye, V., & Mussell, B. (2001). *Aboriginal mental health: 'What works best?'* https://summit.sfu.ca/item/11161

Stolzenburg, S. D., Freitag, S., Evans-Lacko, S., Muelhan, H., Schmidt, S., & Schomerus, G. (2017). The stigma of mental illness as a barrier to self labelling as having a mental illness. *The Journal of Nervous and Mental Disease, 205*(12), 903–909. https://doi.org/10.1097/NMD.0000000000000756

Toronto Mad Pride. (2021). *What is mad pride?* http://www.torontomadpride.com/what-is-mp/

Vandeleur, C. L., Fassassi, S., Castelao, E., Glaus, J., Strippoli, M. P. F., Lasserre, A. M., Rudaz, D., Gebreab, S., Pistis, G., Aubry, J.-M., Angst, J., & Preisig, M. (2017). Prevalence and correlates of DSM-5 major depressive and related disorders in the community. *Psychiatry Research, 250*, 50–58. https://doi.org/10.1016/j.psychres.2017.01.060

Vasiliadis, H.-M., Diallo, F. B., & Rochette, L. (2017). Temporal trends in the prevalence and incidence of diagnosed ADHD in children and young adults between 1999 and 2012 in Canada: A data linkage study. *The Canadian Journal of Psychiatry, 62*(12), 818–826. https://doi.org/10.1177/0706743717714468

Vukic, A., Gregory, D., Martin-Misener, R., & Etowa, J. (2011). Aboriginal and Western conceptions of mental health and illness. *Pimatisiwin: A Journal of Aboriginal and Indigenous Community Health, 9*(1), 65–86.

World Health Organization. (2018). *ICD-11 for mortality and morbidity statistics (ICD-11 MMS): 2018 version*. https://icd.who.int/browse11/l-m/en

Chapter 5

Substance Use, Dependence, and Addictive Behaviour

*Emma Garrod, adapted from original chapter by
Elliot M. Goldner, Emily Jenkins, and Dan Bilsker*

A permanently "drug-free" human culture has yet to be discovered. Like music, language, art, and tool use, the pursuit of altered states of consciousness is a human universal.

—Maya Szalavitz (reporter and author)

Introduction

Substance use refers to the use of psychoactive substances, such as alcohol, plant materials, and other chemicals, which cause noticeable changes in mental function. Substances may be eaten or drunk in pure form or brewed in some type of beverage. They can be taken orally, snorted, inhaled as smoke or vapour, dissolved under the tongue, absorbed through the skin, injected intramuscularly or intravenously, or even inserted into the anus or urethra. The use of psychoactive substances is very common, including that of both **licit substances** (i.e., substances that are not regulated by prevailing laws or regulated substances in compliance with laws and regulations) and **illicit substances** (i.e., substances that are illegal to manufacture, sell, purchase, or consume and that are used in contravention to existing laws and regulations).

In this chapter, we will discuss each of the main classes of psychoactive substances that have a prominent presence and impact in Canada, including alcohol, tobacco, cannabinoids, stimulants, opioids, sedatives, psychedelics, inhalants, and dissociatives. We will examine substance use from individual- and population-based perspectives, revealing the effects that it can have on individuals and reviewing the extent of substance use within the Canadian population. In Chapter 14, we will return to a discussion of the interventions that are available to mitigate the harms of substance use and to treat substance use disorders. In Chapter 17, we will further address issues related to substance use by reviewing important public policy and ethical considerations and discussing how these issues are being grappled with by members of Canadian society.

The Spectrum of Substance Use

Not all substance use is harmful or problematic. Under certain circumstances, substance use is experienced as beneficial to many individuals. Indeed, substance use exists across a wide spectrum, with abstinence at one end and problematic or harmful use at the other (see Figure 5.1).

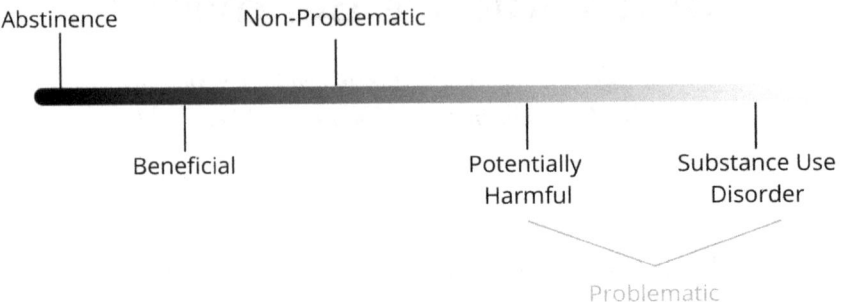

Figure 5.1: The spectrum of substance use. Substance use occurs along a spectrum from abstinence (non-use) at one end through to problematic use at the other.

Source: Adapted from the Centre for Innovation in Campus Mental Health. (n.d.). *Understanding substance use*. https://campusmentalhealth.ca/toolkits/cannabis/cannabis-substance-use/understanding/

For example, the modest use of alcohol is experienced as a pleasure and benefit to those who enjoy an occasional cocktail, glass of wine, or cold beer. For many people, the modest use of alcohol enhances the enjoyment of social events, adds to the taste of food, and helps one to relax and unwind. Of course, some individuals' use of alcohol goes beyond "modest" levels and they can end up experiencing the harmful effects associated with higher levels of alcohol use. There are also some people who respond negatively to even the smallest amounts of alcohol. These are examples of the wide range of responses that people may have to the use of alcohol; this often holds true in relation to other psychoactive substances.

So, how do psychoactive substances exert their effects? Brain cell receptors are stimulated or inhibited by molecules contained in the substance, causing changes in various mental activities. For example, alcohol is quickly transferred from the stomach and small intestine to the bloodstream, where it circulates to the brain. Alcohol (known scientifically as ethanol) is a relatively small molecule (see Figure 5.2) and, consequently, it passes through the blood-brain barrier easily.

Once ethanol molecules reach brain cells, they have a biochemical effect on neurotransmitter function, suppressing the activity of excitatory nerve pathways and increasing the activity of inhibitory nerve pathways. In low doses, the effects of ethanol will often result in feelings of general relaxation and euphoria, but in higher doses, the effects will cause loss of coordination in body movements, lapses

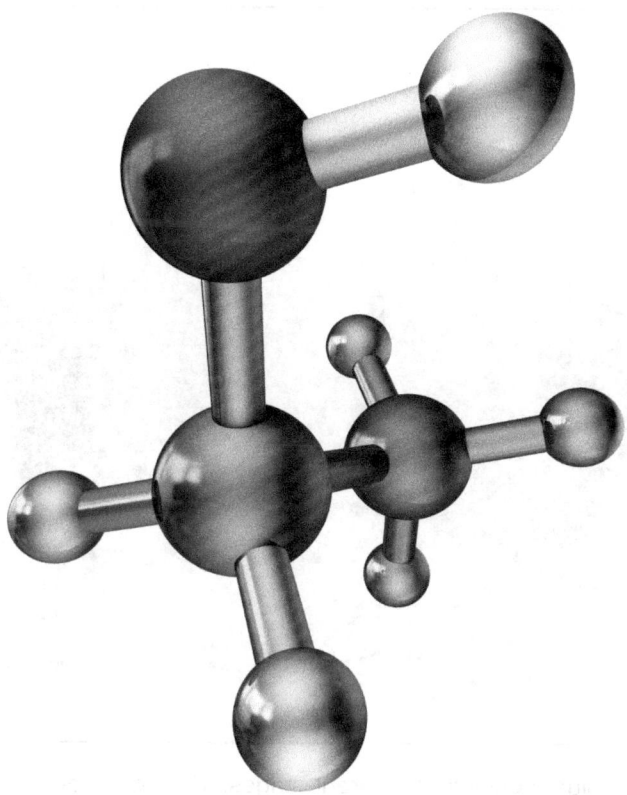

Figure 5.2: Ethanol (alcohol) is a relatively small molecule that passes easily through the blood-brain barrier and affects the actions of various neurotransmitters on brain function.

Source: iStockphoto/Martin McCarthy

in judgment, and a diminished attention span. In very high doses, alcohol can cause sedation, coma, and even death.

Let us look at the effect of opium, another psychoactive substance, on the brain. Opium is derived from the sticky resin of the opium poppy, and once dried, it looks like tar. Opium contains a number of alkaloids (i.e., chemical compounds found in various plants and fungi) that have psychoactive properties. The most active alkaloid is morphine, which is a much larger molecule than ethanol. The effect of morphine and other psychoactive alkaloids found in opium is mediated by their effect on particular receptors, called mu receptors, located on neurons and other cells in the body. Like ethanol, morphine and other opioid alkaloids affect neurotransmitter activity and alter function in many areas of the brain, resulting in analgesia (i.e., pain relief) euphoria, and drowsiness.

We have already discussed the notion of beneficial use of substances, which is the case for many people when they enjoy alcoholic beverages in moderation or a morning coffee that helps energize them at the beginning of the day. In addition,

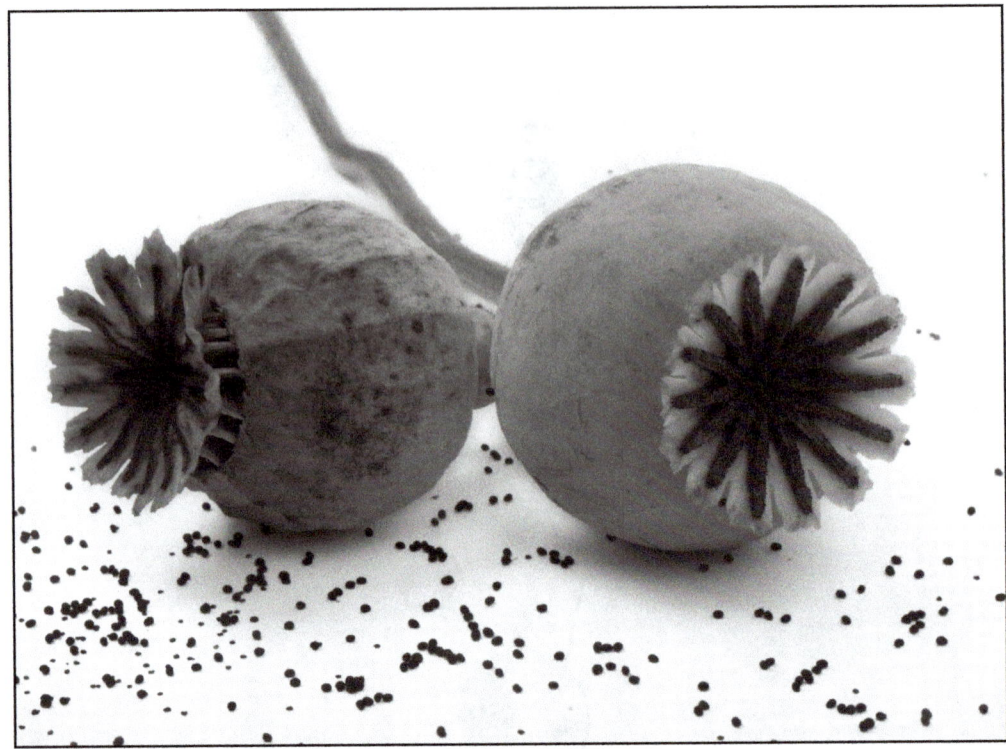

Figure 5.3: Two opium poppies at different stages. The poppy on the left has dumped tasty seeds, used for pastries and sauces. The poppy on the right is at an earlier stage, used to harvest resin for heroin.

Source: iStockphoto/Stephanie Horrocks

psychoactive substances are prescribed by physicians for therapeutic purposes, such as the use of a sedative drug during surgery or the use of an anti-anxiety medication to treat uncomfortable symptoms of an anxiety disorder. Certain plant products (e.g., ayahuasca, a psychoactive brew endemic to the Amazon regions of South America) have been used in therapeutic, health-promoting manners by Indigenous peoples for at least a few thousand years.

However, psychoactive substances can also create much harm as a result of their direct effects on the brain and other organs, or because of indirect effects caused by a variety of physical, social, and psychological factors that can accompany substance use. For example, we are all familiar with the harms caused by smoking tobacco. Inhaling smoke containing tars and other carcinogens results in serious damage to the lungs, heart, and other organs. Yet, for many smokers, the brain's craving for the continued delivery of nicotine, the psychoactive substance contained in tobacco, is strong enough to promote continued use, despite knowledge that tobacco smoking comes with high risk of disease and early death. Note that the main negative effects of tobacco are unrelated to its psychoactive properties; instead, they consist of physical harms that result from smoking it. This is also the case with some other psychoactive substances, in which the mode of delivery results in substantial physical harms. Another example of such indirect harms include the severe infections experienced by people who use intravenous drugs in the absence of sterile supplies.

Diagnostic criteria identify individuals as having a **substance use disorder** when they are engaged in a pattern of behaviour that involves ongoing use of substances despite harms. These harms can involve detrimental physical or mental effects for the individual and can also extend to include negative impacts on the welfare of others. In addition to health problems, adverse consequences of substance use include being unable to meet work, family, or school obligations; interpersonal conflicts; and legal problems. Substance use disorders are implicated in a sizable proportion of personal injuries, motor vehicle accidents, and instances of interpersonal violence.

An important concept in understanding substance use is **dependence**. This refers to a state that develops once someone uses a substance for some period of time and develops physiological changes that make it very difficult to stop use. As a result of regular substance use, certain cell functions accommodate to the presence of the substance in the body. This accommodation is called **tolerance**, and it means that the body will need a higher dose of the substance to create the effects that a smaller dose would have achieved previously. This accommodation also means that if the substance is no longer used, the person may experience **withdrawal**, that is, uncomfortable physical and mental symptoms that result from discontinuation of the drug. The symptoms of withdrawal that develop are related to the effect of the particular substance, and some substances can cause particularly intense withdrawal symptoms. For example, heroin (or diacetylmorphine hydrochloride, as it is known by scientists) is associated with a particularly severe withdrawal syndrome that begins within 24 hours after it is last used. Withdrawal from heroin is usually accompanied by intense physical symptoms, including cold sweats, chills, insomnia, malaise, cramping or aching pains, nausea, vomiting, diarrhea, and fever. For many people who use heroin, withdrawal is so terrible that they are driven to get a "fix" (i.e., a dose) of heroin even when they desire and intend to stop using. The phenomena of tolerance and withdrawal appear to be caused by sustained changes in the release and uptake of neurotransmitters at the synaptic junctions of various cells in the body. For example, repeated use of heroin and other opioids is associated with marked changes in a variety of neurotransmitters that coincide with the emergence of tolerance and withdrawal.

In addition to physiological dependence on psychoactive substances (with the development of tolerance and withdrawal, as described above), **psychological dependence** may occur. This involves experiencing intense cravings, anxiety, irritability, or other feelings of distress when substance use is stopped. Some substances (e.g., stimulants like cocaine) do not have a set of physical withdrawal symptoms but can cause intense psychological symptoms when use is stopped. Although described as a "psychological" dependence, the cravings, anxiety, irritability, and other symptoms may have a physiological basis, caused by the same type of alterations in neurotransmitter function as described above. Yet, as we discussed in Chapter 1, it is unlikely that a purely physiological explanation fully accounts for such phenomena. Undoubtedly, there are many other factors that influence the presence of cravings and other features of psychological dependence. For example, cravings have been found to be much more intense when an individual is exposed to stress or when one is in an environment that is associated with use of the substance (Preston & Epstein, 2011).

Addiction is defined as compulsive use of a substance or substances despite adverse consequences. The meaning and usage of the term "addiction" has changed over time. Originally, the term was synonymous with physiological dependence and, over time, was also used to denote psychological dependence. More recently, the term has been extended beyond its original connection to substance use. Addiction is now used to denote other compulsive behaviours, such as gambling and sexual behaviour, which can also persist despite causing significant adverse consequences. In its popular use, the term also refers to harms to others and often carries the negative connotation of a criminal/moral model of thought about substance use as deviant behaviour. The term "addiction" has been replaced by "substance use disorder" in the medical community (American Psychiatric Association, 2014) because of these stigmatizing associations.

In more severe manifestations, substance use disorders can lead to intense human suffering. Serious health problems can result from the direct harmful effects of certain substances on the body. Indirect harms, such as infections caused by intravenous injection, malnutrition, poverty, racism, criminalization, and substandard living conditions, are also common. Due to the various and intersecting harms associated, people with severe substance use disorders constitute one of the most marginalized populations in Canada (Keller et al., 2013). Attention—at multiple levels—is urgently required to mitigate these harms.

We have discussed the negative consequences that can occur for people with substance use disorders, but the risks and harms associated with substance use are not limited to this population. For example, many people (often teenagers and young people) who are experimenting with substances can end up in harmful circumstances. Serious accidents caused by intoxication rob many young people of their lives or cause lifelong disability or suffering. Indeed, hazardous alcohol use is one of the leading causes of morbidity and mortality among young people worldwide (Gore et al., 2011; World Health Organization, 2018).

Substances Commonly Used in Canada

There are many hundreds of substances used for known psychoactive effects. Here, we will not attempt to catalogue them all. Rather, we will focus on substances that are used by a large proportion of Canada's populations.

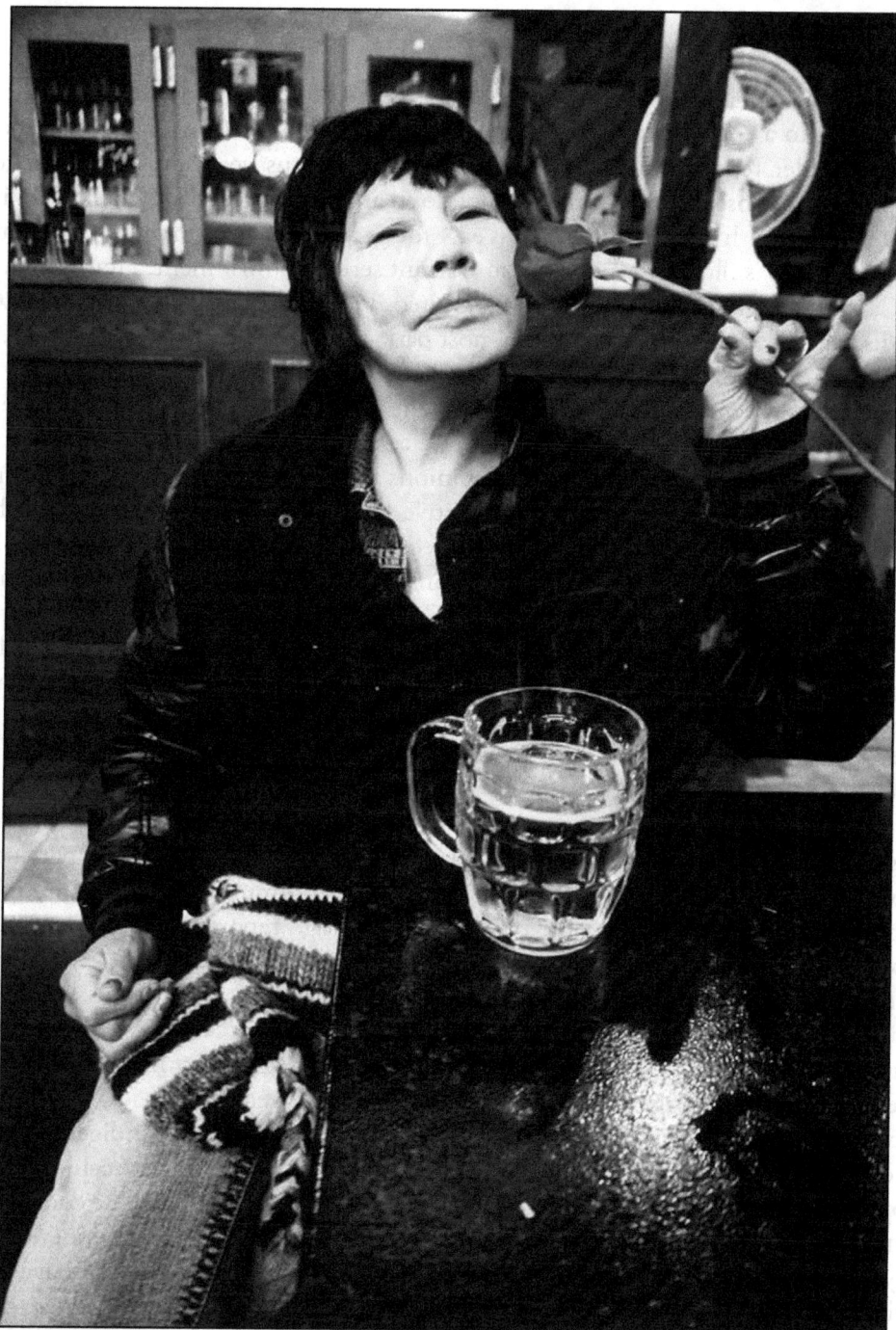

Figure 5.4: This photo was taken in a bar in the Downtown Eastside of Vancouver. This community experiences inequitable harms resulting from substance use and related control and policing efforts.

Source: Chris Sang Yeob Park

Alcohol

For most Canadians, the use of alcohol is accepted as a normal part of our lives. According to a recent national survey, almost 80 percent of Canadians 15 years of age and older report consuming alcohol in the previous year, and approximately 20 percent of those who consume alcohol do so at levels above the low-risk drinking guidelines (Health Canada, 2017). It is easy for us to forget that, in other parts of the world, alcohol is illegal, and its use can warrant serious punishment. However, even in Canada, alcohol was once widely prohibited. From the early 1900s to the 1920s, the use or sale of alcohol was illegal in most parts of the country. In a federal referendum held in 1898, 51 percent voted for prohibition. Prohibition had a majority in all provinces except Quebec, where 81 percent voted against it (possibly because of the French cultural tradition of valuing wine as one of life's great pleasures).

How can we explain such divergent opinions about alcohol? Why do some people and some societies view alcohol in a positive light, while others feel strongly that alcohol should be avoided or even outlawed? In part, this is because of the wide spectrum of human behaviour and the consequences associated with alcohol use. Certainly, the extent of risk and harm to Canadians due to alcohol use is very real and cannot be ignored. Almost 200 disease or injury conditions (e.g., acute alcohol poisoning, cirrhosis of the liver, motor vehicle accidents, falls, and other accidents) are entirely or partially attributable to alcohol use. Moreover, the total burden of disease related to alcohol use in Canada is estimated to be double or triple that of all illicit substances combined.

Some sectors of Canadian society have suffered disproportionately with the negative consequences of alcohol use. Many Indigenous peoples have experienced devastating harm as a result of alcohol use in their communities. Overall, a higher proportion of Indigenous people over 12 years of age report past-year abstinence from alcohol when compared to the rest of the Canadian population (27.4 vs 24.6 percent); however, the prevalence of heavy drinking, alcohol use disorder, and alcohol-related harm is higher. For example, according to Statistics Canada data published in 2019, 25.1 percent of Indigenous individuals report heavy drinking in the past month, compared to 19.6 percent of non-Indigenous Canadians. Further, alcohol-related mortality was estimated to be 5.43 times higher in Indigenous men and 10.11 times higher in Indigenous women than within the non-Indigenous populations of Canada (Statistics Canada, 2019). These statistics must be considered within the context of colonialism and the historical, social, political, economic, and psychological factors and conditions, described further in Chapter 8, that have contributed to profound inequities in the prevalence of substance use harms experienced by Indigenous peoples in Canada. Further to these harms, Indigenous people have reported significant negative experiences, including profound stigma and discrimination when accessing health care, especially in the context of substance use disorders (Goodman et. al, 2017).

> **Box 5.1: Substance Use Stigma and Discrimination towards Indigenous People in British Columbia Health Care Services**
>
> In April 2020, allegations surfaced of a "Price is Right"–style game being played by health care providers in BC emergency departments. This game involved guessing the blood alcohol levels of Indigenous patients who presented for care. These allegations were immediately recognized by the Government of BC as extremely serious and representative of stereotypes related to alcohol use among Indigenous peoples, as well as ongoing stigma and discrimination towards Indigenous peoples in health care. The BC Minister of Health launched an investigation into this "game" and more broadly, the experiences of Indigenous people within the health care system, led by Hon. Dr. Mary Ellen Turpel-Lafond. This investigation sought input from Indigenous peoples, health care providers, and the general public and heard from nearly 9,000 people, resulting in the publication of the report *In Plain Sight* (Turpel-Lafond, 2020).
>
> After extensive inquiry, the investigation concluded that there was no direct evidence of this "game" being played in BC hospitals and that it is not currently being played today. However, inquiry into these allegations surfaced numerous other instances of Indigenous-specific racism, stigma, and discrimination in health care, including related to the stereotype of Indigenous people as "drinkers" and "alcoholics." One Indigenous woman's narrative recounted in the report describes waking up from a brain aneurysm surgery to a nurse commenting, *"You people drink too much,"* and the suggestion that her post-anesthetic side effects of nausea and vomiting were related to alcohol withdrawal. These stories, illuminated by the report, are a call to action to all of us to question our assumptions about alcohol and drugs and challenge societal stereotypes about people who use substances.

Tobacco

The smoking of tobacco in pipes, cigars, and cigarettes has been popular in Canada since Confederation. Although Indigenous peoples used tobacco, this was primarily as a component of ceremonial rituals. The habit of smoking tobacco frequently throughout the day appears to have been initiated in the Americas by European settlers, and the large tobacco-growing industry in the southern United States continues to promote the widespread use of this substance.

As mentioned earlier in this chapter, the psychoactive substance found in tobacco is nicotine. When tobacco is ingested through smoking, chewing, or sniffing, nicotine travels quickly to the brain and acts on receptors there and elsewhere in the body, altering neurotransmitters such as dopamine, and leading to feelings of relaxation, alertness, euphoria, and appetite suppression. Due to nicotine's properties, physiological dependence develops quickly with repeated use; however, psychological dependence appears to be a significant factor in its addictive potential. It is now well-known that tobacco causes substantial harm through damage to organs and can precipitate various forms of cancer and other diseases. Lung diseases, such as cancer and chronic obstructive pulmonary disease, are particularly common, but tobacco also causes heart disease and diseases of the digestive tract and has many other serious detrimental effects on health. The World Health Organization (WHO) estimates that tobacco use causes 6 million deaths per year and considers it to be the leading preventable cause of death worldwide (WHO, 2015). In 2017, 11 percent (3.3 million) of Canadians reported smoking daily and 4 percent (1.3 million) reported smoking occasionally (Health Canada, 2017); this is a dramatic decline in tobacco consumption from previous decades. Various countries are modelling their efforts on Canada's Federal Tobacco Control Strategy (Health Canada, 2012). Still, tobacco smoking is the foremost cause of premature mortality in Canada, with estimated national health care costs in excess of $20 billion annually (Krueger et al., 2014).

Cannabinoids

Cannabis (also commonly referred to as marijuana or weed) has been used medicinally and recreationally for many centuries. Tetrahydrocannabinol (THC) is the main psychoactive ingredient contained in the cannabis plant, but there are many others, including cannabidiol (CBD). Most commonly, the dried buds and leaves of the plant, or a resin (i.e., hashish, which is extracted from the plant), is smoked. However, cannabis can also be vaporized, taken in edible form, and used topically.

THC binds to cannabinoid receptors on cells throughout the brain and influences neurotransmission that causes activation of various brain centres. Common effects include feelings of euphoria, relaxation, altered perception of time, sensory stimulation, and an increased appetite ("the munchies"), though for some people, the effects can also include high levels of anxiety and paranoia. In contrast, CBD does not produce a "high" like THC and can mitigate some of these negative effects, while also having anti-psychotic and anti-inflammatory properties. In the early 1990s, scientists conducting research on cannabis identified that the human body creates its own (i.e., endogenous) neurotransmitters that also bind to the cannabinoid receptors. Anandamide was the first isolated endogenous neurotransmitter; it binds to the cannabinoid receptor and has effects similar to THC. A number of other endogenous cannabinoid neurotransmitters have since been isolated and researchers continue to explore their actions and potential therapeutic uses.

The use of cannabis is widespread in Canada. In 2017, about 11 percent of Canadians aged 15 and older reported using cannabis at least once in the past year. Of those that used cannabis in the previous 3 months, 32 percent reported doing so every day or almost every day and 37 percent of cannabis users indicated doing so for medical reasons (Health Canada, 2017). In an effort to better protect public health and safety, keep cannabis out of the hands of young people, and redirect profits of cannabis sales away from criminal organizations, Canada legalized non-medical cannabis use for adults in October 2018. Adults may now purchase cannabis in several different forms at dispensaries or through government-operated online stores.

While it can be difficult to find reliable and conclusive information about the health risks and benefits of cannabis (Moffat et al., 2013), there is substantial evidence to suggest that it is effective in the management of chronic pain, nausea in patients with cancer, and spasticity in people with multiple sclerosis (National Academy of Sciences, 2017). There is also clear evidence indicating that cannabis use can play a role in the onset of schizophrenia and other psychoses, motor vehicle accidents, respiratory problems (particularly when used heavily and for a long duration), low birth weight (when consumed by pregnant individuals), and problematic use/cannabis use disorder.

A review of scientific evidence indicates that the health harms associated with cannabis use increase alongside frequency of use (Fischer et al., 2011). In an effort to reduce cannabis-related harms, researchers at the Centre for Addiction and Mental Health developed *Canada's Lower-Risk Cannabis Use Guidelines*. These guidelines

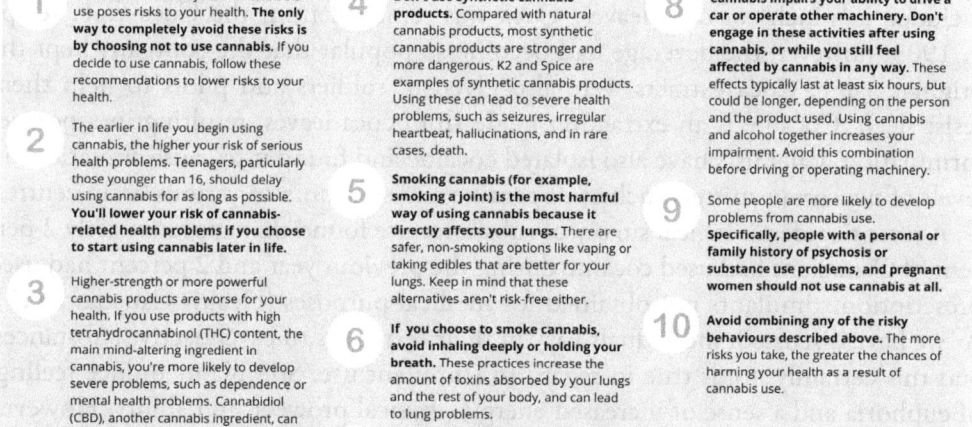

Figure 5.5: Canada's Lower-Risk Cannabis Use Guidelines.

Source: Adapted from Fischer, B., Russell, C., Sabioni, P., van den Brink, W., Le Foll, B., Hall, W., Rehm, J., & Room, R. (2017). Lower-risk cannabis use guidelines: A comprehensive update of evidence and recommendations. *American Journal of Public Health, 107*(8), e1–e12. https://doi.org/10.2105/AJPH.2017.303818

include 10 strategies for using cannabis more safely, including delaying first use, using lower strength products, and avoiding synthetic products (Fischer et al., 2017).

Stimulants

The most commonly used psychoactive substance in Canada is caffeine, a stimulant that has the effect of increasing alertness and temporarily warding off drowsiness. We have already mentioned that coffee and other caffeine-containing drinks are consumed daily by more than 75 percent of adult Canadians. Intake of large amounts of caffeine-containing substances can cause the following symptoms: nervousness, irritability, insomnia, muscle twitches, and palpitations. Frequent use also increases stomach acid and can cause various esophageal and gastrointestinal problems, including peptic ulcers. Most coffee drinkers would find it very difficult to eliminate coffee from their daily routines, and cessation or reduction of coffee intake is likely to result in a withdrawal syndrome characterized by headache, fatigue, nausea, and depressed mood.

For at least a thousand years, Indigenous peoples of South America have been chewing the leaves of the coca plant for its stimulant properties. By the 19th century, European physicians and chemists began to experiment with the extracts of coca leaves for their medicinal and stimulant properties. Various tinctures and mixtures included extracts from the coca plant, and the original recipe for Coca-Cola included a "pinch" of coca leaves. Coca was removed from the Coca-Cola recipe in 1903; however, the beverage had become so popular that the company kept the original name. Coca extracts were also given to soldiers and pilots to help them resist sleep. Cocaine is an extraction made from coca leaves, resulting in a powder formulation. Chemists have also isolated cocaine and found it to cause alterations in levels of neurotransmitters such as dopamine and serotonin in various brain centres.

A recent epidemiological survey of substance use found that approximately 2 percent of Canadians had used cocaine during the previous year and 2 percent had used prescription stimulants not obtained for medical purposes (Health Canada, 2017). As we have discussed, individuals vary in their responses to psychoactive substances, and this certainly holds true in regard to stimulant use. Stimulants induce feelings of euphoria and a sense of increased energy, physical prowess, and ability. However, in high doses or with repeated use, their use is also associated with agitation, aggression, paranoia, and psychosis, as well as cardiovascular risk. Indeed, one of the risks of stimulant use is substance-induced psychosis, which can present similarly to schizophrenia but tends to resolve once the substance is out of the person's system.

Cocaine is taken in various forms using different routes of administration. Snorting (i.e., insufflation) of cocaine powder is a common way of using cocaine. Smoking of either freebase or crack cocaine (chemical preparations of cocaine that vaporize at low temperatures) emerged a few decades ago as a lower-cost form of the substance that delivers a much more immediate and powerful intoxication and induces strong cravings and psychological dependence. Cocaine can also be injected intravenously, which is associated with high rates of serious complications, including infections.

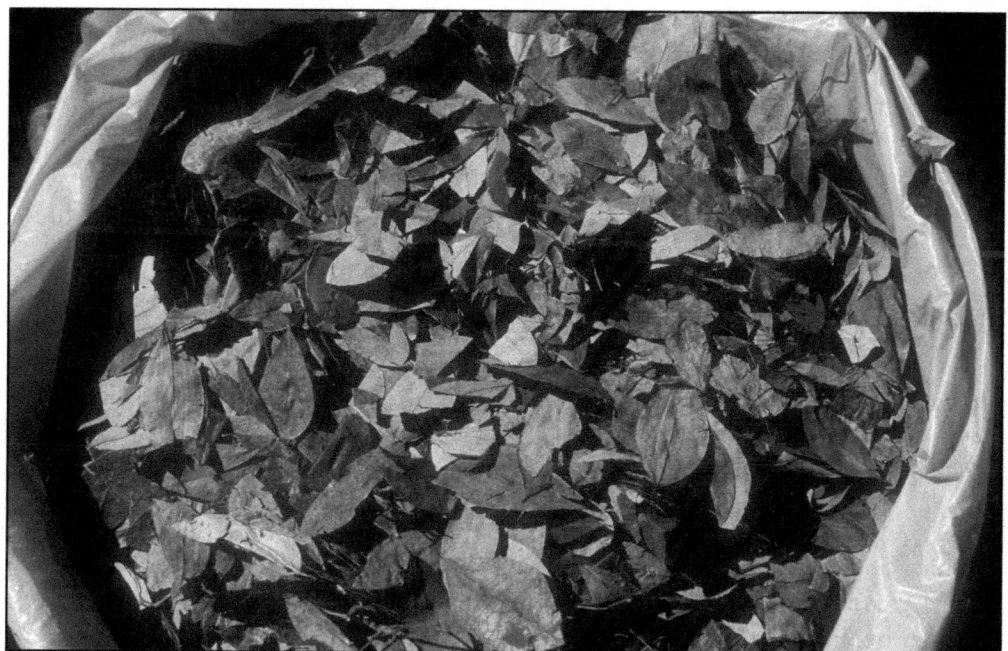

Figure 5.6: Coca leaves for sale in a Peruvian street market.

Source: iStockphoto/Brasil2

Another stimulant that has been in prominent use in Canada is methamphetamine, also known in street terms as "crystal," "meth," and "jib." This substance can be made in illicit laboratories with ingredients that are readily available in household products or over-the-counter medications. Consequently, methamphetamine can be produced and sold cheaply. It is a potent stimulant of the central nervous system, resulting in feelings of euphoria, insomnia, increased sexual interest, increased heart rate, increased body temperature, and loss of appetite. Methamphetamine causes a huge spike in dopamine release, which can lead to compulsive, ongoing use despite consequences. It is of particular concern that methamphetamine has been found to result in structural and functional damage to the brain (Kim et al., 2020). Methamphetamine production and distribution was the focus of the popular television series *Breaking Bad*, in which the main character, Walter White, a science teacher diagnosed with cancer, decided to "cook" meth in order to make money to support his medical treatment. The show demonstrated how the substance is often created, in makeshift laboratories, with one of the initial meth productions taking place in an RV. *Breaking Bad* also portrayed the dangers of production (e.g., the release of toxic chemicals), as well as the violence and crime associated with the drug trade.

Ecstasy or methylenedioxymethamphetamine (MDMA) is similar in chemical structure to amphetamines; however, its psychoactive effects appear unique. In addition to feelings of euphoria, MDMA is often described as increasing feelings of

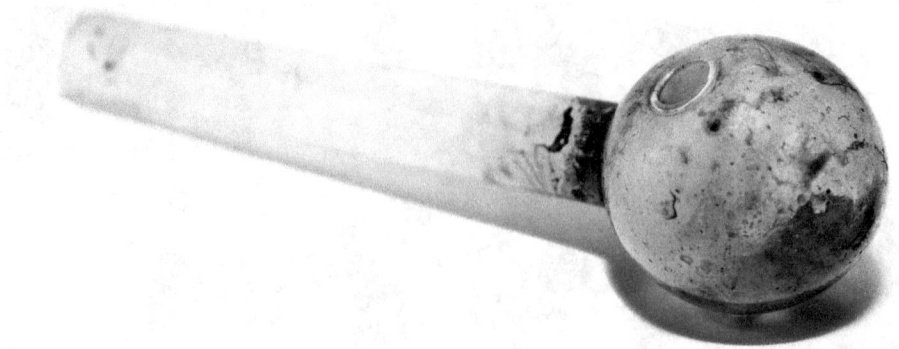

Figure 5.7: Methamphetamine is often smoked using a pipe.

Source: iStockphoto/KarenMower

intimacy and empathy (it is sometimes called "the love drug"). Like other stimulants, MDMA contributes to increased energy and loss of appetite. In recent decades, MDMA became popular at raves and other dance club scenes. Intense hyperthermia (increased body temperature) is a significant risk associated with MDMA, but long-term health risks are unclear. Recently, MDMA has been used for its psychedelic properties to treat post-traumatic stress disorder with promising outcomes.

Opioids

Opioids are psychoactive substances that are either extracted from the opium poppy or are derivatives that are synthesized to have similar chemical structures and properties. Opioids include heroin, morphine, codeine, methadone, oxycodone, hydrocodone, fentanyl, and hydromorphone. Certain types of opioids (e.g., heroin) tend to be injected intravenously or smoked, though others are ingested as pills (e.g., oxycodone). Their potent analgesic (pain-killing) properties have made opioids highly valuable as medicines for many centuries. They can induce intense feelings of euphoria and have high addictive potential, leading to strong physical and psychological dependence. A growing problem in recent years has been the rise of new and more potent opioids in the illicit drug supply. Fentanyl, a synthetic opioid that is up to 100 percent more potent than morphine, has gained much attention due to a significant spike in deaths attributed to the substance. Between January 2016 and March 2021, 22,828 opioid-related deaths occurred in Canada—approximately 10 deaths each day (Government of Canada, 2021). Some individuals are unaware that they are ingesting the drug, which is added to other commonly used opioids or accidentally contaminates other drugs (e.g., cocaine) during production. The rise in fentanyl-related deaths has sparked campaigns across the country to encourage people to know the source of their drugs and to be in the presence of others when using substances (Canadian Community Epidemiology Network on Drug Use, 2015). It has

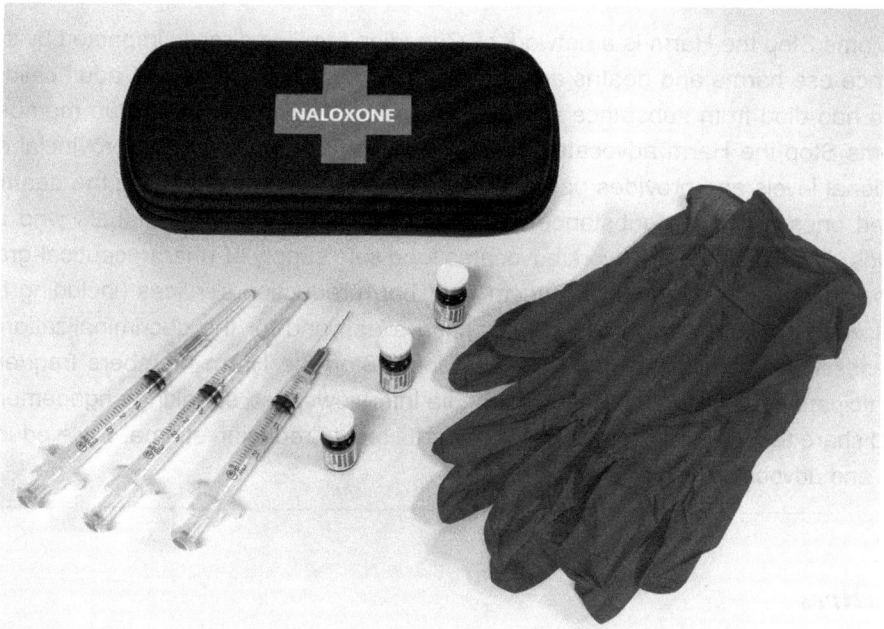

Figure 5.8: Components of a Naloxone kit.

Source: Shutterstock/Tomas Nevesely

also led to the widespread distribution of Naloxone, an opioid antagonist (a drug that blocks the effects of opioids) and thus reverses the effects of opioid overdoses. Anyone using illicit substances should be trained and have access to a Naloxone kit. It is also important that individuals who are physically dependent on opioids are offered opioid agonist medications, such as methadone or buprenorphine-naloxone (Suboxone). These medications can help prevent withdrawal, support people in reducing or stopping their opioid use, and are protective against overdose.

Box 5.2: Moms Stop the Harm: Advocacy Efforts of Families Impacted by Substance Use Related Harms and Deaths

The drug poisoning crisis has had profound and devastating impacts internationally and in Canada. In addition to the thousands of deaths per year due to opioid-related causes, the tainted drug supply (i.e., with fentanyl and other synthetic opioids) contributes to countless non-fatal overdoses requiring immediate medical attention. Although this crisis has been described by researchers, political leaders, and people who use drugs as an "epidemic," the response from the Canadian government has been critiqued as wildly insufficient.

> Moms Stop the Harm is a network of Canadian families directly impacted by substance use harms and deaths and was founded by three mothers of adult children who had died from substance use–related harms. Now with over 2,200 members, Moms Stop the Harm advocates to change current drug policies at provincial and national levels and provides peer support to families who are grieving the death of loved ones related to substance use or currently supporting individuals who use drugs. Specifically, the network advocates for a safe supply of pharmaceutical-grade substances, access to the full spectrum of harm reduction services (including free Naloxone kits and supervised consumption sites), and for the decriminalization of possession of drugs for personal use. Moms Stop the Harm members frequently participate in government meetings, media interviews, and speaking engagements; and share their personal stories as a powerful tool to reducing stigma, while educating and advocating for change.

Sedatives

A wide variety of substances with different chemical structures have psychoactive effects in which sedation is a prominent feature. In general, sedatives depress function in brain centres that govern wakefulness and alertness. Benzodiazepines have strong sedative effects and are used in high doses to induce anesthesia during medical procedures. In lower doses, benzodiazepines, such as lorazepam and diazepam, can be used as anxiolytics (i.e., to reduce anxiety) and as soporifics (sleeping pills). Barbiturates (such as amobarbital and secobarbital) are potent sedatives that are also used as part of general anesthesia but have also been used in a non-prescribed manner. Two other sedatives are flunitrazepam and gamma hydroxybutyrate (GHB). Flunitrazepam (more commonly known by its trade name Rohypnol) is a benzodiazepine tranquilizer that induces sedation, muscle relaxation, confusion, memory loss, dizziness, and impaired coordination. Flunitrazepam has legitimate medical purposes; however, it has become infamous as a drug used in committing sexual assaults and is also known as "the date rape drug" or "roofies." Flunitrazepam is produced as a small white tablet and is colourless, tasteless, and odourless. The effects are almost immediate and can last anywhere from 8 to 24 hours, depending on the dose.

GHB is a central nervous system depressant that is also known as "G" and "liquid ecstasy." Due to its sedating properties at higher doses, GHB is also used by perpetrators of sexual assault. More commonly, GHB is used at lower doses, which produces euphoric and sedative effects, similar to alcohol. Individuals have reported feeling relaxed, happy, and sociable, as well as having an increased libido when using this drug. With frequent use, GHB can cause strong physiological dependence, and cessation can result in some life-threatening withdrawal symptoms that can require medical monitoring. GHB is typically found as an oral solution and can be difficult to dose accurately, leading to significant overdose risk, including coma and death.

Psychedelics

Psychedelics are drugs that can cause significant alterations in sensory perception, emotion, and thought, sometimes leading to experiences that are unusual and outside the bounds of normal consciousness. Psychedelics have been used in the spiritual practices of various cultures for centuries and became popularized in the Western world during the 1960s as part of the counterculture movement. These substances are not typically used in a way that causes dependence or substance use disorders (Bogenschutz & Johnson, 2016).

A wide variety of naturally occurring and synthesized substances are classified as psychedelics. Examples include the peyote cactus, which contains the hallucinogen mescaline, the psilocybin mushroom ("magic mushroom"), as well as ayahuasca, a combination of two different plants that contains N, N-dimethyltryptamine (DMT). Many of these substances have been used by Indigenous peoples in Central and South America for centuries as entheogens, or substances used to bring on spiritual experiences. Lysergic acid diethylamide (LSD) is another psychedelic substance that was synthesized from ergot, a fungus that grows on grains, by Swiss chemist Albert Hoffman. After absorbing a small amount through his skin, Hoffman described seeing through his closed eyes "fantastic pictures, extraordinary shapes with intense, kaleidoscopic play of colors" (Hoffman, 1980).

Box 5.3: Medical Use of Psychedelic Substances

In the 1950s there was a surge in research using psychedelic substances in supervised settings to treat alcohol use disorder and mental illnesses, with encouraging results. Unfortunately, not all research was conducted ethically. A Montreal hospital was the site of one of these unethical studies, which involved psychiatrist Dr. Ewen Cameron, who administered LSD and other psychedelic drugs to patients without obtaining informed consent. These experiments were funded by the US Central Intelligence Agency, because it was interested in Dr. Cameron's theories that he could erase existing memories and "rebuild" the psyche (Collins, 1998). In more recent years, there has been resurgence in the medical use of psychedelic drugs. The psychoactive substances found in magic mushrooms, LSD, ketamine, and MDMA have all been used in the treatment of substance use and mental disorders, including post-traumatic stress disorder (PTSD), depression, and anxiety (Garcia-Romeu et al., 2016). Recently, certain psychedelic substances, such as ketamine, MDMA, and psilocybin, have been authorized for use on a restricted basis by Health Canada for the treatment of PTSD, refractory depression, and other mental illnesses.

Inhalants

Inhalants include many easily accessed substances such as glue, gasoline, paint, butane, and other solvents and can cause intoxication when inhaled. Effects include slurred speech, lack of coordination, euphoria, and dizziness and are relatively brief, lasting only 60 to 90 minutes. Inhalants can cause damage to the central nervous system, lungs, heart, and brain and—in some cases—they can cause sudden death. Due to low cost and accessibility, inhalant use is particularly prevalent among young people who are living in especially marginalized circumstances, such as homeless youth. Studies have indicated that the majority of first-time inhalant use occurs between the ages of 12 and 16 years and that use in adult populations is generally low (Dell et al., 2011).

Dissociatives

Dissociative drugs distort perceptions of sight and sound and cause users to feel a disconnection from reality. Phenylcyclohexyl piperidine, or PCP as it is more commonly known, is one example of a dissociative drug. It causes individuals to feel a sense of numbness and invulnerability. Originally developed as an anesthetic, the medical use of PCP has been discontinued; however, it continues to be produced illicitly. Some users experience psychotic symptoms, such as hallucinations and paranoia. In addition to synthetic dissociative drugs, there are also naturally occurring substances, such as the salvia divinorum herb, that cause dissociative effects. Growing natively in Mexico, salvia leaves are chewed or smoked and cause short and intense hallucinogenic effects, including changes in visual and body perceptions, mood, emotions, and a feeling of detachment from reality.

Box 5.4: ANKORS Harm Reduction Services

In recent years, electronic dance music festivals have become widely popular across North America. One of the largest of these events is the Shambhala Music Festival, which is held on the Salmo River Ranch, located in the West Kootenay region of British Columbia. Shambhala brings together approximately 15,000 music enthusiasts each summer, many of whom are experienced drug users. The large crowds of partiers combined with the use of alcohol and other drugs increases the incidence of bingeing, overdose, and sexual assault. To reduce such negative occurrences, ANKORS, a non-profit organization funded by Interior Health and the Public Health Agency of Canada, offers an array of harm reduction services. One of the main services offered is pill and powder drug-purity testing. Often, the true nature of a drug that people have purchased is not actually what was represented when sold to them. For instance, individuals who thought they purchased ketamine have actually been sold other substances, many of which can be extremely dangerous. Drug tests are offered free of charge and without any repercussion from law enforcement for possession of illicit substances. At the 2019 festival, ANKORS performed 3,067 tests with about 52 percent negative results (i.e., the drug was not what it was sold as or it contained additional substances), which prompted 41 people to dispose of their drugs entirely. With the services that ANKORS provides, along with a medical personnel team, the Shambhala Music Festival has seen just 1 death due to overdose since its establishment 18 years ago.

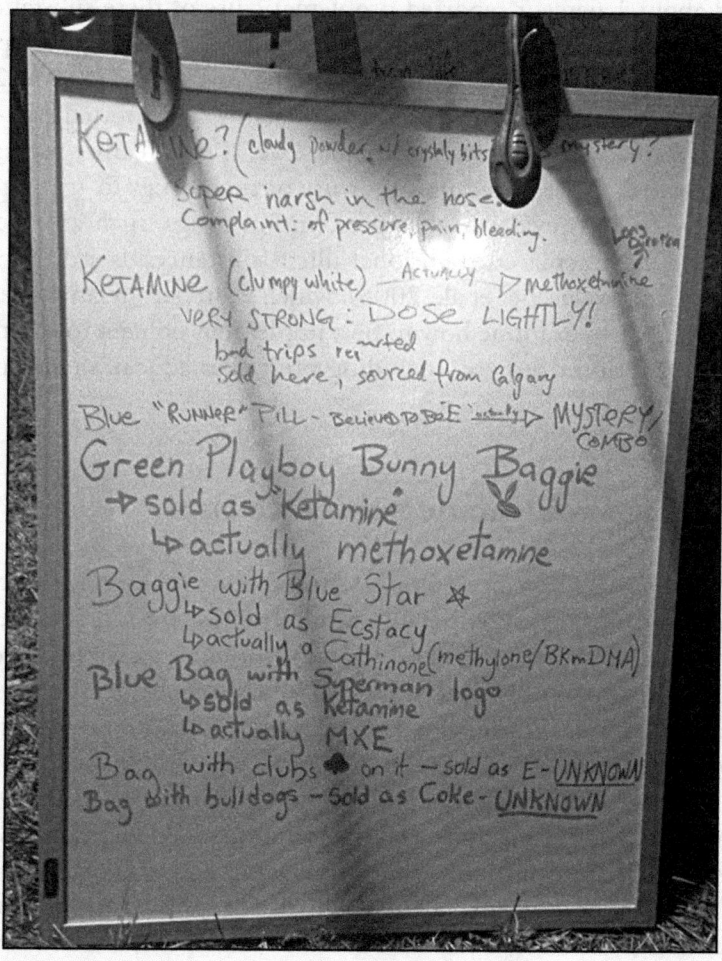

Figure 5.9: A whiteboard outside the ANKORS harm reduction tent at Shambhala Music Festival warns partiers of misrepresented drugs they have found from drug-purity tests.

Source: ANKORS Harm Reduction Project.

Prescription Drug Use

Historically, the use of illicit drugs has garnered the most attention regarding concerns about individual and societal harms. However, there are now indications that the use of psychoactive pharmaceuticals or prescription medications (including opioids, stimulants, and sedatives) has grown to become a significant public health problem. This may be related to increasing access and the perception that prescription medications are safer than illicit drugs. In Canada, 22 percent of respondents to a national survey reported using psychoactive pharmaceuticals in a non-prescribed manner, and about 1 percent reported problematic use of these substances (Health Canada, 2017). Of particular concern is the rising misuse of prescription drugs among youth populations. For example, according to Health Canada (2017) data, 17 percent of individuals between 15 and 19 years of age reported past-year use of psychoactive pharmaceuticals (Health Canada, 2017). In an earlier survey, 4 percent of youth in grades 6–12 reported past-year use of such drugs to "get high" (Health Canada, 2013). There is evidence that prescription drugs, such as oxycodone and hydromorphone, have replaced traditional illicit substances as a drug of choice in major cities in Canada (Fischer et al., 2008), which is, in part, related to accessibility. Efforts are underway to examine how to best implement policies to limit harms that accompany prescription drug use, including prescriber education and prescription monitoring systems.

Understanding Problematic Substance Use

A wide variety of models have been proposed to explain problematic substance use. In 2016, Csiernik classified these theories into four categories: the moral model, biological theories, psychological theories, and sociological theories, as shown in Table 5.1.

One perspective that is now widely scorned by substance use experts is the "moral model." The moral model is a belief system based on a dichotomous moral theory in which people are considered fully and individually responsible for their behavioural choices, which may be either good or bad. Those who choose good behaviour should be praised, whereas those who choose bad behaviour should be punished. Since substance use is a "bad habit," it follows that people who use substances should be punished. Much of the stigma faced by people who use drugs is based on this underlying moral model that labels anyone with a "bad habit" as a "bad person." The dangers of the moral model have become increasingly clear over the years. For example, alcohol prohibition, which was based on the moral model, failed to eliminate drinking. However, this policy did lead to increased criminal activity through black market sales of alcohol, increasing potency, and other harms. Programs in Canada that once required people who use heroin to undergo compulsory treatment were considered unsuccessful and discontinued in the 1970s. The "War on Drugs" waged by the US since the early 1970s has led to the highest incarceration rates in American history,

Table 5.1 Theories of Addiction

Theory Category	Description
The Moral Model	The moral model upholds that any drug use is inherently wrong and sinful, and addiction is a result of poor personal choices. There is no research evidence in support of this theory.
Biological Theories	Biological theories attempt to find a chemical or physiological cause for addiction. • Disease (Medical) model • Neurobiology • Genetic theory • Brain dysfunction theory • Biochemical theories • Allergy theory
Psychological Theories	Psychological theories focus on an individual's behaviour and study how they are learned, modified, and reinforced. • Learning theory • Personality theory • Psychodynamic theory • Humanistic theory • Attachment theory • Rational theory
Sociological Theories	Sociological theories propose that addiction is influenced by sociocultural events and that politics, cultural norms, media, and how drugs are regulated in society should be considered. • Cultural theories • Sub-cultural theories • Deviant behaviour theory • Marxist theory • Availability-control theory • Environmental stress

Source: Adapted from Csiernik, R. (2016). *Substance use and abuse: Everything matters* (2nd ed.). Canadian Scholars.

with little evidence of reduced illicit substance use and no improvement in health or social outcomes. People with problematic substance use are stigmatized and often report negative encounters with the health care system, which affects engagement in treatment and access to care.

Our best understanding of problematic substance use or substance use disorders is that they are shaped by a complex interplay of factors, as illustrated by the diverse concepts and theories presented in Table 5.1. For example, genetics (biological theory) have been shown to account for about 50 percent of alcohol use disorders (Deak et al., 2019). Another factor that is starting to receive more attention is trauma (our understandings of which are drawn from across biological, sociological, and psychological theories). As explored in this chapter, one half to two-thirds of serious substance use challenges are experienced by those with early adverse childhood experiences (Dube et al., 2003). Lastly, understanding and addressing the harms of substance use also requires attention to the social determinants of health. Given the many influences, each person's risk factors and experiences with substance use and treatment will be different.

The Impact of Substance Use in Canada

As we have described, substance use ranges widely from beneficial use at one extreme, to profoundly harmful use at the other. The associated financial costs are extremely high, with both direct health care and criminal justice costs, and indirect losses of productivity resulting from disability and premature death. In 2017, the total annual cost of substance use in Canada was estimated to be $45.98 billion, with alcohol and tobacco use leading contributions to these costs by a wide margin (Canadian Substance Use Costs and Harms Scientific Working Group, 2020).

The extraordinary harm, suffering, and loss that is associated with substance use has led to a variety of efforts and approaches to prevent such negative consequences and to reduce harms to individuals, families, and society. In Chapter 14, this text offers further discussion of the efforts that are in place in Canada to respond to substance use challenges. We will discuss the treatments and interventions that can be offered to individuals to reduce harm and treat substance use disorders. In Chapter 17, we will address the approaches that are taken by governments to minimize substance use and its associated harms at a population level.

Harm Reduction

In the context of substance use, **harm reduction** is a pragmatic approach to health policy, programming, and practice that recognizes that abstinence may not be a realistic or a desirable goal for everyone. It aims to decrease adverse consequences associated with substance use by offering a range of services to support safer use practices. Harm reduction originated within grassroots advocacy organizations, often led by people who use drugs. For example, in the mid-1990s, a peer-led advocacy group in British Columbia called IV Feed opened "Back Alley"—an unofficial and unsanctioned supervised injection site providing daily harm reduction services to over 100 people who used injection drugs (Kerr et al., 2017). While this site was closed after only a year of operation, programs such as Back Alley advanced harm reduction as a crucial and effective response to reducing substance use harms, including infectious disease transmission as well as those associated with the tainted drug supply. Despite a long history of advocacy as well as strong evidence of effectiveness, many harm reduction programs and practices continue to face opposition and controversy across all levels of the Canadian government and within health care settings. Two widely implemented harm reduction approaches—supervised consumption sites and supply distribution and disposal programs—are discussed below.

Supervised Consumption Sites

Supervised consumption sites provide a space where people can use pre-obtained drugs, in the presence of others (usually a peer or health care provider), without fear of arrest. These sites also create an opportunity for service providers to deliver harm reduction supplies, engage in onsite primary care, refer individuals to health care services, and offer education on strategies to reduce risk for overdose. Research has shown that supervised consumption sites reduce the transmission of infectious diseases—through the adoption of safer use practices (Marshall et al., 2011)—and also reduce the incidence of overdose death (Bayoumi & Zaric, 2008). Policy and legislation related to supervised consumption sites is frequently changing, and many provinces and territories do not currently offer this service due to political and social pressures and lack of funding. In the Recommended Websites section at the end of this chapter, we provide information on a Government of Canada (2020) maintained map of currently operating supervised consumption sites, as well as a list of open applications for new sites.

Some supervised consumption sites additionally offer drug checking, a service that allows people to chemically analyze their drugs and receive individualized consultation regarding the contents and any associated risks detected from their sample. The first harm reduction–focused drug checking program was established in 1992 in the Netherlands (Venture et al., 2013). Drug checking has been identified as a crucial service in the context of the drug poisoning crisis, as contamination of drug supplies with extremely potent synthetic opioids (such as fentanyl and carfentanil) has contributed to high numbers of overdoses and deaths among people who use drugs. Illustrating the importance of drug checking, one study conducted in Vancouver, BC, found that 80 percent of drug checks identified contamination with fentanyl (Karamouzian et al., 2018).

Supply Distribution and Disposal Programs

Supply distribution and disposal programs provide people who use drugs with clean supplies and facilitate collection of used supplies. In Canada, needle exchange programs have been around since the late 1980s and provide individuals who use injection drugs with clean supplies to prevent the reuse and sharing of needles. Needle exchange programs are credited with successfully reducing HIV and hepatitis C infections. They also facilitate an opportunity to discuss an individual's drug use, which may help to connect people to health services (Hyshka et al., 2012). Since their inception, supply distribution and disposal programs have expanded to include additional injection equipment, such as sterile cookers, water, and tourniquets, as well as safer smoking kits comprised of tubing, screens, and push sticks.

Your Personal Substance Use

Since problematic substance use is so common, we encourage you to consider whether your own use of substances is generally healthy or whether there are times when you are using substances in ways that produce harms. Whether it be caffeine, alcohol, cannabinoids, or one of the less commonly used substances, remember that people respond differently to the use of various substances. For some people, any substance use can be unhealthy and problematic. If you think there are times when your substance use is potentially unhealthy, we encourage you to review the section in Chapter 14 titled "Personal Mental Health Tool Kit," where we provide some recommendations for maintaining good mental health, including minimizing substance use harms.

Conclusion

Psychoactive substance use is common and widespread within the Canadian population. Psychoactive substances are derived from plant materials or are synthesized by chemical procedures. They exert their effects by binding to various receptors that modulate neuronal transmission in the brain and may result in mental stimulation, sedation, or cause changes in perception, cognition, mood, and behaviour. For the most part, regular use of certain substances (e.g., having caffeinated beverages in the morning or drinking small amounts of alcohol in social circumstances) can be innocuous or even beneficial. However, many people experience substantial harms due to intoxication, physiological or psychological dependence, or accidents.

We have provided brief descriptions of the substances that are most commonly used in Canada and some of the factors that can contribute to problematic use. Additional recommended readings are listed at the end of this chapter for those who would like to pursue further information about the topics introduced or those that we were not able to cover.

Glossary

addiction: The compulsive use of a substance despite its adverse consequences.
dependence: A state that develops once someone has used a substance for some time, in which it becomes very difficult to stop use because of the physiological changes that have occurred.
harm reduction: A pragmatic approach to health policy, programs, and practices that aims to decrease harms associated with substance use by offering safe and supportive alternatives.

illicit substances: Substances that are used in contravention to existing laws and regulations.
licit substances: Substances that are legal to produce, sell, buy, or consume.
psychological dependence: Occurs when an individual experiences intense cravings, anxiety, irritability, or other feelings of distress when substance use is stopped.
substance use disorder: A diagnosis for ongoing use of substances despite detrimental impacts.
tolerance: A state in which the body will need a higher dose of a substance to create the effects that a smaller dose would have previously.
withdrawal: A state in which the body experiences physical and mental symptoms that are often very uncomfortable when a substance is no longer used.

Critical Thinking Questions

1. Substance use can be understood to occur across a wide spectrum. Describe the spectrum and provide examples.
2. What are some of the factors that can contribute to problematic substance use or a substance use disorder?
3. Discuss the concepts of dependence, tolerance, and withdrawal. How are they related?
4. Define substance use disorder and describe the impact it can have on an individual's life and well-being.
5. Select a substance commonly used in Canada and describe its characteristic effects on the human body.

Recommended Readings

Boyd, S. C., Carter, C. I., & MacPherson, D. (2016). *More harm than good: Drug policy in Canada*. Fernwood Publishing.

Csiernik, R. (2016). *Substance use and abuse: Everything matters* (2nd ed.). Canadian Scholars.

Strike, C., & Watson, T. M. (2019). Losing the uphill battle? Emergent harm reduction interventions and barriers during the opioid overdose crisis in Canada. *International Journal of Drug Policy, 71*, 178–182. https://doi.org/10.1016/j.drugpo.2019.02.005

Szalavitz, M. (2017). *Unbroken brain: A revolutionary new way of understanding addiction*. Picador.

Recommended Websites

Canadian Centre on Substance Use and Addiction. www.ccsa.ca/Eng/Pages/default.aspx
Canadian Drug Policy Coalition. https://drugpolicy.ca
Canadian Nurses' Association—Harm Reduction. www.cna-aiic.ca/en/policy-advocacy/harm-reduction
CRACKDOWN Podcast. https://crackdownpod.com
Government of Canada—Substance Use. www.canada.ca/en/health-canada/services/substance-use.html
Government of Canada—Supervised Consumption Sites and Services. https://www.canada.ca/en/health-canada/services/substance-use/supervised-consumption-sites.html
Public Health Agency of Canada—Canada's Opioid Crisis. www.canada.ca/en/services/health/campaigns/drug-prevention.html
Multidisciplinary Association for Psychedelic Studies. https://maps.org

References

American Psychiatric Association. (2014). *Diagnostic and statistical manual of mental disorders* (5th ed.). https://doi.org/10.1176/appi.books.9780890425596
Bayoumi, A. M., & Zaric, G. S. (2008). The cost-effectiveness of Vancouver's supervised injection facility. *Canadian Medical Association Journal, 179*(11), 1143–1151. https://doi.org/10.1503/cmaj.080808
Bogenschutz, M. P., & Johnson M. W. (2016). Classic hallucinogens in the treatment of addictions. *Progress in Neuro-psychopharmacology & Biological Psychiatry, 64*, 250–258. https://doi.org/10.1016/j.pnpbp.2015.03.002
Canadian Community Epidemiology Network on Drug Use. (2015). *Deaths involving fentanyl in Canada 2009–2014.* www.ccsa.ca/Resource%20Library/CCSA-CCENDU-Fentanyl-Deaths-Canada-Bulletin-2015-en.pdf
Canadian Substance Use Costs and Harms Scientific Working Group. (2020). *Canadian substance use costs and harms 2015–2017.* https://csuch.ca/publications/CSUCH-Canadian-Substance-Use-Costs-Harms-Report-2020-en.pdf
Centre for Innovation in Campus Mental Health. (n.d.). *Understanding substance use.* https://campusmentalhealth.ca/toolkits/cannabis/cannabis-substance-use/understanding/
Collins, A. (1998). *In the sleep room: The story of the CIA brainwashing experiments in Canada.* Key Porter Books.
Csiernik, R. (2016). *Substance use and abuse: Everything matters* (2nd ed.). Canadian Scholars.

Deak, J. D., Miller, A. P., & Gizer, I. R. (2019). Genetics of alcohol use disorder: A review. *Current Opinion in Psychology, 27*, 56–61. https://doi.org/10.1016/j.copsyc.2018.07.012

Dell, C. A., Seguin, M., Hopkins, C., Tempier, R., & Lewis, M. (2011). From benzos to berries: Treatment offered at an Aboriginal youth solvent abuse treatment centre relays the importance of culture. *Canadian Journal of Psychiatry, 56*(2), 75–83. https://doi.org/10.1177/070674371105600202

Dube, S. R., Felitti, V. J., Dong, M., Chapman, D. P., Giles, W. H., & Anda, R. F. (2003). Childhood abuse, neglect, and household dysfunction and the risk of illicit drug use: The Adverse Childhood Experiences study. *Pediatrics, 111*(3), 564–572. https://doi.org/10.1542/peds.111.3.564

Fischer, B., Jeffries, V., Hall, W., Room, R., Goldner, E., & Rehm, J. (2011). Lower risk cannabis use guidelines for Canada (LRCUG): A narrative review of evidence and recommendations. *Canadian Journal of Public Health, 102*(5), 324–327. https://doi.org/10.1007/BF03404169

Fischer, B., Rehm, J., Goldman, B., & Popova, S. (2008). Non-medical use of prescription opioids and public health in Canada: An urgent call for research and interventions development. *Canadian Journal of Public Health, 99*(3), 182–184. https://doi.org/10.1007/BF03405469

Fischer, B., Russell, C., Sabioni, P., van den Brink, W., Le Foll, B., Hall, W., Rehm, J., & Room, R. (2017). Lower-risk cannabis use guidelines: A comprehensive update of evidence and recommendations. *American Journal of Public Health, 107*(8), e1–e12. https://doi.org/10.2105/AJPH.2017.303818

Garcia-Romeu, A., Kersgaard, B., & Addy, P. H. (2016). Clinical applications of hallucinogens: A review. *Experimental and Clinical Psychopharmacology, 24*(4), 229–268. https://doi.org/10.1037/pha0000084

Goodman, A., Fleming, K., Markwick, N., Morrison, T., Lagimodiere, L., Kerr, T., & Western Aboriginal Harm Reduction Society. (2017). "They treated me like crap and I know it was because I was Native": The healthcare experiences of Aboriginal peoples living in Vancouver's inner city. *Social Science and Medicine, 178*, 87–94. https://doi.org/10.1016/j.socscimed.2017.01.053.

Gore, F. M., Bloem, P., Patton, G. C., Ferguson, J., Joseph, V., Coffey, C., Sawyer, S. M., & Mathers, C. D. (2011). Global burden of disease in young people aged 10–24 years: A systematic analysis. *The Lancet, 377*(9783), 2093–2102. https://doi.org/10.1016/S0140-6736(11)60512-6

Government of Canada. (2020). *Supervised consumption sites and services.* https://www.canada.ca/en/health-canada/services/substance-use/supervised-consumption-sites.html

Government of Canada. (2021). *Opioid- and stimulant-related harms in Canada.* https://health-infobase.canada.ca/substance-related-harms/opioids-stimulants/

Health Canada. (2012). *Federal tobacco control strategy.* www.hc-sc.gc.ca/ahc-asc/alt_formats/pdf/performance/eval/ftcs-evaluation-sflt-eng.pdf

Health Canada. (2013). *Youth Smoking Survey.* https://www.canada.ca/en/health-canada/services/publications/healthy-living/summary-results-youth-smoking-survey-2012-2013.html

Health Canada. (2017). *Canadian Tobacco, Alcohol and Drugs Survey: Summary of results for 2017.* https://www.canada.ca/en/health-canada/services/canadian-tobacco-alcohol-drugs-survey/2017-summary.html

Hoffman, A. (1980). *LSD: My problem child.* McGraw-Hill.

Hyshka, E., Strathdee, S., Wood, E., & Kerr, T. (2012). Needle exchange and the HIV epidemic in Vancouver: Lessons learned from 15 years of research. *International Journal of Drug Policy, 23*(4), 261–270. https://doi.org/10.1016/j.drugpo.2012.03.006

Karamouzian, M., Dohoo, C., Forsting, S., McNeil, R., Kerr, T., & Lysyshyn, M. (2018). Evaluation of a fentanyl drug checking service for clients of a supervised injection facility, Vancouver, Canada. *Harm Reduction Journal, 15,* Article 46. https://doi.org/10.1186/s12954-018-0252-8

Keller, C., Goering, P., Hume, C., Macnaughton, E., O'Campo, P., Sarang, A., Thomson, M., Vallee, C., Watson, A., & Tsemberis, S. (2013). Initial implementation of Housing First in five Canadian cities: How do you make the shoe fit, when one size does not fit all? *American Journal of Psychiatric Rehabilitation, 16*(4), 275–289. https://doi.org/10.1080/15487768.2013.847761

Kerr, T., Mitra, S., Kennedy, M. C., & McNeil, R. (2017). Supervised injection facilities in Canada: Past, present, and future. *Harm Reduction Journal, 14,* Article 28. https://doi.org/10.1186/s12954-017-0154-1

Kim, B., Yun, J., & Park, B. (2020). Methamphetamine-induced neuronal damage: Neurotoxicity and neuroinflammation. *Biomolecules & Therapeutics (Seoul), 28*(5), 381–388. https://doi.org/10.4062/biomolther.2020.044

Krueger, H., Turner, D., Krueger, J., & Ready, A. E. (2014). The economic benefits of risk factor reduction in Canada: Tobacco smoking, excess weight and physical inactivity. *Canadian Journal of Public Health, 105,* e69–e78. https://doi.org/10.17269/cjph.105.4084

Marshall, B. D., Milloy, M. J., Wood, E., Montaner, J. S., & Kerr, T. (2011). Reduction in overdose mortality after the opening of North America's first medically supervised safer injecting facility: A retrospective population-based study. *The Lancet, 377*(9775), 1429–1437. https://doi.org/10.1016/S0140-6736(10)62353-7

Moffat, B. M., Jenkins, E. K., & Johnson, J. L. (2013). Weeding out the information: An ethnographic approach to exploring how young people make sense of the evidence on cannabis. *Harm Reduction Journal, 10,* Article 34. https://doi.org/10.1186/1477-7517-10-34

National Academies of Sciences, Engineering, and Medicine. (2017). *The health effects of cannabis and cannabinoids: The current state of evidence and recommendations for research.* The National Academies Press. https://doi.org/10.17226/24625

Preston, K. L., & Epstein, D. H. (2011). Stress in the daily lives of cocaine and heroin users: Relationship to mood, craving, relapse triggers, and cocaine use. *Psychopharmacology, 218*, 29–37. https://doi.org/10.1007/s00213-011-2183-x

Statistics Canada. (2019). *Health indicator profile, by Aboriginal identity and sex, age-standardized rate, four year estimates* (Table 13-10-0099-01). https://www150.statcan.gc.ca/t1/tbl1/en/tv.action?pid=1310009901

Turpel-Lafond, M. E. (2020). *In plain sight: Addressing Indigenous-specific racism and discrimination in BC health care, full report.* https://engage.gov.bc.ca/app/uploads/sites/613/2020/11/In-Plain-Sight-Full-Report.pdf

Venture, M., Noijen, J., Bücheli, A., Isvy, A., van Huyck, C., Martins, D., Nagy, C., & Schipper, V. (2013). *Drug checking service: Good practice standards.* Nightlife Empowerment & Well-being Implementation Project (NEWIP). http://newip.safernightlife.org/pdfs/standards/NEWIP_D_standards-final_20.12-A4.pdf

World Health Organization. (2015). *Tobacco: Key facts.* www.who.int/mediacentre/factsheets/fs339/en/

World Health Organization. (2018). *Fact sheet—Alcohol.* https://www.who.int/news-room/fact-sheets/detail/alcohol

Chapter 6

Trauma, Violence, and Mental Health

Nancy Clark, Allie Slemon, and Emily Jenkins

Trauma is not what happens to you, it's what happens inside you as a result of what happened to you.
—Dr. Gabor Maté (Canadian physician, author, and speaker)

Introduction

Before progressing further in our examination of mental health in forthcoming chapters, we will first draw attention to the relationship between trauma, violence, and mental health. Building a base knowledge about trauma and violence and engaging with the concepts of Trauma and Violence Informed Practice, or TVIP, should be considered as "universal precautions." That is, we should understand the impacts of trauma and apply principles of TVIP in *all* health care interactions, regardless of whether someone has a known trauma history. This is similar to how we would use personal protective equipment in all patient care interactions to prevent the transmission of infectious diseases, regardless of whether the individual has a known communicable condition.

In this chapter, we explore trauma and violence as they relate to mental health and illness and discuss how mental health services can support people who have encountered these circumstances. We introduce **TVIP**—an approach to understanding the connections between trauma, violence, and health; and to fostering physical and emotional safety for all people, including those who have a history of these experiences (Government of Canada, 2018). TVIP serves as an ethical guide towards reducing potential harms and promoting mental health in diverse care settings. Indeed, without TVIP, we risk contributing to inaccurate mental health diagnoses, inappropriate treatment, and *retraumatization*, an experience in which feelings and memories of a traumatic event are triggered (Haskell, 2011; Sweeney et al., 2016).

Fully integrating TVIP into our health care organizations will require fundamental changes in how these systems are designed and how practitioners engage with key policy and practice principles (Government of Canada, 2018). However, anyone can adopt TVIP as a personal framework to guide their interactions with others and their work with people who are experiencing mental health challenges. In this chapter, we consider TVIP as the starting point for addressing experiences of trauma—individual and collective. Moreover, we encourage you to utilize this framework as you continue your journey through this textbook.

To begin, we will provide an introduction to trauma and violence, exploring their occurrence at individual and societal levels. We then examine the linkages between trauma, violence, and mental health. Following this, we will introduce the mental health challenges that arise as a direct result of experiences with trauma and violence, and we discuss some of the treatment options and community trauma supports available. Finally, we present an overview of the EQUIP Health Care TVIP framework and illustrate how TVIP policies and guidelines can be used to avoid harms and support mental health recovery and overall well-being.

Trauma and Violence

Trauma is defined as "an experience that overwhelms an individual's ability to cope" and can lead to feelings of fear, shame, and powerlessness (Canadian Centre on Substance Abuse, 2014). The concept of trauma can be best understood through consideration of three elements: *exposure* to harmful events, the *experience* of these events, and the *effects* of these events (BC Ministry of Children and Family Development, 2017). There are many different types of harmful events that may constitute a trauma exposure, including accidents, natural disasters, war, sudden loss, and child abuse or neglect. The experience and effects of these events vary from person to person. Some individuals may not experience any trauma response following an exposure to a potentially traumatizing incident, while others will have considerable and long-lasting effects. The US Department of Veterans Affairs and Department of Defense has identified three types of factors that are associated with experiencing prolonged reactions to trauma or trauma-related disorders (see Table 6.1).

Although they are different concepts, the Government of Canada (2018) acknowledges the importance of including violence in discussions about trauma, due to the connection between the two experiences. Indeed, trauma can be understood as a *response* to violence or to another type of distressing event. The World Health Organization (WHO; 2002) defines **violence** as:

> the intentional use of physical force or power, threatened or actual, against oneself, another person, or against a group or community, that either results in or has a high likelihood of resulting in injury, death, psychological harm, maldevelopment, or deprivation.

Table 6.1 Risk Factors for Trauma-Related Disorders

Type	Factors
Pre-Traumatic Factors	• Ongoing life stress • Lack of social support • Young age at time of trauma • Pre-existing psychological conditions or substance misuse *or* family history of psychological conditions • History of traumatic events or abuse • History of PTSD
Peri-Traumatic or Trauma-Related Factors	• Severe trauma • Physical injury to self or others • High-risk trauma (e.g., combat, killing another person, torture, rape, assault) • High perceived threat to life of self or others • Mass trauma • History of peri-traumatic dissociation
Post-Traumatic Factors	• Ongoing life stress • Lack of positive social support • Bereavement or traumatic grief • Major loss of resources • Negative social support (blaming environment) • Poor coping skills • Distressed spouse or children

Source: Adapted from Defense Centers of Excellence for Psychological Health & Traumatic Brain Injury. (2013). *Posttraumatic stress disorder pocket guide: To accompany the 2010 VA/DoD clinical practice guideline for the management of post-traumatic stress.* U.S. Department of Veterans Affairs. https://www.healthquality.va.gov/guidelines/MH/ptsd/PTSDPocketGuide23May2013v1.pdf

Examples of violence that have been linked to trauma include, but are not limited to, domestic violence, sex/gender-based violence, childhood abuse and neglect, civil war, and intimate partner violence. The health impacts of violence are far reaching and can include psychological as well as physiological symptoms and conditions.

Although violence is a part of the human condition and "embedded in the structures of most ... societies" (Kirmayer et al., 2007), it may not always be visible or explicit. For example, it may manifest through **microaggressions**, which are subtle, everyday insults or indignities that reflect stigmatizing and discriminatory views held in society. **Stigma** can be defined as "a mark of disgrace" or an "attribute that is deeply discrediting" (Link & Phelan, 2001) and results in a person being "disqualified from full social acceptance" (Goffman, 1963). For the most part, stigma results from stereotypes (i.e., beliefs—positive or negative—about the overly generalized characteristics of a group or population) and prejudicial attitudes (i.e., unreasonable negative opinions or attitudes about a particular group or member of a group that are not grounded in reason and are resistant to rational influence). **Discrimination** occurs when our stereotypes and prejudices are acted upon and involves behaviours that exclude, subordinate, and disadvantage others on the basis of gender, ethnicity,

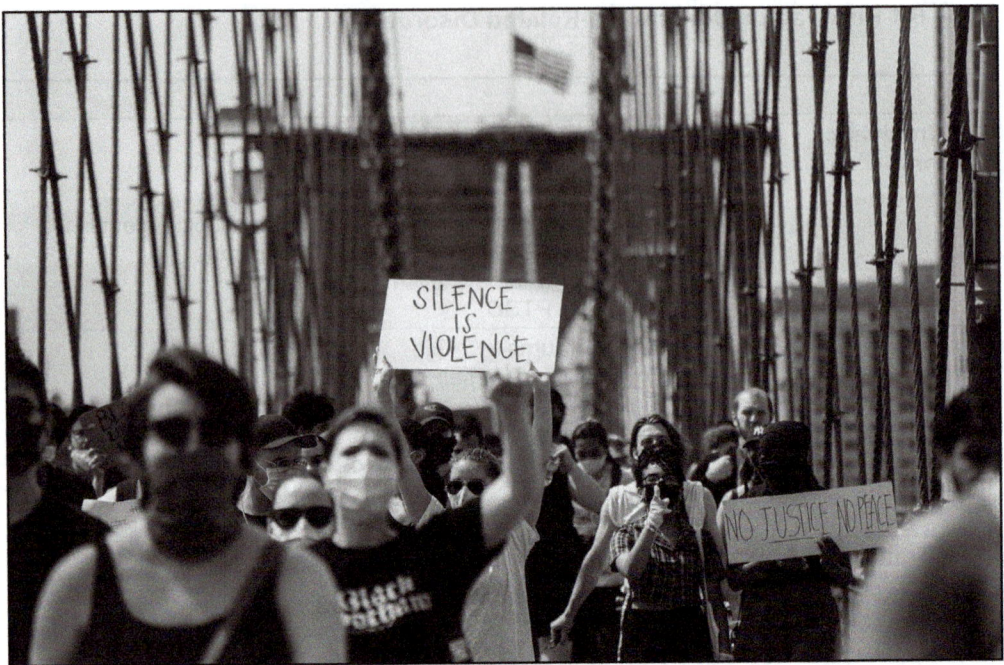

Figure 6.1: Protesters march in support of the Black Lives Matter movement in response to discrimination and violence towards Black people across the globe.

Source: Pexels/Life Matters

age, disability, or other aspects of a person's identity (Young, 2008). When these patterns of stigma and discrimination are integrated into the fabric of our society—including social, political, and economic systems—it can be understood as **structural violence** (Farmer, 2004; Galtung, 1969). While discriminatory acts occur at the interpersonal level (i.e., between individuals or groups), structural violence recognizes how stigma and discrimination operate at the societal level.

Box 6.1: The Role of Structural Violence in the National Crisis of Missing and Murdered Indigenous Women and Girls

In Canada, violence against Indigenous women and girls has been recognized as a national crisis. Indigenous women and girls are 12 times more likely to be murdered or go missing than other women and experience significantly higher rates of violence, including intimate partner violence, family violence, and violence perpetrated by strangers (Brownridge et al., 2017; TAKEN, 2021). However, there is limited media reporting on violence against Indigenous women and girls, while coverage of violence against white women and children is prominent (Gilchrist, 2010). Indigenous

> people and activists have been speaking up about this violence—and the lack of media and societal attention to this issue—for decades. However, it was not until 2015 that the Government of Canada launched a National Inquiry into Missing and Murdered Indigenous Women and Girls.
>
> The final report of the National Inquiry was released in 2019 and acknowledged the disproportionate rates of interpersonal violence experienced by Indigenous women and girls. However, the report predominantly focused on the ways that *structural* violence has contributed to this crisis. For example, the report identifies that people who perpetrate violence against Indigenous women and girls (including assault, exploitation, and sex trafficking) "count on society's turning a blind eye" with minimal media reporting, police investigation, or legal prosecuting of these crimes. Findings from the report reinforce that stigma, discrimination, and social and economic inequities are all forms of structural violence that directly impact Indigenous peoples and also create conditions that lead to increases in interpersonal violence. Therefore, addressing this crisis requires attention not only to individual events but also to the root causes of violence. This involves acknowledging the historical and intergenerational trauma experienced by Indigenous peoples and incorporating a TVIP approach "into all policies, procedures, and practices of solutions" (National Inquiry into MMIWG, 2019).

Historical Events Shaping Our Understandings of Trauma

According to Kirmayer et al. (2007), our present views about trauma have been shaped by three sets of historical events:

1. The wars and genocides of the 20th century and the clinical and moral challenges they have raised.
2. The inclusion of trauma-related disorders in official psychiatric classifications of diseases.
3. The increasing public and professional recognition of the prevalence and long-term effects of childhood abuse.

During World War I, the term "shell shock" was used to describe the trauma experienced by soldiers during and after the war. While trauma is an "essentially timeless" human experience, the recognition of the physical and psychological impacts of war was a crucial event in the gradual process of understanding trauma and its effects (Loughran, 2012). While shell shock was used to describe the traumatic effects of war from World War I onwards, the language and diagnosis of trauma-related disorders, such as post-traumatic stress disorder (PTSD), was not established until after the end of the Vietnam War in 1975. It is important to note that the concepts of shell shock and PTSD both arose in a particular historical, political, and cultural context, within which it was understood that experiences of trauma follow a violent traumatic event, such as fighting in a war. However, the International Classification of Diseases-11 (ICD-11, which you were introduced to in Chapter 4) provides a definition of PTSD that recognizes that traumatic events are not always associated with violence. In this publication, PTSD is described as involving the re-experience and avoidance of "an extremely threatening or horrific event or series of events," with longstanding symptoms causing significant distress and impairment of functioning (WHO, 2019).

Another important event shaping our understandings of trauma was the recognition of **adverse childhood experiences** (ACEs). ACEs are potentially traumatic events occurring in childhood (0–17 years) that may be distressing and can result in persistent adverse impacts on an individual across the life course (National Center

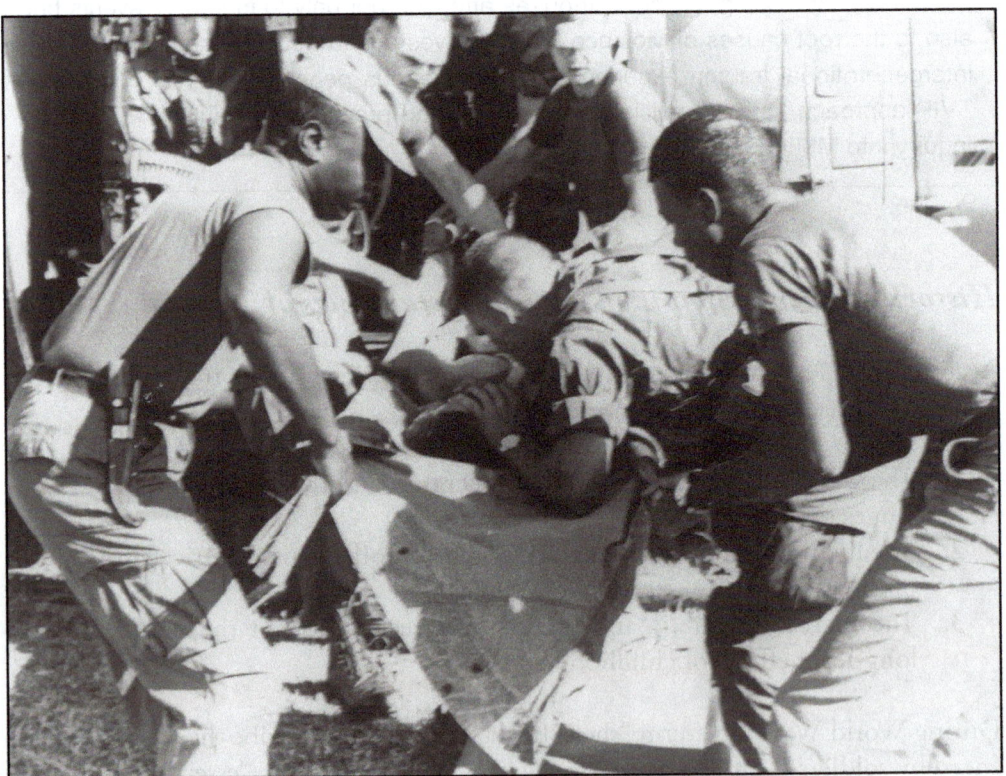

Figure 6.2: The traumatic effects of war on soldiers contributed to the establishment of the classification of PTSD following the end of the Vietnam War. Traumatic experiences of war, including witnessing injury and death, contributed to an estimated PTSD prevalence of 20–30 percent among Vietnam War veterans.

Source: Unsplash/The New York Public Library

for Injury Prevention and Control, 2019). ACEs include experiencing violence, abuse, or neglect; witnessing violence in the household or community; exposure to other challenges within the home environment such as parental mental illnesses or problematic substance use; or having a family member in jail (Centers for Disease Control and Prevention, 2021; Felitti et al., 1998). Public Health Ontario estimates that approximately two-thirds of people living in Canada have experienced at least one type of ACE (Public Health Ontario, 2020). ACEs have been described as "highly interrelated," that is, if someone is exposed to one form of ACE, it is likely that they will also be exposed to others (McDonald et al., 2015). Across the general population, 16 percent (1 in 6 people) have experienced 4 or more types of ACE (Centers for Disease Control and Prevention, 2021). ACEs contribute to significant physical and mental health challenges later in life and have been linked to depression, problematic substance use, heart disease, cancer, and respiratory diseases (Hughes et al., 2017). While treatments are available to address some of the poor health outcomes related to ACEs, experts note that the most important strategy we can draw on is prevention. This includes building stronger supportive environments and community contexts to enhance access to the social determinants of good health.

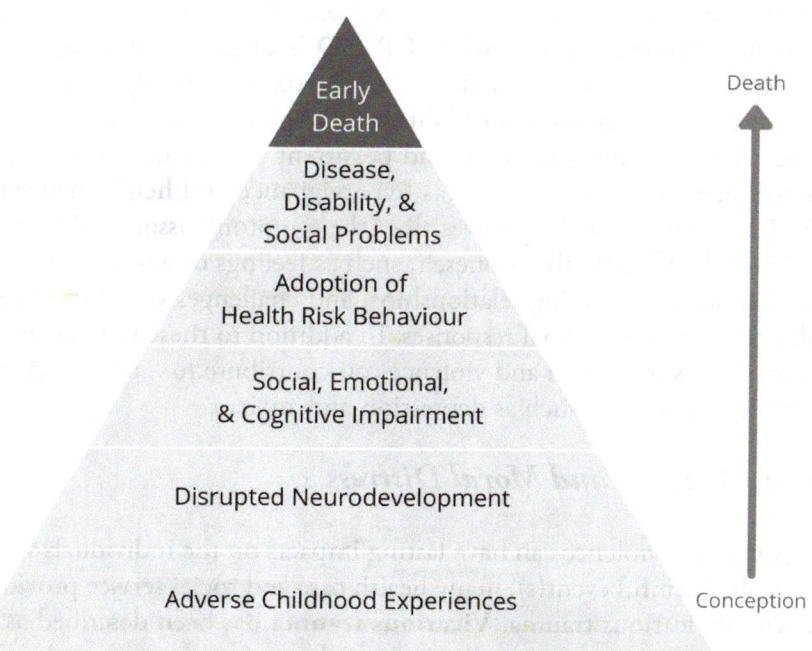

Figure 6.3: The ACEs pyramid illustrates how experiencing ACEs contributes to health consequences across the lifespan.

Source: Adapted from the Centers for Disease Control and Prevention.

Trauma, Violence, and Mental Health

Understanding trauma and violence is particularly important in the mental health field. People with mental health challenges are more likely to experience violence at the *individual* level, including microaggressions and violent assaults (Khalifeh et al., 2015). Additionally, structural violence is a common experience among people with mental health challenges, particularly those with more severe and persistent mental illnesses and substance use disorders. Structural violence operates to create exclusion and may result in discrimination in housing, employment, and access to health care and other services. Further, structural violence contributes to the criminalization of people with mental health challenges, resulting in an overrepresentation of people with mental illnesses in the prison system. Structural violence and its indirect effects are not always easy to see, but it has profound impacts on the lives of people who experience mental health challenges.

In addition to the connections between violence (at multiple levels) and mental ill health, there are also important linkages between trauma and mental health. As we explored in the discussion of ACEs, traumatic events in childhood can contribute to experiences of depression, anxiety, and problematic substance use later in life (Negriff, 2020). Moreover, the ICD-11 recognizes two mental health disorders as directly resulting from traumatic experiences: **post-traumatic stress disorder** (PTSD) and complex post-traumatic stress disorder (CPSTD). PTSD is associated with a discrete traumatic event, while CPTSD is diagnosed in people with more chronic exposures to trauma. PTSD is characterized by re-experiencing the traumatic event through flashbacks or nightmares, avoidance of thoughts or memories associated with the traumatic event, and persistent perceptions of a current threat. This contributes to behaviours such as hypervigilance and heightened startle reaction (WHO, 2019). CPTSD involves all of the symptoms associated with PTSD, as well as diminished beliefs about oneself, such as feelings of worthlessness, shame or guilt, difficulties in sustaining relationships, and challenges with "affect regulation" or moderating one's emotional responses. In addition to these trauma-specific diagnoses, experiences of trauma and violence can contribute to—or exacerbate—other mental health challenges, such as depression and anxiety.

Vicarious Trauma and Moral Distress

While trauma and violence can have lasting impacts on the individuals who directly encounter the harmful event(s), many health care and social service providers report experiences of vicarious trauma. **Vicarious trauma** has been described as "harmful changes that occur in professional's views of themselves ... as a result of exposure to graphic and/or traumatic material life events of their clients" (Baird & Kracen, 2006). This experience can result in emotional residue and burnout, and providers may experience hopelessness, detachment, and low self-esteem. Recently, vicarious trauma has also been documented within community samples. For example, a recent study on the university protests in Hong Kong in late 2019 showed that those who witnessed the events, or who were repeatedly exposed to images and video of the events on social media, experienced symptoms of vicarious trauma, including increased stress and anxiety, disturbed sleep, and feelings of helplessness (Turnbull et al., 2020).

Experiences of witnessing and hearing others' experiences of trauma may also contribute to "moral distress." This concept has emerged in the recent scientific literature and describes the suffering experienced by health care professionals when they "[lack] the necessary resources to provide attentive, competent, and ethical care" (Musto & Schreiber, 2012). The situations that are seen to constrain moral action and contribute to moral distress include a perceived lack of support from health care leadership, feeling unheard by colleagues, being unable to act in accordance with values, and having concerns left unaddressed—situations which, unfortunately, are prevalent in mental health settings, as they are often underfunded and undervalued (Mental Health Commission of Canada, 2012).

Individuals who provide mental health care services need a sound understanding of the impact that the work can have on their own mental health and require coping strategies to deal with the stress and potential vicarious trauma that accompanies the role. Ideally, health care professionals put provisions in place to promote or safeguard their mental health, including regular contact with colleagues and mentors. Professional associations often provide confidential services and supports to help members who are experiencing difficulties. Unfortunately, some health care professionals are reluctant to disclose mental health or substance use challenges, due to concerns that they could lose credibility or have their privileges to practice suspended.

Treatment Approaches

There are a variety of specialized services and related therapies that have been developed to treat trauma-related disorders, with the aim to build skills for emotional regulation, reduce the adverse impacts of trauma on day-to-day life, and enhance overall quality of life. These include psychotherapeutic interventions such as exposure-based therapies and cognitive-based therapies, both of which involve varying degrees of exposure to traumatic stimuli (e.g., in real life, or through imagined or narrative formats) alongside cognitive restructuring (i.e., reframing beliefs connected to the traumatic event) and relaxation exercises (American Psychological Association, 2017). A common, more alternative form of trauma-related psychotherapy is eye movement desensitization and reprocessing (EMDR). This therapy aims to alter the way that memories of traumatic events are stored in the brain, reducing heightened emotions and vivid flashbacks (Wilson et al., 2018). Other strategies, such as art or dance therapy, interpersonal therapy, trauma-sensitive yoga, and traditional healing methods, are also beneficial for many people who have experienced trauma and violence.

While psychotherapeutic approaches are considered "first line" treatments for PTSD, individuals may continue to experience distressing symptoms even after treatment. In some cases pharmacotherapy may be used, most notably, antidepressant medications (e.g., selective serotonin reuptake inhibitors [SSRIs]) or Prazosin, an alpha blocker medication that has shown mixed effects in the treatment of PTSD-related nightmares. The search for new and effective approaches to treating symptoms of PTSD has led to recent advances in psychedelic-assisted psychotherapy, including the use of MDMA, ketamine, psilocybin (magic mushrooms), lysergic acid diethylamide (LSD), and cannabinoids (Krediet et al., 2020). These treatments must be used with caution to avoid side effects or re-traumatization and should be guided by a trained professional who assists the individual in "integrating" their mind and body following a shift in consciousness initiated by psychedelic use.

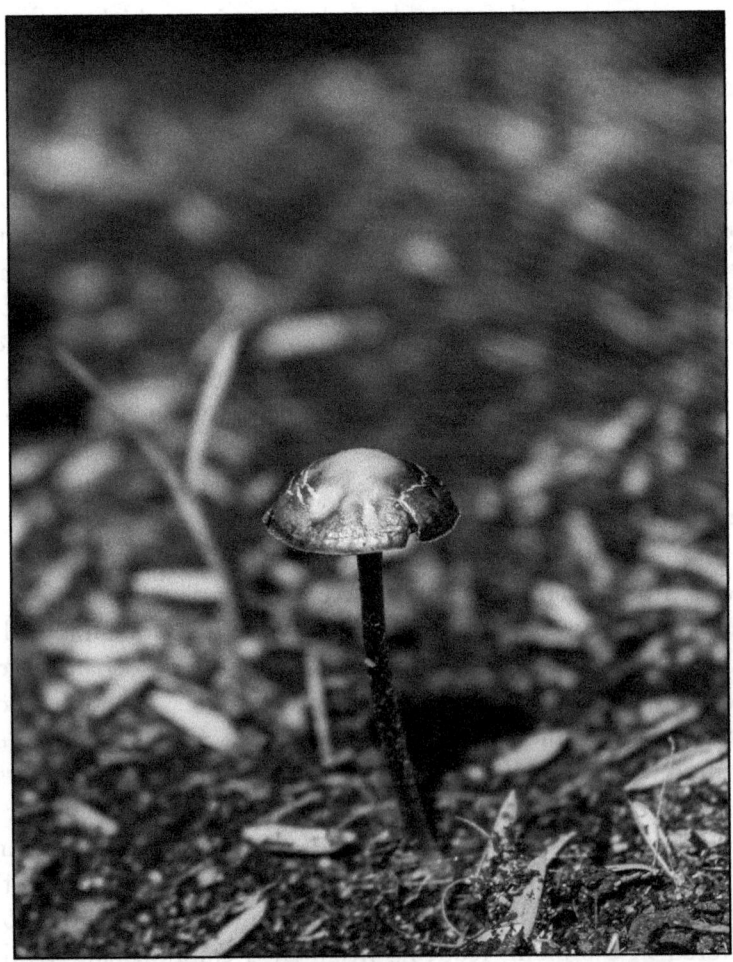

Figure 6.4: Psilocybin mushrooms may be used as an alternative therapy for PTSD.

Source: Pexels/Loifotos

A TVIP Framework for Practice

Now that you are familiar with the concepts of trauma and violence as well as their impacts on mental health at an individual and population level, we will now move to a discussion of TVIP. A key aspect of a TVIP approach is that it aims to promote physical and emotional safety, regardless of whether there is a known trauma history (Government of Canada, 2018). EQUIP Health Care is a research-based program housed at the University of British Columbia, School of Nursing, that has been influential in advancing the science and practice of TVIP for health and social service providers as well as within health care organizations (EQUIP Health Care, 2017). EQUIP's TVIP framework includes four key elements:

1. Building awareness and understanding
2. Emphasizing safety and trust
3. Adapting language
4. Considering trauma as a risk factor

Building awareness and understanding involves recognizing the high prevalence of trauma in the general population and the particular impacts of these events on populations that experience structural violence. This also entails understanding the relationship between trauma, violence, and mental health. Emphasizing safety and trust reinforces that we do not need to know whether an individual has experienced trauma and/or violence in order to create safe and welcoming spaces. Adopting practices such as ensuring privacy and confidentiality and communicating clearly about expectations and procedures are part of a TVIP approach. Adapting language is also important in an effort to avoid perpetuating microaggressions and stigma. This involves reframing problematic terms, such as "drug abusers" or "addicts," and instead adopting person-first language, such as "people who use drugs." Another example would be to move from terms such as "schizophrenic" to "a person experiencing schizophrenia." Additionally, recognizing the widespread and enduring impacts of ACEs, as described earlier in this chapter, is an important first step to appreciating trauma as a risk factor. Understanding the potential health impacts of trauma can help support early prevention efforts and avoid "blaming" individuals for particular trauma responses or coping behaviours, such as substance use or high-risk sexual behaviours. Further, a TVIP approach can contribute to identifying and transforming policies and practices that unintentionally contribute to re-traumatization and harm. As mentioned at the outset of this chapter, an ultimate goal is to support health care organizations in adopting TVIP principles at a systems level, which will take time. However, there are a variety of ways that you can incorporate TVIP into your everyday encounters. For inspiration, see Table 6.2, which describes principles for TVIP at both organizational and individual levels.

Table 6.2: Principles for TVIC at Organizational and Individual Levels

Principle	Organizational Strategies	Provider Practices

1. Understand trauma, violence, and its impacts on people's lives and behavior	• Develop structures, policies, processes (e.g., hiring practices) to build culture based on understanding of trauma and violence
	• Staff training on health effects of violence/trauma and vicarious trauma
		• Be mindful of potential histories and effects ("red flags")
		• Handle disclosures appropriately:
		  • Believe the experience
		  • Affirm and validate
		  • Recognize strengths
		  • Express concern for safety and well-being

2. Create emotionally and physically safe environments for all clients and providers	• Create a welcoming space and intake procedures; emphasize confidentiality and client/patient priorities • Seek client input about safe and inclusive strategies • Support staff at risk of vicarious trauma (e.g., peer support, check-ins, self-care programs)	• Take a non-judgemental approach (make people feel accepted and deserving) • Foster connection and trust • Provide clear information and predictable expectations about programming
3. Foster opportunities for choice, collaboration, and connection	• Have policies and processes that allow for flexibility and encourage shared decision-making and participation • Involve staff and clients in identifying ways to implement services/programs	• Provide appropriate and meaningful options/real choices for treatment/care • Consider choices collaboratively • Actively listen and privilege the person's voice
4. Use a strengths-based and capacity-building approach to support clients	• Allow sufficient time for meaningful engagement • Program options that can be tailored to people's needs, strengths, and contexts	• Help people identify strengths • Acknowledge the effects of historical and structural conditions • Teach skills for recognizing triggers, calming, and centring

Source: Adapted from EQUIP Health Care. (n.d.). *Principles of TVIC—Organizational and individual provider levels*. https://equiphealthcare.ca/resources/tvic-workshop/

Conclusion

Trauma and violence manifest through a wide variety of experiences, which can involve everything from one-time exposures to traumatic events, through to longer-term or ongoing adversities such as those stemming from ACEs, or secondary experiences of trauma such as vicarious trauma. The mental health impacts of trauma can include trauma-specific diagnoses, such as PTSD or CPTSD, and trauma may also result in depression or anxiety. Many treatment approaches have been developed to help individuals address the effects of trauma and include psychotherapy, pharmacological treatments, and alternative and more emergent interventions such as the therapeutic use of psychedelics. Beyond treatment for individuals who have experienced trauma and violence, TVIP is an important framework to guide delivery of mental health services and practices. TVIP can be applied as a "universal precaution" for all people seeking health or social services and can support creating a welcoming, safe, and supportive environment.

Glossary

adverse childhood experiences: Potentially traumatic events occurring in childhood (0–17 years) that can be distressing and have impacts on individuals that may persist for years.

discrimination: Behaviours that act on stereotypes and prejudices and involve actions that exclude, subordinate, and disadvantage others on the basis of gender, ethnicity, age, disability, or other aspects of a person's identity.

microaggressions: Subtle, everyday incidents or indignities that can contribute to the experience of trauma.

post-traumatic stress disorder: Re-experiencing and avoidance of an extremely threatening or horrific event or series of events, with longstanding symptoms causing significant distress and impairment of functioning.

stigma: A mark or sign of disgrace, infamy, or reproach when a person is identified by a label that sets the person apart and links them to undesirable stereotypes that result in unfair treatment and discrimination.

structural violence: Structural violence occurs when stigma and discrimination are enacted through the systems of our society.

trauma: An event or experience that overwhelms one's capacity to cope and that can contribute to feelings of fear, shame, and powerlessness.

Trauma and Violence Informed Practice (TVIP): An approach to practice and policy of understanding the connections between trauma, violence, and health, and fostering physical and emotional safety.

vicarious trauma: The challenging emotions that may be experienced by people who provide health and social services as they witness and listen to accounts of other people's traumatic experiences.

violence: The intentional use of physical force or power, threatened or actual, against oneself, another person, or against a group or community that either results in or has a high likelihood of resulting in injury, death, psychological harm, maldevelopment, or deprivation.

Critical Thinking Questions

1. What are the key differences between trauma and violence?
2. How can structural violence contribute to trauma and poor mental health outcomes?
3. Describe several ways that experiencing trauma and violence can affect mental health.
4. Why is TVIP considered a "universal precaution"?

Recommended Readings

Gerber, M. R. (Ed.). (2019). *Trauma-informed healthcare approaches: A guide for primary care.* Springer.

Klinic Community Health Centre. (2013). *Trauma-informed: The trauma toolkit.* https://trauma-informed.ca/wp-content/uploads/2013/10/Trauma-informed_Toolkit.pdf

Linklater, R. (2014). *Decolonizing trauma work: Indigenous stories and strategies.* Fernwood Publishing.

Perry, B. D., & Winfrey, O. (2021). *What happened to you? Conversations on trauma, resilience, and healing.* Flatiron Books.

Poole, N., & Greaves, L. (2012). *Becoming trauma informed.* Centre for Addiction and Mental Health (CAMH).

van der Volk, B. (2014). *The body keeps the score: Brain, mind, and body in the healing of trauma.* Penguin Books.

Recommended Websites

Alberta Health Services—Trauma Informed Care Learning Modules. www.albertahealthservices.ca/info/page15526.aspx

EQUIP Health Care—TVIC Workshop. www.equiphealthcare.ca/resources/tvic-workshop

Government of British Columbia—Trauma-Informed Practice: Webinars. www2.gov.bc.ca/gov/content/health/managing-your-health/mental-health-substance-use/child-teen-mental-health/trauma-informed-practice-resources

Government of Canada—Trauma and Violence-Informed Approaches to Policy and Practice. https://www.canada.ca/en/public-health/services/publications/health-risks-safety/trauma-violence-informed-approaches-policy-practice.html

Trauma-Informed Care Implementation Resource Center. www.traumainformedcare.chcs.org

References

American Psychological Association. (2017). *Clinical practice guideline for the treatment of PTSD*. https://www.apa.org/ptsd-guideline/ptsd.pdf

Baird, K., & Kracen, A. C. (2006). Vicarious traumatization and secondary trauma stress: A research synthesis. *Counselling Psychology Quarterly, 19*(2), 181–188. https://doi.org/10.1080/09515070600811899

British Columbia Ministry of Children and Family Development. (2017). *Healing families, helping systems: A trauma-informed practice guide for working with children, youth and families*. https://www2.gov.bc.ca/assets/gov/health/child-teen-mental-health/trauma-informed_practice_guide.pdf

Brownridge, D. A., Taillieu, T., Afifi, T., Chan, K. L., Emery, C., Lavoie, J., & Elgar, F. (2017). Child maltreatment and intimate partner violence among Indigenous and non-Indigenous Canadians. *Journal of Family Violence, 32*(6), 607–619. https://doi.org/10.1007/s10896-016-9880-5

Canadian Centre on Substance Abuse. (2014). *Trauma-informed care*. https://www.ccsa.ca/sites/default/files/2019-04/CCSA-Trauma-informed-Care-Toolkit-2014-en.pdf

Centers for Disease Control and Prevention. (2021). *Adverse childhood experiences (ACEs)*. https://www.cdc.gov/violenceprevention/aces/index.html

Defense Centers of Excellence for Psychological Health & Traumatic Brain Injury. (2013). *Posttraumatic stress disorder pocket guide: To accompany the 2010 VA/DoD clinical practice guideline for the management of post-traumatic stress*. U.S. Department of Veterans Affairs. https://www.healthquality.va.gov/guidelines/MH/ptsd/PTSDPocketGuide23May2013v1.pdf

EQUIP Health Care. (2017). *Trauma-and-violence-informed care (TVIC): A tool for health & social service organizations and providers*. www.equiphealthcare.ca

EQUIP Health Care. (n.d.). *Principles of TVIC—Organizational and individual provider levels*. https://equiphealthcare.ca/resources/tvic-workshop/

Farmer, P. (2004). An anthropology of structural violence. *Current Anthropology, 45*(3), 305–324.

Felitti, V. J., Anda, R. F., Nordenberg, D., Williamson, D. F., Spitz, A. M., Edwards, V., & Marks, J. S. (1998). Relationship of childhood abuse and household dysfunction to many of the leading causes of death in adults: The Adverse Childhood Experiences (ACE) Study. *American Journal of Preventive Medicine, 14*(4), 245–258. https://doi.org/10.1016/S0749-3797(98)00017-8

Galtung, J. (1969). Violence, peace, and peace research. *Journal of Peace Research, 6*(3), 167–191. https://doi.org/10.1177/002234336900600301

Gilchrist, K. (2010). "Newsworthy" victims? Exploring differences in Canadian local press coverage of missing/murdered Aboriginal and White women. *Feminist Media Studies, 10*(4), 373–390. https://doi.org/10.1080/14680777.2010.514110

Goffman, E. (1963). *Stigma: Notes on the management of spoiled identity*. Simon & Schuster.

Government of Canada. (2018). *Trauma and violence-informed approaches to policy and practice*. https://www.canada.ca/en/public-health/services/publications/health-risks-safety/trauma-violence-informed-approaches-policy-practice.html

Haskell, L. (2012). A developmental understanding of complex trauma. In N. Poole & L. Greaves (Eds.), *Becoming trauma informed* (pp. 9–27). Centre for Addiction and Mental Health.

Herman, J. L. (1992). *Trauma and recovery: The aftermath of violence*. Basic Books.

Hughes, K., Bellis, M. A., Hardcastle, K. A., Sethi, D., Butchart, A., Mikton, C., Jones, J., & Dunne, M. P. (2017). The effect of multiple adverse childhood experiences on health: A systematic review and meta-analysis. *The Lancet Public Health, 2*(8), e356–e366. https://doi.org/10.1016/S2468-2667(17)30118-4

Khalifeh, H., Johnson, S., Howard, L. M., Borschmann, R., Osborn, D., Dean, K., Hogg, H. J., & Moran, P. (2015). Violent and non-violent crime against adults with severe mental illness. *The British Journal of Psychiatry, 206*(4), 275–282. https://doi.org/10.1192/bjp.bp.114.147843

Kirmayer, L. J., Lemelson, R., & Barad, M. (2007). *Understanding trauma: Integrating biological, clinical, and cultural perspectives*. Cambridge University Press.

Krediet, E., Bostoen, T., Breeksema, J., van Schagen, A., Passie, T., & Vermetten, E. (2020). Reviewing the potential of psychedelics for the treatment of PTSD. *International Journal of Neuropsychopharmacology, 23*(6), 385–400). https://doi.org/10.1093/ijnp/pyaa018

Link, B. G., & Phelan, J. C. (2001). Conceptualizing stigma. *Annual Review of Sociology, 27*(1), 363–385. https://doi.org/10.1146/annurev.soc.27.1.363

Loughran, T. (2012). Shell shock, trauma, and the First World War: The making of a diagnosis and its histories. *Journal of the History of Medicine and Allied Sciences, 67*(1), 94–119. https://doi.org/10.1093/jhmas/jrq052

McDonald, S., Kingston, D., Bayrampour, H., & Tough, S. (2015). Adverse childhood experiences in Alberta, Canada: A population based study. *Medical Research Archives*, (3). https://esmed.org/MRA/mra/article/view/142

Mental Health Commission of Canada. (2012). *Changing directions, changing lives: The mental health strategy for Canada*. https://www.mentalhealthcommission.ca/wp-content/uploads/drupal/MHStrategy_Strategy_ENG.pdf

Musto, L., & Schreiber, R. S. (2012). Doing the best I can do: Moral distress in adolescent mental health nursing. *Issues in Mental Health Nursing, 33*, 137–144. https://doi.org/10.3109/01612840.2011.641069

National Center for Injury Prevention and Control. (2019). *Preventing adverse childhood experiences (ACEs): Leveraging the best available evidence.* https://www.cdc.gov/violenceprevention/pdf/preventingACES.pdf

National Inquiry into Missing and Murdered Indigenous Women and Girls. (2019). *Final report.* https://www.mmiwg-ffada.ca/final-report/

Negriff, S. (2020). ACEs are not equal: Examining the relative impact of household dysfunction versus childhood maltreatment on mental health in adolescence. *Social Science & Medicine, 245,* 112696. https://doi.org/10.1016/j.socscimed.2019.112696

Public Health Ontario. (2020). *Adverse childhood experiences (ACEs): Interventions to prevent and mitigate the impact of ACEs in Canada.* Queen's Printer for Ontario. https://www.publichealthontario.ca/-/media/documents/a/2020/adverse-childhood-experiences-report.pdf?la=en

Sweeney, A., Clement, S., Filson, B., & Kennedy, A. (2016). Trauma-informed mental healthcare in the UK: What is it and how can we further its development? *Mental Health Review Journal, 21*(3), 174–192. https://doi.org/10.1108/MHRJ-01-2015-0006

TAKEN. (2021). *Infographic.* https://www.takentheseries.com/infographic/

Turnbull, M., Watson, B., Jin, Y., Lok, B., & Sanderson, A. (2020). Vicarious trauma, social media and recovery in Hong Kong. *Asian Journal of Psychiatry, 51,* 102032. https://doi.org/10.1016/j.ajp.2020.102032

Wilson, G., Farrell, D., Barron, I., Hutchins, J., Whybrow, D., & Kiernan, M. D. (2018). The use of eye-movement desensitization reprocessing (EMDR) therapy in treating post-traumatic stress disorder—A systematic narrative review. *Frontiers in Psychology, 9,* 923. https://doi.org/10.3389/fpsyg.2018.00923

World Health Organization. (2002). *World report on violence and health: Summary.* https://www.who.int/violence_injury_prevention/violence/world_report/en/summary_en.pdf

World Health Organization. (2019). *International Statistical Classification of Diseases and Related Health Problems, 11th Revision.* www.who.int/classifications/icd/en/

Young, I. M. (2008). Structural injustice and the politics of difference. In T. Christiano & J. Christman (Eds.), *Contemporary debates in political philosophy* (pp. 362–384). Wiley-Blackwell.

Chapter 7

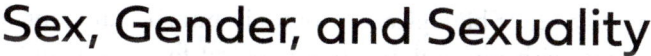

Sex, Gender, and Sexuality

> Both men and women should feel free to be sensitive. Both men and women should feel free to be strong ... It is time that we all perceive gender on a spectrum, not as two opposing sets of ideas.
>
> —Emma Watson (British actress)

Introduction

In this chapter, we discuss issues related to sexual health as well as the relationship between sex, gender, and mental health. Sex and gender are separate concepts that are both central to every person's identity; however, there is a lot of confusion in society about the distinctions between these terms. This chapter begins by defining sex and gender and describing the wide variation in gender identity, gender expression, and sexual orientation that exist across the human population. We will then move to an exploration of the sexual disorders that have an impact on mental health, including trends in mental health for women, men, and trans people, illuminating gender as an important underlying facet of mental health and illness.

Sex and Gender

The majority of people in the Western world identify as either men or women; however, many historical and contemporary cultures and societies recognize more than two categories and describe alternative identities (Lubbe, 2012). The first distinction to be made is between **sex**, assigned at birth based on biological characteristics of a person's reproductive system and other features, and **gender**, a person's identity and expression of roles and behaviours in a social and cultural context. A definition of these terms has been developed by researchers affiliated with the Canadian Institutes of Health Research's Institute of Gender and Health (2018):

> "Sex" and "gender" are often used interchangeably, despite having different meanings:
>
> Sex refers to a set of biological attributes in humans and animals. It is primarily associated with physical and physiological features including chromosomes, gene expression, hormone levels and reproductive/sexual anatomy. Sex is usually categorized as female or male but there is variation in the biological attributes that comprise sex and how those attributes are expressed.
>
> Gender refers to the socially constructed roles, behaviours, expressions and identities of girls, women, boys, men, and gender- and sexually-diverse people. It influences how people perceive themselves and others, how they act and interact and the distribution of power and resources in society. Gender identity is not confined to a binary (girl/woman vs. boy/man) nor is it static; it exists along a continuum and can change over time. There is considerable diversity in how individuals and groups understand, experience and express gender through the roles they take on, the expectations placed on them, relations with others and the complex ways that gender is institutionalized in society.

Genetic Basis of Sex

A person's sex is assigned at birth and is determined by the karyotype (i.e., chromosomal complement) that includes sex chromosomes of either XX (female) or XY (male). Although relatively rare, variations in sex chromosomes include the following: single X chromosome (Turner syndrome), XXY (Klinefelter syndrome), XXX (Triple X), XYY, or other sex chromosome configurations. The presence of one or the other of these sex chromosome configurations puts into play a series of characteristic biological differences that begin during fetal development and continue through life, such as development of different reproductive organs, external genitalia, breast growth, and hormone production. Usually, the presence of a Y chromosome initiates the development of male reproductive and hormonal features.

Intersex is an umbrella term used to describe people born with sex characteristics (including sex chromosomes, genitals, and hormones) that do not fit within binary "male" or "female" categories. The Intersex Society of North America (n.d.) describes intersex as "a socially constructed category that reflects real biological variation." This means that while variations in sex chromosomes and other characteristics exist, intersex is also an *identity*. It is important to note that the "male," "female," and "intersex" categories that have been constructed lie along a continuum and that there is great diversity in opinion regarding which biological variations are considered reflective of being intersex. For example, people with an XXY sex chromosome composition may be considered biologically intersex, though individuals may identify as intersex, male, or female (Herlihy & Gillam, 2011).

Gender Identity and Gender Expression

Gender refers to both gender identity (how a person feels internally) and gender expression (how a person expresses their gender publicly). **Gender identity** has been defined as "one's innermost concept of self as male, female, a blend of both, or neither—how individuals perceive themselves and what they call themselves" (Human Rights Campaign, 2019). Gender identity is distinct from sex, and an individual's gender identity can be different from their sex assigned at birth. **Gender expression** is an individual's public presentation of their gender, including through behaviour and appearance. A person's name and pronoun use are considered aspects of gender expression.

The term **transgender** refers to people within a wide range of gender identities and expressions that differ from their assigned sex at birth. The term **trans** is frequently used as an umbrella term for both transgender and other nonbinary gender identities and expressions, such as genderfluid, genderqueer, or gender neutral (agender). Individuals whose gender identity aligns with their assigned sex at birth are referred

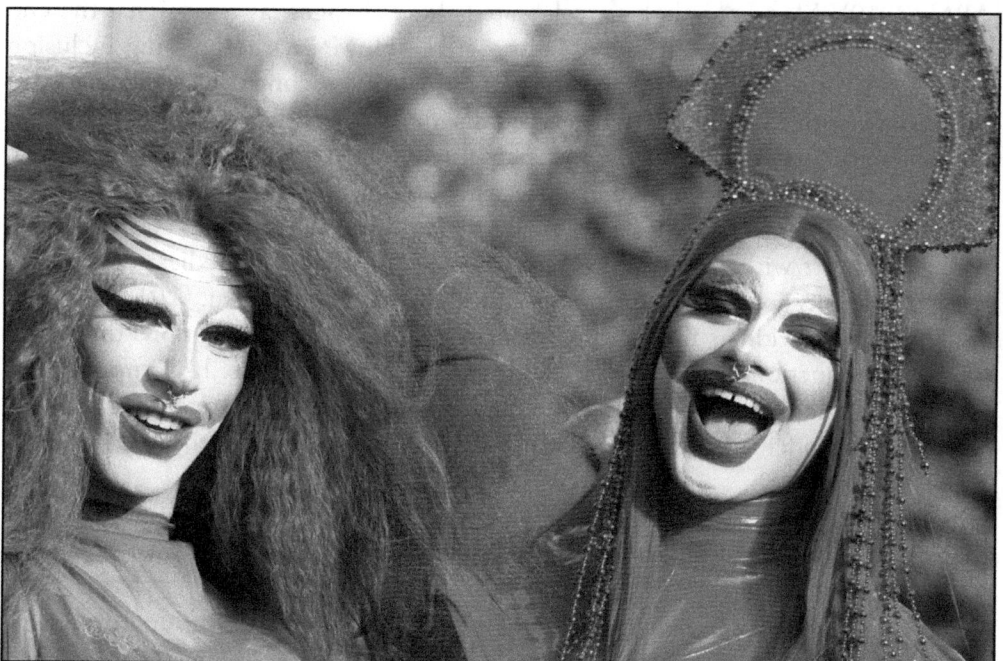

Figure 7.1: Two drag queens at a Pride parade. Drag is a form of art and performance where people use clothing, makeup, and other props to support their gender expression. Many drag queens are gay men who experience drag as an important part of their identity, developing a drag persona with a unique name, personality, and mannerisms.

Source: Unsplash/Sandy Millar

to as **cisgender**. In this textbook, the use of terms such as "women" and "men" are inclusive of people who identify as trans women and trans men. "Cisgender women" is used when describing people who identify as women and were assigned female at birth, and "cisgender men" is used when describing those who identify as men and were assigned male at birth. Currently, there are very few accurate population-level estimates of how many Canadians identify as trans, though estimates from the United States suggest approximately 0.6 percent (Waite & Denier, 2019). Beginning in 2019, Statistics Canada first included questions on both sex at birth and gender in their census test and other population surveys, which will produce more accurate estimates.

The feeling of incongruence between gender and assigned sex at birth can cause significant emotional distress for trans individuals and, for many years, was classified as a mental disorder in the ICD and the DSM. The ICD has recently removed "gender identity disorder" and moved the condition of "gender incongruence" from the mental disorders category to the sexual health conditions category. Similarly, the DSM-5 removed "gender identity disorder" and replaced it with "gender dysphoria" in an attempt to focus the diagnosis on experiences of distress that may arise from the conflict between felt gender and assigned sex (American Psychiatric Association [APA], 2019). Many people have celebrated these changes, as they signal the end of trans identities being considered "disordered." However, the ongoing inclusion in the DSM of a diagnosis related to gender identity is controversial in the trans community, with many believing that the diagnosis of gender dysphoria continues to pathologize trans individuals and perpetuate stigma towards this population (Davy & Toze, 2018). Recommended treatment for gender incongruence/dysphoria involves a wide range of approaches for reducing distress, including counselling to increase comfort with one's lived gender identity, or pursuing medical options for physical and physiological transition (APA, 2019; Coleman et al., 2012). For example, some individuals may choose to use hormones and medications that affect hormone production or to undergo gender-confirming surgeries. It is important to note that not all trans individuals will pursue medical or surgical treatment and may express their gender through other means such as hairstyle and clothing.

> **Box 7.1: Two-Spirit Identity**
>
> Since time immemorial, many Indigenous populations across North America have acknowledged a Two-Spirit identity. People who are Two-Spirit are neither men nor women in a binary sense of sex and gender but hold both male and female "spirits" or identities within themselves. Two-Spirit is an Indigeous-specific identity that is complex and does not easily translate into current Western understandings of gender; however, it can be understood as capturing diversity in gender identity, gender expression, and/or sexual orientation. Today, some Two-Spirit people may also identify

as part of the lesbian, gay, bisexual, transgender, queer, and Two-Spirit (LGBTQ2+) spectrum, while others may identify only as Two-Spirit and not with Western sex and gender identities.

Hunt (2016) describes that, in many Indigenous cultures prior to colonization, "Two-Spirit individuals carried unique responsibilities that were vital to the nations' collective well-being and survival, including as teachers, knowledge keepers, healers, herbalists, child minders, spiritual leaders, interpreters, mediators and artists." In most Indigenous groups, Two-Spirit people were respected, and their identities were not viewed as deviant or immoral. However, colonial processes led to Western ideas about sex and gender being projected onto Indigenous peoples, and discrimination against Two-Spirit people became commonplace. Today, many Indigenous communities are working to decolonize understandings of sex and gender and to reclaim the Two-Spirit identity as central to Indigenous culture (Driskill, 2010).

Gender Roles and Mental Health

Gender roles are different from gender identity and expression and involve the socially constructed collection of values, attitudes, beliefs, and behaviours that are thought of as masculine or feminine. For example, child rearing is often considered to be a feminine undertaking, or "women's work," though in contemporary society many families are rejecting these gender roles and striving for equality in parenting responsibilities. Gender roles, in conjunction with biological sex, have important implications for mental health. For example, widely held stereotypes of masculinity in our society often pressure men to adopt "strong and silent" behavioural styles, including stoicism and independence. Personal belief that men should adhere to such gender norms has been shown to predict less favourable attitudes towards seeking help for mental health challenges (Seidler et al., 2016). It is concerning that gender stereotypes may influence men's willingness to seek help, as this may negatively impact their mental health status and opportunities for receiving treatment.

Box 7.2: Gender Role Development in Children

Often, we see children adopt conventional, stereotypical gender roles at a young age: for example, boys playing with trucks and building blocks, and girls playing with dolls and cooking sets. These observed play behaviours have historically been thought to reflect natural and innate differences and were attributed to inherent personality traits in males versus females. However, these behaviours are also now understood to be reflective of gender roles that are socially constructed and perpetuated through adult behaviours towards children, peers' play behaviour and preferences, and the influence of the media and advertising (Brown & Stone, 2018). Through their play and social interactions, children internalize and establish gender roles.

In another example, women are often stereotypically portrayed as more "emotional" than men, and in fact, adult women cry five times more often than men. Interestingly, researchers have found that these differences in crying behaviour do not emerge until puberty; until the ages of 11 or 12, girls and boys cry at about the same rate (Frey, 1985). Why does this difference appear at puberty? Some theories link these changes to hormonal differentiation that occurs during this developmental stage. Yet more recent research suggests that the establishment of gender roles and gender stereotyping may begin as young as three months and develop over the life course: adults have been shown to make assumptions about babies' sex based on the pitch of their cries (Reby et al., 2016). Theories drawing on this type of research evidence suggest that psychological and sociocultural factors—not simply biological variation—influence adolescent boys and girls to behave differently from each other.

Sexual Orientation

Sexual orientation is defined as an enduring pattern of emotional, romantic, and/or sexual attractions to men, women, or both/any gender and refers to "a person's sense of identity based on those attractions, related behaviours, and membership in a community of others who share those attractions" (American Psychological Association [APA], 2008). Sexual orientation is understood as a continuum, with some people experiencing attraction exclusively to those of the "opposite" sex/gender, some experiencing attraction exclusively to those of the same sex/gender, and some experiencing attraction to people of a variety of sex and gender identities. A wide range of terms have been used to describe categories of sexual orientation. Heterosexuality, or being "straight," involves enduring patterns of attraction to a sex/gender different from one's own. Attraction to the same sex/gender has historically been termed homosexuality, though this label is now considered outdated and stigmatizing. More commonly used and accepted is the LGBTQ2+ acronym: lesbian, gay, bisexual, transgender, and queer, and Two-Spirited, with the "+" representing a wide array of additional identities that fall under this umbrella. Other such identities that describe sexual orientations include "pansexuality," sometimes used to refer to patterns of attraction to any or all sexes/genders, and "asexuality," which describes a spectrum of lower sexual attraction. People who identify as asexual—or "ace"—may experience romantic interest or may also identify as "aromantic," experiencing lower romantic attraction. Despite intensive scientific study of human development and various speculative theories that have come and gone, we have not yet been able to understand how or why individuals develop particular sexual attractions, though recent research suggests that a combination of genetic, social, and environmental factors shape our attractions (Ganna et al., 2019).

For many decades, any sexual orientation other than heterosexuality was considered to be a mental disorder. This may be surprising, but it seemed obvious to psychiatrists of the 1940s and 1950s, whose views were consistent with widespread social prejudice towards people with LGBTQ2+ identities. In the 1960s, social activists in the gay rights movement argued against the pathologizing of non-heterosexual identities, and in 1973, homosexuality was removed as a diagnosis in the prevailing psychiatric diagnostic system in North America (the DSM-II). There remained a diagnosis of sexual orientation disorder, defined by psychological distress over one's orientation, (i.e., those who were extremely unhappy about their non-heterosexual orientation would be considered to have a mental disorder and, thus, be appropriate for psychiatric intervention). The use of this diagnosis was based on the belief endorsed by prominent psychiatrist Dr. Robert Spitzer, who claimed that LGBTQ2+ identities could be cured if people were motivated to change their sexual orientation. More recently, Dr. Spitzer has apologized to the LGBTQ2+ community and acknowledged that his studies were deeply flawed (Carey, 2012). However, such research continues to be falsely claimed as "evidence" for the dangerous practice of conversion therapy, which purports to be able to change LGBTQ2+ individuals' sexual orientation to heterosexual. Throughout history, many psychiatric and psychological treatments have been applied in efforts to change LGBTQ2+ orientation. None have been successful. Such "treatments" have generally involved psychotherapy, though other extreme and unethical strategies have been attempted:

> In electric shock aversion therapy, electrodes were attached to the wrist or lower leg and shocks were administered while the patient watched photographs of men and women in various stages of undress. The aim was to encourage avoidance of the shock by moving to photographs of the opposite sex. It was hoped that arousal to same sex photographs would reduce, while relief arising from shock avoidance would increase interest in opposite sex images. (Smith et al., 2004)

In December 2021, the House of Commons passed legislation to ban conversion therapy in Canada. Despite the proliferation of similar bans in other regions, conversion therapy continues to be practised in many places in the world, resulting in harmful psychological effects for LGBTQ2+ people (Drescher et al., 2016).

The historical characterization of non-heterosexual sexual orientations as mental disorders in psychiatric diagnostic systems highlights the well-known challenges with the validity of psychiatric diagnosis, which was discussed in Chapter 4. This characterization also demonstrates the substantial role that social norms and ideologies contribute to the way in which "disorder" is conceptualized. Although the mental health field does not currently view LGBTQ2+ identities as disordered, such identities are associated with mental health challenges that can result from stigma and experiences of discrimination. People who are LGBTQ2+ have been condemned by religious systems, vilified by societies, and portrayed by ideological movements as inferior. At the extreme, German Nazis massacred hundreds of thousands of individuals believed to have a non-heterosexual orientation. Today, LGBTQ2+ individuals continue to experience significant stigma, with incidences of violence and discrimination occurring all too often. Gender identity and gender expression were not added to the Canadian *Human Rights Act* as prohibited grounds for discrimination until 2017, illustrating the work still needed to redress stigma and discrimination towards LGBTQ2+ individuals at a societal level.

As well as experiencing the harms of stigma in broader society, LGBTQ2+ individuals may experience self-stigma as well as rejection by family or friends if they openly express their sexual orientation or gender identity. This results in high levels of anxiety and depression as well as elevated suicide rates (Gonzales & Henning-Smith, 2017; Steele et al., 2017). In fact, recent reports identify that LGBTQ2+ youth are up to 15 times more likely to have considered suicide or made suicide attempts compared to their heterosexual peers (Blais et al., 2015). Further, 75 percent of Canadian transgender youth report engaging in self-harm in the past year, while one-third have attempted suicide (Stigma and Resilience Among Vulnerable Youth Centre, 2018). It is important to realize that individuals may present to clinical services with depressive or anxiety disorders without indicating the central role of stress and conflict about sexual/gender identity or orientation.

People who identify as LGBTQ2+ have been the recipients of profound prejudice and discrimination. Cruelty and harm experienced by LGBTQ2+ individuals often springs from ignorance, fear, and the need to feel superior to others. Through increasing education, exposure, and awareness, Canadians have gradually become more accepting and less stigmatizing of LGBTQ2+ individuals. In great part, this is the result of efforts by LGBTQ2+ communities to fight prejudice, build pride, and advocate for appropriate rights and freedoms.

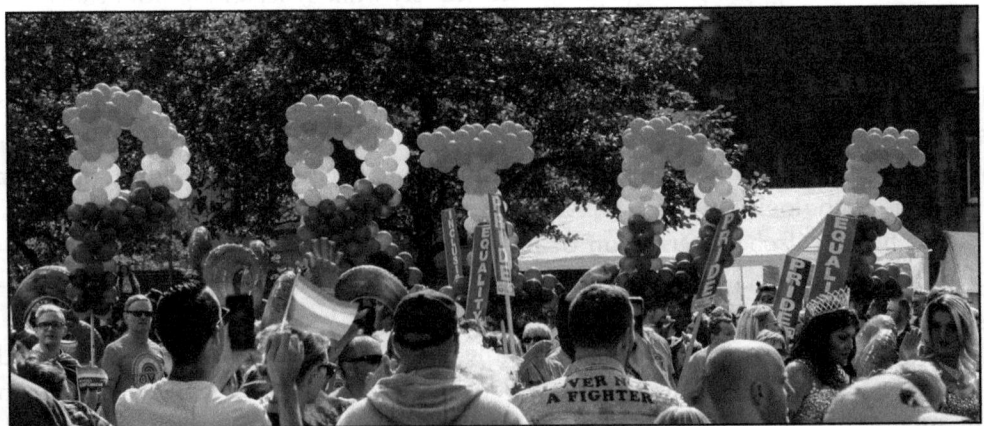

Figure 7.2: The annual Pride events celebrate LGBTQ2+ culture, and they serve as venues for social activism (e.g., fighting for legal rights, such as gay marriage).

Source: Unsplash/Toni Reed

Sexual Activity and Sexual Dysfunction

Survival and continuation of the human species is dependent on large numbers of people having sexual intercourse and procreating. Evolutionary biologists theorize that as a means to ensure that this happens, sexual intercourse, for most people, is experienced as highly pleasurable. There is a wide range in the particular preferences individuals may have in the type and style of sexual activity they enjoy. For example, some people experience fascination with particular items of clothing or derive sexual pleasure from roleplaying dominance and submission in sexual relationships. Most of these sexual behaviours are viewed as individual traits and preferences and part of the wide spectrum of human sexuality. However, some people have strong sexual attractions that lead to harm or difficult personal circumstances, and these are considered to be mental disorders known as **paraphilias**. These are often characterized by an inability to resist strong impulses, may involve participation of non-consenting or underaged individuals, and can interfere with social relationships. Paraphilias, such as exhibitionism and pedophilia, frequently result in criminal charges and severe consequences.

The ICD-11 (World Health Organization [WHO], 2019) describes sexual dysfunctions as a broad category of disorders that "comprise the various ways in which adult people may have difficulty experiencing personally satisfying, non-coercive sexual activities." Some of these disorders describe difficulties characterized by diminished sexual desire and lack of sexual enjoyment. Such disorders have received greater clinical and research attention for women than for men. It may be that men have been more reluctant to acknowledge loss of sexual desire, given societal expectations of men's sexual virility. It may also be that patriarchal expectations of women's sexual availability for pleasuring men have led to women being frequently and inappropriately diagnosed with disorders of "low libido" (Taylor, 2015). It is important for clinicians to carefully assess the underlying reasons for seeking treatment for sexual dysfunction and to remember that there is a wide range of what can be considered "normal" sexual activity and interest. For individuals who experience significant distress associated with sexual dysfunction, treatment is usually psychological in nature but may also involve pharmacological treatments (Parish & Hahn, 2016).

Other forms of sexual dysfunction are described as sexual arousal dysfunctions (e.g., erectile dysfunction or absence of genital response) and orgasmic dysfunction (e.g., anorgasmia, premature ejaculation, and substantial delay in achieving orgasm or ejaculation; WHO, 2019). Erectile dysfunction has received much focus in recent years with the marketing of medications such as Viagra and Cialis, which are effective treatments in about half of the cases of erectile dysfunction (Chen et al., 2015). However, evidence indicates that prevention of erectile dysfunction is possible through maintaining a generally positive level of overall health, including getting enough physical exercise, minimizing the use of tobacco and alcohol, and maintaining a low level of blood cholesterol. The disorder of "compulsive sexual behaviour" is also described in the ICD (WHO, 2019) and, in recent years, has often been referred to in the popular press and media as "sexual addiction." However, the nature and validity of the construct of sexual addiction is neither universally accepted nor endorsed. A variety of private therapists and treatment programs have sprung up to provide treatment for sexual addiction, and various self-help groups, such as Sexaholics Anonymous, can be found in North America.

Sexual dysfunction is often associated with depression and anxiety, whether caused by these mental health problems (e.g., depression often triggers a reduction in desire, and anxiety can impair erectile function) or causing them (e.g., the experience of sexual dysfunction and associated discouragement, self-doubt, or relationship challenges may trigger mood problems). Ironically, antidepressant medications often cause forms of sexual dysfunction as side effects! The rate of antidepressant-induced sexual dysfunction is in the range of 7 to 73 percent across different studies and drug types, a strikingly high rate for this problematic set of symptoms (Reichenpfader et al., 2014). Sexual side effects, such as reduced sex drive or inability to achieve orgasm, are one of the most common reasons for self-discontinuation of antidepressants.

Romantic Love

Some social psychologists and evolutionary biologists have described romantic love as a "device" for ensuring successful mating, child rearing, and the continuation of humanity (Fletcher et al., 2015). Others have argued that this understanding is heteronormative (i.e., it implies that heterosexuality is dominant, normal, and ideal) and ignores central aspects of romantic love, such as caring, intimacy, comfort, passion, security, and attachment (Thorne et al., 2019). Romantic love is also associated with the release of neurotransmitters and hormones such as dopamine, serotonin, and oxytocin, all responsible for feelings of happiness and pleasure. People can share romantic love with one person or with many people, either at one time or over the course of their lives. In a 2007–2008 Global Sex Survey, Canadians reported having a lifetime average of 10 to 23 sexual partners (Lunau, 2009). **Monogamy** can be defined as having only one romantic or sexual partner at a time. **Polyamory** refers to having consensual, ethical relationships with more than one partner at a time. Polyamory is different from infidelity, which involves being unfaithful to a partner and is considered a breach of trust.

Gendered Experiences of Mental Health Challenges

Women's Mental Health

Epidemiological studies have consistently found that compared to men, women are more likely to be diagnosed with the most common mental illnesses, that is, anxiety and depression. For example, an analysis of data from the Canadian Community

Health Survey—Mental Health found that 4.9 percent of women and only 2.8 percent of men reported past-year major depressive disorder (Patten et al., 2015). What accounts for this difference in prevalence? Some researchers and clinicians point to genetic and hormonal factors, such as the potential role of fluctuating estrogen levels throughout the menstrual cycle, in contributing to depression and anxiety symptoms (Albert, 2015). These differences may also reflect an absence of gender considerations in the development of diagnostic classifications and criteria, which ultimately, can influence prevalence estimates, help-seeking behaviour, diagnosis, and treatment (Johnson & Stewart, 2010). Further, there is some evidence that physicians are biased towards diagnosing depression in women over men, even when given the same symptom report (WHO, 2015). Gender roles likely account for differences in prevalence and in how mental health challenges are experienced, diagnosed, and treated. For women, symptoms of emotional distress may be more socially acceptable to discuss, and women may be more likely to be socialized to recognize feelings such as sadness, hopelessness, or anxiety. An even more extreme example of gender disparity in mental health diagnosis can be illustrated through the disparities in eating disorders, where 90 percent of Canadians who are diagnosed with anorexia nervosa or bulimia nervosa are women (Statistics Canada, 2015a). Though genetic factors are thought to play a role in the development of eating disorders, many researchers also attribute this difference to the substantial pressures of beauty norms, social expectations, and media portrayals of women.

Environmental factors and life events that disproportionately affect women—including violence against women and pregnancy—also have a profound influence on women's mental health. Violence against women is a major mental health concern in Canada and globally. Surveys conducted through Statistics Canada have found that 87 percent of all sexual assaults are committed against women (Statistics Canada, 2017a) and that 79 percent of individuals who experience intimate partner violence are women (Statistics Canada, 2018). Women who have experienced physical violence have increased rates of depression, anxiety, and post-traumatic stress disorder (PTSD). Symptoms of violence-related PTSD include chronic fear, nightmares, and flashbacks in which the violence is re-experienced. As discussed in Chapter 6, exposure to violence in childhood also strongly predicts the development and severity of mental health challenges later in life. Violence against women has a cumulative effect on mental health: women who have experienced violence in both childhood and adulthood are between four and seven times more likely to have depression than women who have never experienced violence (Ouellet-Morin et al., 2015).

Pregnancy, while generally considered a positive and happy life event, also significantly impacts mental health. Mental health problems, such as depression, anxiety, and even psychosis can be triggered during the pregnancy, childbirth, and the post-partum period. This is partially related to biological and hormonal changes during and following pregnancy, which may have negative impacts on mood. Additionally, there are multiple psychological and behavioural changes that accompany these life events and may impact mental health, such as the sudden increase in responsibility associated with parenting, limitations in contact with friends or colleagues, and loss of workplace involvement that are central to many new parents' identities. In some circumstances, these losses and new stressors may be associated with a sense of shame (e.g., for not feeling unreservedly happy as a new parent) and guilt over perceived inadequacy in the parenting role. The incidence of postpartum depression is estimated to be 12 percent among mothers (Shorey et al., 2018); however, it is also important to note that co-parents can experience depression in the pregnancy and postpartum, with rates as high as 8.4 percent (Cameron et al., 2016).

Men's Mental Health

While it is widely documented that men are diagnosed with depression at much lower rates than women, experts in men's mental health suggest that this may not be because men are truly less likely to experience the illness. Rather, this disparity may be the product of diagnostic criteria that do not adequately capture men's symptoms of depression, as well as a tendency for men to be reluctant to seek mental health care (Seidler et al., 2016). Despite low reported rates of depression among men, death by suicide (which is highly correlated with a diagnosis of depression) is much more common among men than women—about three times higher, in fact (Public Health Agency of Canada, 2019). Figure 7.3 shows the age- and gender-specific incidence rate of suicide in Canada, based on data from 2016. As you can see, the rates of suicide are far greater for males than for females across all age categories. Further,

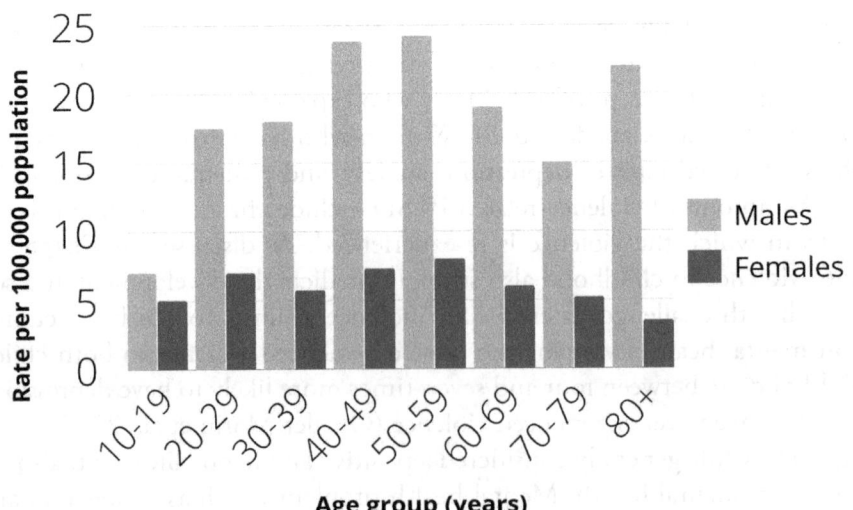

Figure 7.3: Suicide rates in Canada, 2016.

Source: Adapted from Public Health Agency of Canada. (2019). *Suicide in Canada: Key statistics*. https://www.canada.ca/en/public-health/services/publications/healthy-living/suicide-canada-key-statistics-infographic.html

suicide rates increase steadily with age until peaking among men in their late fifties. They then decrease slightly until they rise again among men aged 80 years and older. Although men have significantly higher rates of death by suicide than do women, it should be noted that women attempt suicide three to four times as often as men (Statistics Canada, 2017b).

Suicide in men has been described as a "silent epidemic" (Ogrodniczuk et al., 2018). There is a low degree of public awareness regarding the magnitude of this problem and relatively few preventive or research efforts specifically targeting male suicide. As a result, men often experience difficulty recognizing their own symptoms of depression and remain reluctant to seek help. In comparison to women, men also tend to lack social support, which has been implicated as another important factor in male suicide. Men's self-identified strategies for managing suicidal thoughts include opening up to others about their emotions and reframing help-seeking as "masculine" (Oliffe et al., 2012).

Men also have much higher rates of problematic alcohol and drug use compared to women (Statistics Canada, 2015b). In relation to problematic substance use, men experience a wide range of serious mental health challenges, including depression, anxiety, and psychotic episodes (e.g., in the context of withdrawal). Among the global population, 2.2 percent of women's deaths are attributable to alcohol, compared to 6.8 percent of all men's deaths (Griswold et al., 2018). For the population of men aged 15–49, this rate is even higher, with 12.2 percent of all deaths attributable to alcohol. Although we have a limited understanding of the reasons for men's greater propensity towards problematic substance use, it may well be that gendered expectations of men as stoic, independent, and even-keeled play a role. Substance use may serve as a coping strategy for feelings of distress related to life stressors or as a form of self-medication for more serious mental health challenges such as depression or anxiety. Reducing stigma about men's mental health and supporting men in understanding and coping with difficult emotions could have enormous health and social benefits.

Trans People's Mental Health

Trans individuals (including people who identify as transgender, nonbinary, gender-fluid, genderqueer, gender neutral, and other gender identities that fall outside of the binary male or female identities) experience numerous threats to good mental health. Rates of depression, anxiety, problematic substance use, and eating disorders are much higher for trans people compared to the general population (Dhejne et al., 2016). Indeed, research has identified that up to 88 percent of trans people have experienced depression, either presently or in the past (McNeil et al., 2012). In adolescent populations, trans youth are substantially more likely to experience depressive symptoms than cisgender youth. The Canadian Trans Youth Health Survey identified that two-thirds of trans youth aged 14–18 seriously considered suicide in the past year, and three-quarters engaged in past-year self-harm (Veale et al., 2017).

One of the greatest contributors to poor mental health in the trans population is the effects of stigma and discrimination. Although gender identity is now a prohibited grounds for discrimination in Canada, trans people continue to experience discrimination in everyday life, including in employment, housing, and health care. Violence and hate crimes committed against trans people because of their gender identity is also common, with 20 percent of trans individuals reporting this experience. This has damaging effects on mental health and is associated with depression, anxiety, and PTSD (Bauer & Scheim, 2015). Having strong social support is a protective factor for trans people and can help to mitigate the risk of developing mental health challenges (Pflum et al., 2015). However, due to interpersonal discrimination and stigma, many people who come out as trans risk losing important social connections, including with family, friends, and coworkers. Further, many trans people report experiencing social exclusion in communities and barriers to participating in social activities.

Given the high prevalence of mental health challenges faced by the trans population in Canada, it is crucial that mental health services are available, accessible, and safe. Unfortunately, experiences of anticipated and actual discrimination within the health care system often results in trans people avoiding or being refused care. For example, a study in Ontario identified that while 11 percent of the general population had an unmet health care need in the past year, this rose to 44 percent among the trans population (Giblon & Bauer, 2017). Strategies that clinicians can use to make health care spaces safer for trans individuals include using correct names and pronouns and, as detailed in Chapter 6, adopting principles of Trauma and Violence Informed Practice. It is also important to note that not all mental health challenges in the trans population relate to trans identity. Therefore, clinicians must avoid making assumptions and instead conduct thorough assessments to correctly identify precipitating factors.

Conclusion

Sex and gender must be differentiated and understood as unique contributors to our identities. Sexual identity is distinct from gender identity and gender expression and, when these identities do not align with dominant societal norms, people are often subjected to profound stigma and discrimination. Efforts by the LGBTQ2+ people to enhance public awareness and education have contributed to some improvement in society's embracing of diversity. However, discrimination in health care and in everyday life continues to impact the mental health of LGBTQ2+ people.

As a product of the intersecting influences of biology, gender roles, and stigma and discrimination, those who identify as men, women, or trans tend to experience different types of mental health challenges. Women tend to have higher rates of depression and anxiety. Men tend to have higher rates of problematic substance use and are more likely to die by suicide. Trans people tend to have higher rates of several mental illnesses compared to both men and women, including greater levels of suicidal thinking and self-harm. Despite these overall trends, individual experiences of mental health and illness vary widely.

Glossary

cisgender: Describes individuals whose gender identity corresponds to their assigned sex at birth.

gender: Differentiated from sex, a person's identity and expression of roles and behaviours in a social and cultural context.

gender expression: An individual's public presentation of their gender, including through behaviour and appearance.

gender identity: An individual's personal sense of knowing which gender they belong to or the way they see themselves.

gender roles: The socially constructed collection of values, attitudes, beliefs, and behaviours that are thought of as masculine or feminine.

intersex: An umbrella term used to describe people born with sex characteristics that do not fit within binary "male" or "female" categories.

monogamy: Having only one romantic partner at a time.

paraphilias: Mental disorders involving strong sexual attraction that lead to harm or result in disabling problems or circumstances.

polyamory: Refers to having consensual, ethical relationships with more than one partner at a time.

sex: Category of male, female, or intersex assigned at birth based on biological attributes of a person's reproductive system and other features.

sexual orientation: The enduring pattern of emotional, romantic, and/or sexual attractions to other people, and a person's sense of identity based on those attractions, related behaviours, and membership in a community of others who share those attractions.

trans: An umbrella term for both transgender and other gender identities and expressions, such as genderfluid, genderqueer, or agender (no gender).

transgender: People with a wide range of gender identities and expressions that differ from their assigned sex at birth.

Critical Thinking Questions

1. What is the difference between sex and gender?
2. How is gender identity related to mental health?
3. Describe the mental health challenges of particular relevance to women, men, and trans people.
4. Is LGBTQ2+ identity considered a mental disorder? Explain.

Recommended Readings

Castle, D. J., & Abel, K. M. (2016). *Comprehensive women's mental health*. Cambridge University Press.

Chang, S. C., Singh, A. A., & dickey, l. m. (2018). *A clinician's guide to gender-affirming care: Working with transgender and gender nonconforming clients*. Context Press.

Fine, C. (2010). *Delusions of gender: How our minds, society, and neurosexism create difference*. W.W. Norton & Company.

Fugère, M. A., Leszczynski, J. P., & Cousins, A. J. (2015). *The social psychology of attraction and romantic relationships*. Red Globe Press.

Yarbrough, E. (2018). *Transgender mental health*. American Psychiatric Association Publishing.

Recommended Websites

HeadsUpGuys. https://headsupguys.org

It's Pronounced Metrosexual—The Genderbread Person. www.itspronouncedmetrosexual.com/2018/10/the-genderbread-person-v4

Movember—Men's Health. https://ca.movember.com/mens-health/mental-health

Trans PULSE Project. http://transpulseproject.ca

Women's Health Research Network. www.cwhn.ca

World Health Organization—Gender and Women's Mental Health. www.who.int/mental_health/prevention/genderwomen/en

References

Albert, P. R. (2015). Why is depression more prevalent in women? *Journal of Psychiatry and Neuroscience, 40*(4), 219–221. https://doi.org/10.1503/jpn.150205

American Psychiatric Association [APA]. (2019). *What is gender dysphoria?* https://www.psychiatry.org/patients-families/gender-dysphoria/what-is-gender-dysphoria

American Psychological Association [APA]. (2008). *Answers to your questions: For a better understanding of sexual orientation and homosexuality*. https://www.apa.org/topics/lgbt/orientation.pdf

Bauer, G. R., & Scheim, A. I. (2015). *Transgender people in Ontario, Canada: Statistics for the Trans PULSE Project to inform human rights policy*. Trans PULSE Project Team. http://transpulseproject.ca/wp-content/uploads/2015/06/Trans-PULSE-Statistics-Relevant-for-Human-Rights-Policy-June-2015.pdf

Blais, M., Bergeron, F. A., Duford, J., Boislard, M. A., & Hébert, M. (2015). Health outcomes of sexual-minority youth in Canada: An overview. *Adolescencia & Saude, 12*(3), 53–73.

Brown, C. S., & Stone, E. A. (2018). Environmental and social contributions to children's gender-typed toy play: The role of family, peers, and media. In E. S. Weisgram & L. M. Dinella (Eds.), *Gender typing of children's toys: How early play experiences impact development* (pp. 121–140). American Psychological Association.

Cameron, E. E., Sedov, I. D., & Tomfohr-Madsen, L. M. (2016). Prevalence of paternal depression in pregnancy and the postpartum: An updated meta-analysis. *Journal of Affective Disorders, 206,* 189–203. https://doi.org/10.1016/j.jad.2016.07.044

Canadian Institutes of Health Research. (2018). *Science is better with sex and gender: Strategic plan 2018–2023.* http://www.cihr-irsc.gc.ca/e/documents/igh_strategic_plan_2018-2023-e.pdf

Carey, B. (2012, May 18). Psychiatry giant sorry for backing gay "cure." *New York Times.* https://www.nytimes.com/2012/05/19/health/dr-robert-l-spitzer-noted-psychiatrist-apologizes-for-study-on-gay-cure.html

Chen, L., Staubli, S. E. L., Schneider, M. P., Kessels, A. G., Ivic, S., Bachmann, L. M., & Kessler, T. M. (2015). Phosphodiesterase 5 inhibitors for the treatment of erectile dysfunction: A trade-off network meta-analysis. *European Urology, 68*(4), 674–680. https://doi.org/10.1016/j.eururo.2015.03.031

Coleman, E., Bockting, W., Botzer, M., Cohen-Kettenis, P., DeCuypere, G., Feldman, J., Fraser, L., Green, J., Knudson, G., Meyer, W. J., Monstrey, S., Adler, R. K., Brown, G. R., Devor, A. H., Ehrbar, R., Ettner, R., Eyler, E., Garofalo, R., Karasic, D. H., ... Zucker, K. (2012). Standards of care for the health of transsexual, transgender, and gender-nonconforming people, version 7. *International Journal of Transgenderism, 13*(4), 165–232. https://doi.org/10.1080/15532739.2011.700873

Davy, Z., & Toze, M. (2018). What is gender dysphoria? A critical systematic narrative review. *Transgender Health, 3*(1), 159–169. https://doi.org/10.1089/trgh.2018.0014

Dhejne, C., Van Vlerken, R., Heylens, G., & Arcelus, J. (2016). Mental health and gender dysphoria: A review of the literature. *International Review of Psychiatry, 28*(1), 44–57. https://doi.org/10.3109/09540261.2015.1115753

Drescher, J., Schwartz, A., Casoy, F., McIntosh, C. A., Hurley, B., Ashley, K., Barber, M., Goldenberg, D., Herbert, S. E., Lothwell, L. E., Mattson, M. R., McAfee, S. G., Pula, J., Rosario, V., & Tompkins, A. (2016). The growing regulation of conversion therapy. *Journal of Medical Regulation, 102*(12), 7–12. https://doi.org/10.30770/2572-1852-102.2.7

Driskill, Q.-L. (2010). Doubleweaving Two-Spirit critiques: Building alliances between Native and queer studies. *GLQ: A Journal of Lesbian and Gay Studies, 16*(1–2), 69–92. https://doi.org/10.1215/10642684-2009-013

Fletcher, G. J. O., Simpson, J. A., Campbell, L., & Overall, N. C. (2015). Pair-bonding, romantic love, and evolution: The curious case of *homo sapiens. Perspectives on Psychological Science, 10*(1), 20–36. https://doi.org/10.1177/1745691614561683

Frey, W. (1985). *Crying: The mystery of tears*. HarperCollins.

Ganna, A., Verweji, K. J. H., Nivard, M. G., Maier, R., Wedow, R., Busch, A. S., Abdellaoui, A., Guo, S., Sathirapongsasuti, J. F., 23andMe Research Team, Lichtenstein, P., Lundström, S., Långström, N., Auton, A., Harris, K. M., Beecham, G. W., Martin, E. R., Sanders, A. R., Perry, J. R. B., ... Zietsch, B.P. (2019). Large-scale GWAS reveals insights into the genetic architecture of same-sex sexual behavior. *Science, 365*(6456), e7693. https://doi.org/10.1126/science.aat7693

Giblon, R., & Bauer, G. R. (2017). Health care availability, quality, and unmet need: A comparison of transgender and cisgender residents of Ontario, Canada. *BMC Health Services Research, 17*, Article 283. https://doi.org/10.1186/s12913-017-2226-z

Gonzales, G., & Henning-Smith, C. (2017). Health disparities by sexual orientation: Results and implications from the Behavioral Risk Factor Surveillance System. *Journal of Community Health, 42*(6), 1163–1172. https://doi.org/10.1007/s10900-017-0366-z

Griswold, M. G., Fullman, N., Hawley, C., Arian, N., Zimsen, S. R., Tymeson, H. D., Venkateswaran, V., Tapp, A. D., Forouzanfar, M. H., Salama, J. S., Abate, K. H., Abate, D., Abay, S. M., Abbafati, C., Abdulkader, R. S., Abebe, Z., Aboyans, V., Abrar, M. M., Acharya, P., ... Gakidou, E. (2018). Alcohol use and burden for 195 countries and territories, 1990–2016: A systematic analysis for the Global Burden of Disease Study 2016. *The Lancet, 392*(10152), 1015–1035. https://doi.org/10.1016/S0140-6736(18)31310-2

Herlihy, A. S., & Gillam, L. (2011). Thinking outside the square: Considering gender in Klinefelter syndrome and 47, XXY. *International Journal of Andrology, 34*, e348–e349. https://doi.org/10.1111/j.1365-2605.2010.01132.x

Human Rights Campaign. (2019). *Sexual orientation and gender identity definitions*. https://www.hrc.org/resources/sexual-orientation-and-gender-identity-terminology-and-definitions

Hunt, S. (2016). *An introduction to the health of Two-Spirit people: Historical, contemporary and emergent issues*. National Collaboration Centre for Indigenous Health. https://static1.squarespace.com/static/5914bffaf5e231cfb6ab6c6b/t/5aecaf3a03ce647a-b6e19a0e/1525460801855/RPT-HealthTwoSpirit-Hunt-EN%281%29.pdf

Intersex Society of North America. (n.d.). *What is intersex?* www.isna.org/faq/what_is_intersex

Johnson, J., & Stewart, D. E. (2010). DSM-V: Toward a gender sensitive approach to psychiatric diagnosis. *Archives of Women's Mental Health, 13*(1), 17–19. https://doi.org/10.1007/s00737-009-0115-0

Lubbe, C. (2012). LGBT parents and their children: Non-Western research and perspectives. In A. E. Goldberg & K. R. Allen (Eds.), *LGBT-Parent Families* (pp. 209–223). Springer.

Lunau, K. (2009, June 29). Are we blushing yet? *Macleans*. https://www.macleans.ca/news/canada/are-we-blushing-yet/

McNeil, J., Bailey, L., Ellis, S., Morton, J., & Regan, M. (2012). *Trans mental health study 2012*. http://worldaa1.miniserver.com/~gires/assets/Medpro-Assets/trans_mh_study.pdf

Ogrodniczuk, J., Oliffe, J., & Beharry, J. (2018). HeadsUpGuys: Canadian online resource for men with depression. *Canadian Family Physician, 64*, 93–94.

Oliffe, J. L., Ogrodniczuk, J. S., Bottorff, J. L., Johnson, J. L., & Hoyak, K. (2012). "You feel like you can't live anymore": Suicide from the perspectives of Canadian men who experience depression. *Social Science and Medicine, 74*(4), 506–514. https://doi.org/10.1016/j.socscimed.2010.03.057

Ouellet-Morin, I., Fisher, H. L., York-Smith, M., Fincham-Campbell, S., Moffitt, T. E., & Arseneault, L. (2015). Intimate partner violence and new-onset depression: A longitudinal study of women's childhood and adult histories of abuse. *Depression and Anxiety, 32*(5), 316–324. https://doi.org/10.1002/da.22347

Parish, S. J., & Hahn, S. R. (2016). Hypoactive sexual desire disorder: A review of epidemiology, biopsychology, diagnosis, and treatment. *Sexual Medicine Reviews, 4*(2), 103–120. https://doi.org/10.1016/j.sxmr.2015.11.009

Patten, S. B., Williams, J. V. A., Lavorato, D. H., Wang, J. L., McDonald, K., & Bulloch, A. G. M. (2015). Descriptive epidemiology of major depressive disorder in Canada in 2012. *The Canadian Journal of Psychiatry, 60*(1), 23–30. https://doi.org/10.1177/070674371506000106

Pflum, S. R., Testa, R. J., Balsam, K. F., Goldblum, P. B., & Bongar, B. (2015). Social support, trans community connectedness, and mental health symptoms among transgender and gender nonconforming adults. *Psychology of Sexual Orientation and Gender Diversity, 2*(3), 281–286.

Public Health Agency of Canada. (2019). *Suicide in Canada: Key statistics*. https://www.canada.ca/en/public-health/services/publications/healthy-living/suicide-canada-key-statistics-infographic.html

Reby, D., Levréro, F., Gustafsson, E., & Mathevon, N. (2016). Sex stereotypes influence adults' perception of babies' cries. *BMC Psychology, 4*, Article 19. https://doi.org/10.1186/s40359-016-0123-6

Reichenpfader, U., Gartlehner, G., Morgan, L. C., Greenblatt, A., Nussbaumer, B., Hansen, R. A., Van Noord, M., Lux, L., & Gaynes, B. N. (2014). Sexual dysfunction associated with second-generation antidepressants in patients with major depressive disorder: Results from a systematic review with network meta-analysis. *Drug Safety, 37*(1), 19–31. https://doi.org/10.1007/s40264-013-0129-4

Seidler, Z. E., Dawes, A. J., Rice, S. M., Oliffe, J. L., & Dhillon, H. M. (2016). The role of masculinity in men's help-seeking for depression: A systematic review. *Clinical Psychology Review, 49*, 106–118. https://doi.org/10.1016/j.cpr.2016.09.002

Shorey, S., Chee, C. Y. I., Ng, E. D., Chan, Y. H., Tam, W. W. S., & Chong, Y. S. (2018). Prevalence and incidence of postpartum depression among healthy mothers: A systematic review and meta-analysis. *Journal of Psychiatric Research, 104*, 235–248. https://doi.org/10.1016/j.jpsychires.2018.08.001

Smith, G., Bartlett, A., & King, M. (2004). Treatments of homosexuality in Britain since the 1950s—An oral history: The experience of patients. *British Medical Journal, 328*, Article 427. https://doi.org/10.1136/bmj.328.427.37984.442419.EE

Statistics Canada. (2015a). *Eating disorders.* https://www150.statcan.gc.ca/n1/pub/82-619-m/2012004/sections/sectiond-eng.htm

Statistics Canada. (2015b). *Mental health and substance use disorders in Canada.* https://www150.statcan.gc.ca/n1/pub/82-624-x/2013001/article/11855-eng.htm

Statistics Canada. (2017a). *Self-reported sexual assault in Canada, 2014.* https://www150.statcan.gc.ca/n1/pub/85-002-x/2017001/article/14842-eng.htm

Statistics Canada. (2017b). *Suicide rates: An overview.* https://www150.statcan.gc.ca/n1/pub/82-624-x/2012001/article/11696-eng.htm

Statistics Canada. (2018). *Police-reported intimate partner violence in Canada, 2017.* https://www150.statcan.gc.ca/n1/pub/85-002-x/2018001/article/54978/02-eng.htm

Steele, L. S., Daley, A., Curling, D., Gibson, M. F,. Green, D. C., Williams, C. C., & Ross, L. E. (2017). LGBT identity, untreated depression, and unmet need for mental health services by sexual minority women and trans-identified people. *Journal of Women's Health, 26*(2), 116–127. https://doi.org/10.1089/jwh.2015.5677

Stigma and Resilience Among Vulnerable Youth Centre. (2018). *2SLGBTQIA+ students in British Columbia: 12 evidence-based facts.* http://apsc-saravyc.sites.olt.ubc.ca/files/2019/08/SARAVYC_LGBTQ-Students-in-BC_Fact-Sheet-Infographic_FINAL.pdf

Taylor, C. (2015). Female sexual dysfunction, feminist sexology, and the psychiatry of the normal. *Feminist Studies, 41*(2), 259–292. https://doi.org/10.15767/feministstudies.41.2.259

Thorne, S. R., Hegarty, P., & Hepper, E. G. (2019). Equality in theory: From a heteronormative to an inclusive psychology of romantic love. *Theory & Psychology, 29*(2), 240–257. https://doi.org/10.1177/0959354319826725

Veale, J. F., Watson, R. J., Peter, T., & Saewyc, E. M. (2017). The mental health of Canadian transgender youth compared with the Canadian population. *Journal of Adolescent Health, 60*(1), 44–49. https://doi.org/10.1016/j.jadohealth.2016.09.014

Waite, S., & Denier, N. (2019). A research note on Canada's LGBT data landscape: Where we are and what the future holds. *Canadian Review of Sociology, 56*(1), 93–117. https://doi.org/10.1111/cars.12232

World Health Organization. (2015). *Gender and women's mental health.* www.who.int/mental_health/prevention/genderwomen/en/

World Health Organization. (2019). *International Statistical Classification of Diseases and Related Health Problems, 11th Revision.* www.who.int/classifications/icd/en/

Chapter 8

Culture, Ethnicity, and Mental Health

*Victoria Smye, adapted from original chapter by
Elliot M. Goldner, Emily Jenkins, and Dan Bilsker*

I do not want my house to be walled in on all sides and my windows to be stuffed. I want the cultures of all the lands to be blown about my house as freely as possible. But I refuse to be blown off my feet by any.
—Mahatma Ghandi (political and spiritual leader in
India during India's independence movement)

Introduction

Since our health is influenced so strongly by the society and cultural practices in which we are immersed, it is important for us to take a careful look at the impact of cultural factors on mental health. Our cultural identities can serve both to promote good mental health and to expose us to certain risks for mental health challenges. When we develop mental health challenges, our cultural identities may also shape the ways in which mental illnesses are expressed and experienced as well as the manner in which we tend to heal and restore good mental health and wellness. Throughout this book, we have used well-being to describe a state of being content, healthy, and happy; however, here we use the similar term *wellness* to reflect the language used by many Indigenous people to describe the interconnected emotional, physical, mental, and spiritual aspects of wellness (First Nations Health Authority, 2021). In this chapter, we will first tackle the difficult task of defining terms such as "culture," "race," and "ethnicity." As social constructs that categorize and ascribe *difference*, these terms are often confused and used interchangeably, with little consistency when any one term is applied (McConaghy, 2000; Reimer Kirkham & Anderson, 2002). We will then consider how these concepts interact with mental health and illness within Canadian society, with a particular focus on Indigenous peoples and communities. Throughout this chapter, we use the term *Indigenous peoples* to include First Nations, Inuit, and Métis, without regard to their separate origins and identities. The term

"First Nation" replaces the term "Indian," and "Inuit" replaces the term "Eskimo," the terms that were used in earlier times. The terms "Indian" and "Eskimo," however, continue to be used in federal legislation and policy, for example, the *Indian Act*, and in government reports and statistical data.

Culture

What is this thing called **culture**? Many tend to think of culture in terms of ethnic groupings, such as Chinese, Mexican, or First Nations, often referred to as ethnocultural groups. However, cultural groups may instead be divided into different types of social groups for example, by age, sexual orientation, gender identity, language, and/or by a particular profession such as teaching, medicine, nursing or law, and/or by athletic groups—to name several. Most of us identify with a number of such cultural groups; consequently, we usually have multiple cultural identities. Given this multiplicity of cultural identity, "culture" is also understood as "a complex network of meanings shaped by historical, social, economic, and political processes" (Smye & Browne, 2002). Therefore, culture is dynamic and ever-changing—it is relational. In a similar vein, Stuart Hall—sociologist, cultural theorist, and political activist—put forward the perspective that culture is "experience lived, experience interpreted, experience defined" (Slack & Grossberg, 2016).

Canada is home to a multicultural society. With the highest per capita immigration rate of any country in the world, Canada has emerged to be a pluralistic nation that has embraced multiculturalism as an official policy of its government. Praised by some as "the most successful pluralist society on the face of our globe" and "a model for the world," Canada has been considered to be successful at breaking down many intercultural barriers (Stackhouse, 2013). However, not all people see Canadian multiculturalism policy as highly successful. Canadian history has been marked by tension and conflict among the three main ethnocultural groups that existed during the country's early years: Indigenous peoples and French and English Canadians. And as we will discuss later in this chapter, many Indigenous people in Canada continue to experience profound negative consequences, including mental health challenges, as a result of historical intercultural conflict and racism in the form of colonialism and neocolonialism.

Race

Although humans have been studied more intensively than any other creature, there has been profound disagreement about whether humans should be classified as a single species or as 2, 3, 4, 5, or even as 60 different races or subspecies (Darwin, 1871). Many prominent researchers, including Charles Darwin, have identified themselves to be "monogenist" on the question of race, believing that humans are of the same species and finding race to be an arbitrary distinction.

In 1776, German scientist and classical anthropologist Johann Blumenbach, in *On the Natural Varieties of Mankind*, contended that humanity could be divided into five different races. Can you guess what these might be? They were Caucasian, Negroid, Mongoloid, Malayan, and American. Blumenbach based his classification of races on skin colour, craniology (the size and shape of a person's head), and other physical characteristics.

The notion of different human races often assumes that human evolution entailed a branching of evolutionary lines and is similar to the idea of subspecies. However, over recent decades, the notion of distinct races has generally been rejected, and most scientists agree that the concept of race has no validity, that is, "race" is a social category without biological meaning (Graves, 2015). Currently, the predominant scientific notion is that human variation is distributed along a continuum, and scientists have generally abandoned belief in the existence of discrete racial groups. However, although the concept of distinct "races" has generally been rejected, the notion of racism remains important.

Racism

Racism can be defined as a set of attitudes and behaviours in which social groups are identified, separated, treated as inferior or superior, and given disparate access to power and other valued resources. It is a process of differentiation, integrally linked to other social processes of differentiation and identity formation such as sexism, ageism, homophobia, and classism. Over three decades ago, Kimberlé Crenshaw coined the term **intersectionality** to describe the complex intersection of these social categorizations that create overlapping systems of discrimination and oppression. Basically, intersectionality is a lens for seeing the ways in which various forms of inequality often operate together and exacerbate each other to create inequity (Crenshaw, 2017). **Racialization** is a process of social differentiation or racial categorization by which people are labelled based on particular physical characteristics or arbitrary ethnocultural or racial categories, and then acted on in accordance with beliefs related to those labels. All of these processes of differentiation are grounded in an effort to distance us from the "other" and to create "power over" structures.

Racist behaviours and attitudes exist throughout the world, and there are many notorious instances of racism that serve to remind us of the bleakest and most horrific depths to which humankind has plummeted. The kidnapping, abuse, and subjugation of African people for use as slaves in Europe and the Americas is an example of the extreme harm that has been committed through racist beliefs and behaviours. In Canada, Indigenous peoples have suffered as a result of racist beliefs and practices, experiencing genocide and expropriation of their land and resources. Today, colonialism and neocolonialism, underpinned by racism, continue in the form of policies and processes that contribute to health inequities. For example, the *Indian Act (1876)* continues as the formal basis for policy regarding First Nations, Inuit, and Métis peoples in Canada. The deeply rooted racist ideologies that were foundational in the construction of "Indian" social policy remain—what might be deemed as an enactment of **structural violence** (Farmer, 2003; Gerlach et al., 2017; Smye & Oudshoorn, under review). As introduced in Chapter 6, structural violence refers to the existence of unequal power, restricted access to resources, and systematic oppression resulting in the denial of basic needs. It has been defined as "a host of offensives against human dignity, including extreme and relative poverty, social inequalities ranging from racism to gender inequality, and the more spectacular forms of violence" (Farmer, 2003).

Recently disclosed racism and discrimination data in Canada have brought renewed attention to the harms of Indigenous-specific systemic racism. Examples include the horrific death of an Indigenous woman in a Quebec hospital, Ms. Joyce Echaquan; the investigation into emergency department staff playing "games" to guess blood alcohol levels of Indigenous patients in British Columbia (discussed in Chapter 5); and the decade-plus-long investigation into the tragic death of an Indigenous man, Mr. Brian Sinclair, who had a urinary tract infection and waited for 34 hours without being seen in a Manitoba emergency department (Azpiri, 2020; Brian Sinclair Working Group, 2017; Lowrie & Malone, 2020; Turpel-Lafond, 2020).

How can we explain the capacity for racist beliefs to incite large sectors of the population to condone violent and cruel behaviour to fellow human beings? In Chapter 3, we discussed how psychoanalytic theory proposed that there is a part of our minds that is unconscious, that is, hidden from our conscious awareness. One of the early psychoanalytic theorists, Alfred Adler, proposed that much of human striving can be understood as an attempt to overcome the inferiority complex and increase one's sense of personal power and self-esteem. Racism is likely a manifestation of this drive among humans to feel superior, and the lack of compassion and capacity for cruelty that is often attached to racism demonstrates the fallibility of human thought, emotion, and behaviour when influenced by these drives and motivations.

Labelling theory, which was developed as part of the discipline of criminology, states that deviance is caused when individuals who are labelled internalize the label, eventually leading them to take on the traits and behaviours that conform to the label. Thus, when people are repeatedly told that they are inferior in some way, this commonly becomes internalized and accepted as being true, even by those who have become the objects of derision. As noted in Chapter 6, mental health stigma operates in a similar way, that is, when stigma becomes internalized (self-stigma), it can have deleterious effects (Corrigan et al., 2016).

People who are victimized by racist attitudes and behaviours may experience profound mental health challenges. Post-traumatic stress disorder (PTSD) symptoms commonly occur, as do many other mental health challenges. Later in this chapter, we examine how First Nations, Inuit, and Métis people in Canada have been subjected to profound and prolonged racist attitudes and behaviour, and we discuss the impact this has had on mental health and illness for many Indigenous peoples and communities. In her discussion of the *unique* features of Indigenous health equity (IND-equity), Downey (2020) draws attention to the impact colonialism and racism have on the health and wellness of First Nations, Inuit, and Métis people and communities and the need to address the social, political, and historical determinants of mental health (e.g., structural violence). Indeed, the development of an anti-racist/anti-oppression stance is key to recognizing and addressing the inequities experienced by Black, Indigenous, and other Persons of Colour—inequities supported by institutional structures and systems underpinned by white normativity.

Understanding the relationship between culture and mental health helps us see the promise of equity-oriented care practices for enhancing the work that health care professionals do in multicultural contexts. Equity-oriented interventions involve directing resources to those with the greatest needs and are associated with positive health outcomes, including better quality of life, less chronic pain, and fewer depressive and post-traumatic stress symptoms over time. Canadian researchers have identified three *intersecting* dimensions of equity-oriented health care: cultural safety, Trauma and Violence Informed Practice (TVIP), and harm reduction (Browne et al., 2018; Ford-Gilboe et al., 2018). Culturally safe care moves beyond identifying the importance of acknowledging and respecting cultural differences between people (i.e., cultural awareness and cultural sensitivity) to explicitly address inequitable power relations, racism, discrimination, and ongoing impacts of historical and current inequities in the health care encounter. As introduced in Chapter 6, TVIP refers to practices that explicitly address the intersection and cumulative effects of interpersonal (e.g., child abuse, intimate partner violence) and structural (e.g., poverty, stigma) forms of violence on people's lives and health. Harm reduction, also discussed in Chapter 5, focuses on introducing practices that mitigate harms, not only related to substance use but to the historical, sociocultural, and political factors related to *responses* to substance use.

Ethnicity

Ethnicity refers to a common history, language, and set of rituals that create a form of common identity shared by a group of people. The shared heritage may include preferences for music, food, clothing styles, and perceived common values. Ethnicity may be linked to a particular national origin, such as Italian, Korean, or Irish ethnicity, but may also be linked to other religious or geographical histories, such as Jewish or First Nations ethnicity. Ethnicity is clearly linked to health inequities, particularly as it intersects with multiple forms of disadvantage, such as racialization, discrimination, and poverty (Browne et al., 2014). In today's sociopolitical context, even collecting ethnicity data in clinical contexts may prompt harm, particularly for racialized, vulnerable patients (Varcoe et al., 2009). The quality of ethnicity data collected within health care organizations is often unreliable, particularly for people from racialized or visible minority groups who are most at risk, seriously limiting the usefulness of the data. Quality measures for collecting data reflecting ethno-cultural identity in specific health care organizations may be warranted, but only if mechanisms exist or are developed for linking ethnicity with measures of perceived discrimination, stigmatization, income level, and other known contributors to inequities. Methods for linking these kinds of data, however, remain underdeveloped or non-existent in most health care organizations (Browne et al., 2014).

Prominent attention to different ethnicities has often been a result of racist behaviour and attitudes, and many countries have seen tragic conflict, war, and terrible cruelty inflicted on this basis, as discussed above. However, in a country such as Canada, in which the population is comprised of people from so many ethnic backgrounds, ethnic identity often becomes an important value to people who feel a sense of pride about the history of their family origins and ancestors and wish to preserve their ethnic heritage.

According to the 2016 Census, 7,540,830 people (21.9 percent of the population) are or have ever been a landed immigrant or permanent resident in Canada, close to the 22.3 percent recorded during the 1921 Census, the highest level since Confederation. Canada had 1,212,075 new immigrants (3.5 percent of the population) who had permanently settled in Canada from 2011 to 2016. The majority (60.3 percent) of these new immigrants were admitted under the economic category, 26.8 percent were admitted so that they could join family already in the country, and 11.6 percent were admitted to Canada as refugees. In 2016, the majority (61.8 percent) of newcomers were born in Asia (including the Middle East), with Africa ranking second at 13.4 percent, ahead of European immigrants. Toronto, Vancouver, and Montreal are still the places of residence of over half of all immigrants and recent immigrants to Canada, though more immigrants are also now settling in the Prairies and in the Atlantic provinces. Immigrants and their descendants play a significant role in shaping and enriching the ethnic, cultural, and linguistic landscape of the Canadian population, as well as making a substantial contribution to the social and economic development of the country (Statistics Canada, 2017).

Acculturation

Acculturation refers to the gradual adoption of elements of the dominant culture and society by minority groups, such as by immigrants and refugees. **Acculturative stress** refers to the difficulties immigrants face in relation to the process of adapting to the host society; adapting to Western society can pose many challenges for immigrants and refugees. These challenges intersect with economic factors as well as the experience of racialization and can contribute to and/or exacerbate mental ill health (George et al., 2015).

There is large variability in terms of the impact of acculturative stress on mental health related to, for example, country of origin, age, gender, sexual orientation, employment opportunities, education, neighbourhood of re-location, language acquisition (English and French), transportation issues, and access to culturally safe/appropriate (mental) health services. For example, it is common for young people to acculturate at a faster rate than their parents or grandparents, due to their high adaptability and their immersion in Canadian culture at schools and among their new peers. These differing rates of acculturation may lead to conflict among family members. Parents may be concerned that their children will lose important traditional values and practices. Children may see their parents as being out of step with current society, and they often resent restrictions or demands placed on them to adhere to "old world" cultural practices. However, it also has been found that children with parents who have adapted well to Canada, while also maintaining their traditional beliefs and practices, tend to do better after migration than children whose parents have completely assimilated (George et al., 2015). Generally, tensions associated with the migration experience resolve over time as all family members move through a gradual acculturation process. However, some tensions are so severe that they create entrenched conflict, often causing depression or anxiety and, in extreme circumstances, erupting into interpersonal violence and/or family breakdown (Souto et al., 2019).

Acculturation can sometimes be particularly difficult for children and youth who feel rejected by their peers. Newly arrived immigrant youth are sometimes ridiculed or belittled on the basis of their language skills, clothing styles, or other perceived shortcomings, and they become easy targets for bullying by other young people. Some immigrant youth join street gangs as a means of building a defence against such racist behaviour. Of course, gang membership generally involves a negative and violent group identity that most often leads to greater difficulties and tragic circumstances. Many communities in Canada are developing social programs that will assist young people in the acculturation process and ease their path.

It is not only youth who experience mental health challenges as a result of difficulties in their acculturation. Many adults encounter daunting challenges, such as difficulties communicating in a new language, the absence of familiar social supports, and loss of previous occupational or professional status. Some older adults who immigrate have particular difficulty establishing social networks and may end up isolated and depressed (Souto et al., 2019).

We need to recognize the multiple and intersecting oppressions faced by immigrants and the community contexts in which they live. Such an orientation illuminates the ways in which race, class, gender, age, sexual orientation, and newcomer status work simultaneously to marginalize immigrant and refugee groups. Moreover, efforts are required to respond to the vulnerability of immigrants during the settlement process and provide them with resources to improve and expand their social networks. Research findings underline the importance of incorporating social determinants of health into a holistic health promotion intervention and to advocate for more effective policies to facilitate newcomer settlement (Souto et al., 2019).

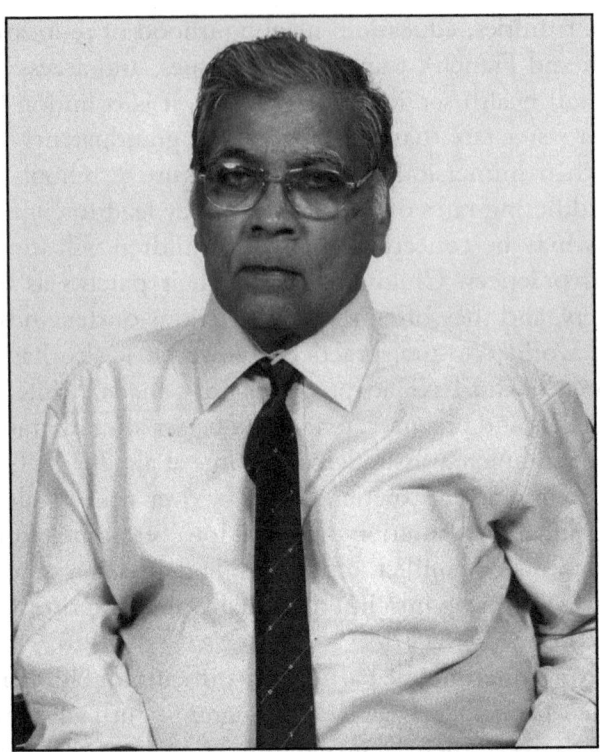

Figure 8.1: Some adults who immigrate experience challenges. The following is the story of a man who immigrated from Fiji as told by his granddaughter: "This is a photo of my grandfather, Manilal Gulab. He immigrated here with his wife from Fiji in 1992 after both his daughters married Canadian citizens. He had a very good life back home where he owned a shop that repaired broken watches, and he had a large and tightly knit social network. Once he moved here, he was diagnosed with Parkinson's disease, which made his transition increasingly difficult over the years as he adapted to cultural changes. Over time, his level of disability heightened and impacted his mental health. His inability to gain employment greatly affected his lifestyle. This is an example of how immigrants face many challenges and are at a greater risk of mental health challenges associated with life changes and unexpected challenges that may arise."

Source: Jessica Kumar, Photographer

Mental Health of Immigrants and Refugees

Most new immigrants to Canada make a good adjustment and maintain good mental and physical health. A phenomenon known as the "healthy immigrant effect" refers to the long-standing finding that shows immigrants to have a better health status than the general population born in a country (Vang et al., 2015). This is thought to be the result of standard immigration policies that screen out people with illnesses, allowing only a relatively healthy group of people to be admitted. Such policies are sometimes waived in relation to individuals designated as refugees, who have a very high likelihood of experiencing mental health challenges.

In Canada, the legal definition of a refugee is "[a person who] owing to a well-founded fear of being persecuted for reasons of race, religion, nationality, membership of a particular social group, or political opinion, is outside the country of his nationality, and is unable to or, owing to such fear, is unwilling to avail himself of the protection of that country" (United Nations Refugee Agency, 1951). Many refugees have experienced horrific persecution, torture, and violence, including physical, psychological, or sexual abuse, before arriving in Canada. Therefore, special attention needs to be paid to the unique needs, experiences, and strengths of refugees to foster their mental health.

The actual rates of mental health and illnesses or substance use disorders for any immigrant, racialized, ethnocultural, or refugee group depend on a complex interplay between risks and resilience (McKenzie, 2019). As noted in the Mental Health Commission of Canada report by Agic et al. (2016), "[m]ental health promotion, resilience, the building of social support, and prevention of mental illness through good planning of resettlement, education, and action on the social determinants of health are fundamental aspects of a good strategy."

However, when compared to majority groups in the Canadian population, immigrants and people belonging to ethnic minority groups are less likely to receive mental health treatment. Reasons for reduced access include language or cultural barriers, fears or feelings of shame about mental illnesses that deter seeking help, and mistrust of officials or professionals due to bad experiences in the past (i.e., a lack of cultural safety). Additionally, the concept of having help available for mental health challenges through the health care system may be unfamiliar, and some people may be unaware of such assistance or may tend to seek help through traditional healers instead. Mental health literacy is an important point for consideration for these populations. Indeed, among ethnocultural communities in which mental health challenges are stigmatized, treatment by health care providers is often only initiated once there has been a profound deterioration of the individual's condition.

Mental Health of Migrant Agricultural Workers

Recently, the COVID-19 pandemic has shone a light on the mental health of migrant workers. In 2018, roughly 72 percent of the 69,775 temporary migrant agricultural labourers arriving in Canada participated in the Seasonal Agricultural Workers Program (SAWP). Despite having legal status in Canada, these individuals are often systematically excluded from community life and face barriers when accessing health and social services. Migrant agricultural workers' experiences of segregation and isolation are complex and multifaceted. Several studies indicate that

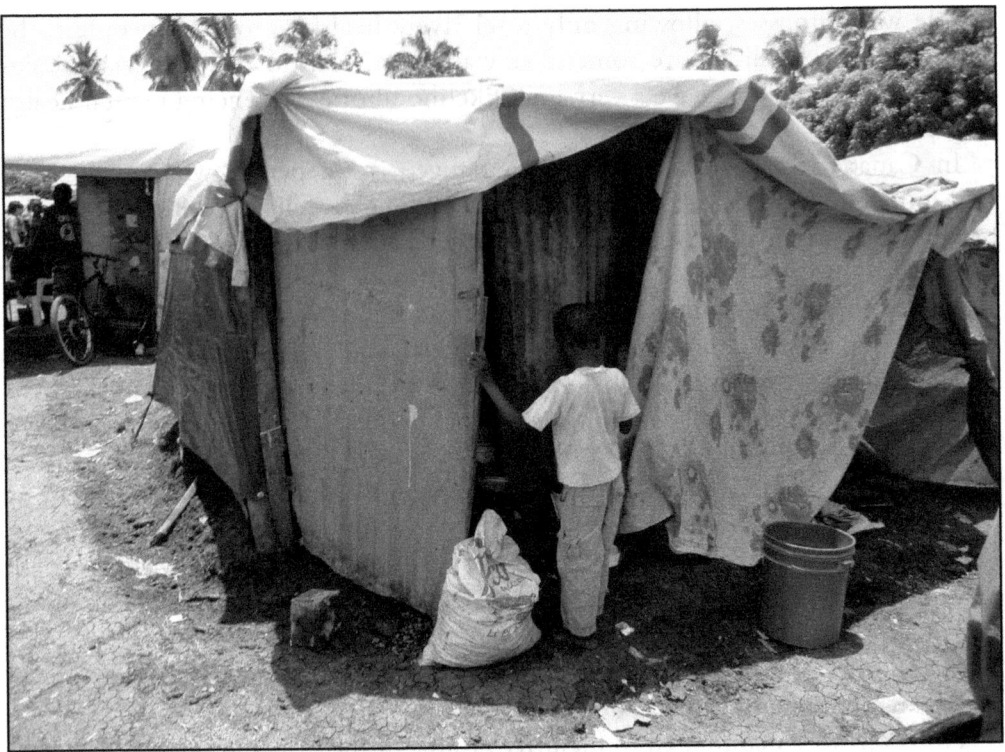

Figure 8.2: A boy living in a refugee camp after a major earthquake in Haiti. Poor living conditions and inadequate access to basic needs in refugee camps contribute to considerable mental health challenges.

Source: Gina Kim, Photographer

migrant agricultural workers are largely restricted to the farm due to geographic, linguistic, and workplace restrictions (Caxaj et al., 2020). Thus, it is not surprising that the mental health of this group of people has been negatively impacted (Basok & George, 2020).

Indigenous Peoples in Canada

Indigenous peoples living in Canada currently comprise approximately 4.9 percent of the country's total population. In some provinces and territories, Indigenous peoples constitute a much larger proportion: in Manitoba, 18 percent; Saskatchewan, 16 percent; in Yukon, 23 percent; in the Northwest Territories, 51 percent; and in Nunavut, 86 percent (Statistics Canada, 2017).

Archaeologists estimate that Indigenous peoples lived in the Americas for somewhere between 10,000 and 17,000 years before Europeans first arrived on the continent. During this lengthy period, many societies thrived and developed. Those living in the coastal areas of Canada sustained themselves by fishing the bountiful oceans, whereas inland societies oriented their lifestyle to agriculture or to hunting various animals, such as moose, caribou, and bison. Many different languages were spoken, and a wide variety of distinctive cultural groups developed, with unique artistic, linguistic, social, and musical traditions.

Following the arrival of Europeans in Canada, Indigenous peoples underwent forced colonization. Broadly, **colonization** is the invasion, dispossession, forced assimilation, and subjugation of peoples by the dominant force/power for the political and economic benefit of the colonizing country—processes that remain active today. From the 15th century onward, European nations (e.g., Britain, Belgium, France, Portugal, and Spain) built colonies in the Americas, Africa, Asia, and Oceania.

Another devastating impact of the arrival of European settlers came in the form of repeated waves of disease that decimated Indigenous communities. Since they

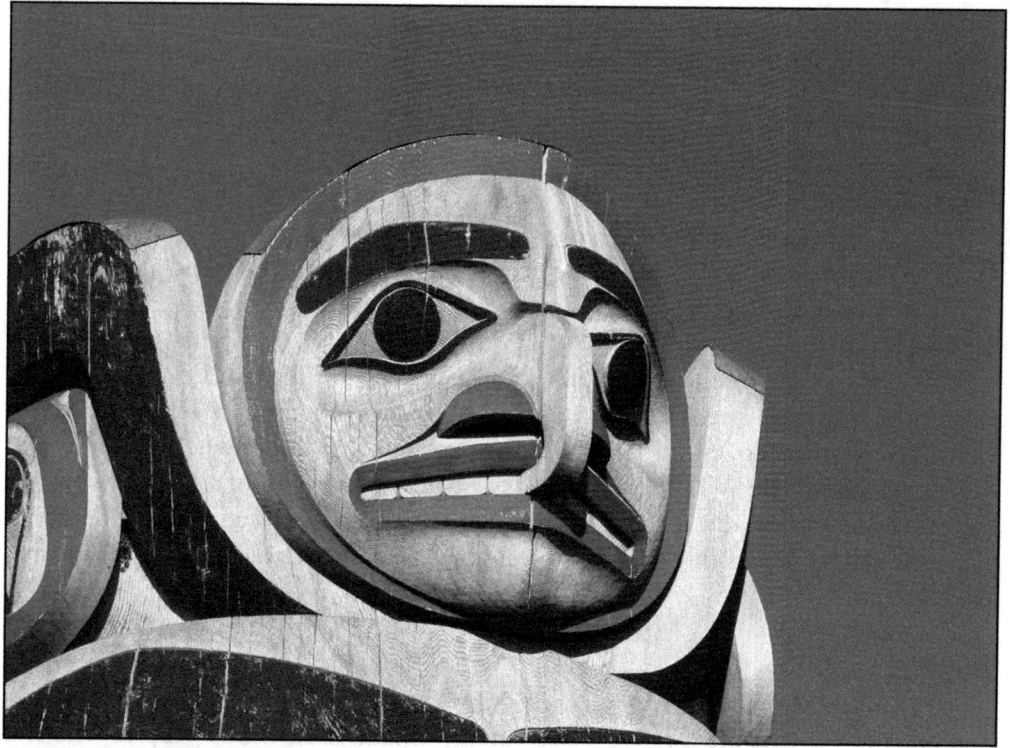

Figure 8.3: The Indigenous population in Canada is comprised of a culturally and linguistically diverse group of peoples. For many Indigenous communities, traditional arts such as the carving shown here are a means to commemorate histories and important events.

Source: iStockphoto/Miranda1066

had no immunity to infectious diseases such as smallpox, measles, influenza, and whooping cough transmitted by Europeans and by the animals brought by settlers, Indigenous peoples succumbed in huge numbers. Without the immunological defences that Europeans had developed over centuries of exposure to these illnesses, Indigenous peoples became very sick and often died when they became infected. Historical accounts describe heart-wrenching circumstances in which up to 90 percent of the population of villages and communities died over short periods of time in the areas that were most severely affected. It has been described as "the greatest human catastrophe in history, far exceeding even the disaster of the Black Death of medieval Europe" (Cook, 1998). Such profound loss of family, friends, and community is inconceivable (Daschuk, 2013).

In the wake of these tragic historical events that harmed Indigenous peoples across Canada, there has been a growing strengthening and revitalization among many of these peoples and communities. Steps have been taken towards self-determination, and advances have been made in the negotiation of Indigenous rights and freedoms. Many First Nations, Inuit, and Métis people have become tired of the repeated recounting of the challenges faced by their communities and, instead, call upon non-Indigenous Canadians to become allies in their strengthening and advancement. We will return to a discussion of the issues being addressed by Indigenous peoples in Canada after the following brief description of the three major groupings of people who are now recognized.

First Nations

The term "First Nations" refers to the original inhabitants of the land and has been in use in Canada since the 1970s and 80s, replacing the previous term "Indian." Section 35 of the *Constitution Act of 1982* declares that Aboriginal (Indigenous) peoples in Canada include Indian (First Nations), Inuit, and Métis peoples. Currently, there are more than 630 First Nations governments or bands across Canada, constituting all Indigenous peoples in Canada other than Inuit and Métis, discussed below. Table 8.1 provides a brief description of a few of the many First Nations in Canada to give a sense of their diversity. According to Statistics Canada's 2016 Census of Population results, 1,954,470 Canadians self-identified as First Nations.

Inuit

The Inuit in Canada are a group of culturally similar Indigenous peoples who live throughout most of Northern Canada in the territory of Nunavut, Nunavik in the northern third of Quebec, Nunatsiavut and NunatuKavut in Labrador, and in various parts of the Northwest Territories, particularly around the Arctic Ocean, in the Inuvialuit Settlement Region. Inuit people also live in Greenland and Alaska. In

Table 8.1: Brief description of a few First Nations across Canada

Tseshaht (pronounced see-sha-ought)	The Tseshaht people live on the west coast of Vancouver Island, British Columbia, and are one of the 14 Nations that make up the Nuu-chah-nulth Tribal Council. Historically, the Tseshaht people were whalers and fishers, and their lives revolved around their territories on both land and water. The Tseshaht First Nation reserve land is now a vibrant community with a membership of over 900 and an active and progressive natural resources–based economy, primarily with its abundant fisheries and well-developed forestry interests. The Tseshaht community is involved in many initiatives, from construction to forestry, from social development to education, from the fisheries to mental health, and is quickly moving toward self-sufficiency. The people of Tseshaht remain proud of their heritage and work as a community to preserve their traditional values and the teachings of the past.
Kainai (Blood Tribe)	The Kainai are proud members of the Blackfoot Confederacy, which includes the Peigan, Siksika, and South Peigan (Blackfeet). The Blood Tribe has a population of over 10,000, occupying approximately 1423.7 square km near the Rocky Mountains. The buffalo sustained the Kainai for untold generations. The Bloods cultivated and maintained an attitude of independence and fierce pride in their identity as Kainai. This spirit allowed them to successfully resist the efforts of governments, the churches, and other European agencies whose policies and practices could have an adverse impact on their cultural identity and legal rights. Today, the Blood Tribe continues to draw strength from the past as it strives to realize a unique vision for the future.
Moose Cree	The Cree are the largest group of First Nations in Canada, with over 200,000 members and 135 registered bands. The Moose Cree First Nations people live on Moose Factory, an island in Ontario's James Bay. The community operates various public utilities, health and social services, education and child care, and law enforcement services and runs a tourism wilderness program and a Cree cultural interpretative centre.
Mi'kmaq	**Mi'kmaq** are considered to be the largest of the First Nations traditionally occupying what are now Canada's eastern Maritime Provinces (Nova Scotia, New Brunswick, and Prince Edward Island) and parts of the present US states of Maine and Massachusetts. Because their Algonquian dialect differed greatly from that of their neighbours, it is thought that the Mi'kmaq may have settled the area later than other tribes in the region. The nation has a population of about 170,000 (including 18,044 members in the recently formed Qalipu First Nation in Newfoundland). According to the 2016 Census, 8,870 people are listed as speaking Mi'kmaq but numbers have been estimated at approximately 11,000.

Canada, sections 25 and 35 of the *Constitution Act of 1982* classify the Inuit as a distinctive group of Aboriginal Canadians who are not included under either the First Nations or the Métis. Previously, the term "Eskimo" was used to refer to an Inuit person. However, this term is considered pejorative by many Inuit people and consequently has fallen into disfavour.

Traditionally, the Inuit were fishers and hunters, and many Inuit individuals still hunt seals, whales, caribou, walruses, and other animals. The inventive adaptations that Inuit people made in order to live in the climate of the far North are well known. These include the carving of ice to build igloo homes, the use of dogs to pull sleds across the snow and ice, and the creation of nimble boats using sealskins (which are now known as kayaks and, in adapted form, are used throughout the world). According to Statistics Canada's 2016 Census of Population results, 65,025 Canadians self-identified as Inuit.

Métis

The Métis are descendants of unions between persons of European origin and Indigenous persons. Beginning in the 17th century, Métis communities began to develop through marriages of Indigenous people to Scottish, French, and other European settlers. However, it is generally recognized that being Métis is more than having mixed Indigenous and European heritage—rather, the Métis have a distinct collective identity, languages, traditions, and spiritual practices unique from Indigenous or European roots.

Controversy exists regarding who should be considered Métis, and legal definitions have not yet been adopted. Although Canada's constitution recognizes Métis people as one of the three distinctive groups of Indigenous peoples, no description of the Métis is given. Through case law, the Supreme Court of Canada has stipulated that a person may qualify under the legal definition of Métis only when they can be shown to self-identify as Métis, demonstrate an ancestral connection to a historic Métis community, and provide evidence of acceptance by the Métis community. According to Statistics Canada's 2016 Census of Population results, 587,545 Canadians self-identified as Métis.

Forced Assimilation of Indigenous Peoples: Residential Schools, the Welfare System, and Incarceration

Over much of Canada's history, policy-driven efforts were undertaken to force the assimilation of Indigenous peoples into the dominant society that was developed by European settlers in Canada. The systematic subjugation of Indigenous peoples has its origins in the colonial laws and policies enacted upon Indigenous peoples in 1876 through the *Indian Act*. While this framework was built on the pretext of assisting "Indians," the underlying intention was to civilize and eliminate "Indians," and despite several amendments, this *Act* is still in existence today. The assimilationist intent of the *Indian Act (1876)* was pursued at many levels: Indigenous lands were appropriated and reserves established; residential schools were instituted with the goal of indoctrinating children into the dominant culture (a collaborative effort between church and state); and cultural spiritual practices were outlawed (Brant Castellano et al., 2008).

One of the most egregious of "Indian" policies was the forced removal of Indigenous children from their families and communities to send them to residential schools. Indigenous children were removed from their families and required to live in residence at schools that were run by religious organizations, such as the Catholic, Anglican, and Presbyterian Churches of Canada. The residential schools generally took in children between the ages of 5 and 16 years of age. Adding to the harm caused to both children and parents by this forced dislocation, the children were pressured to abandon their traditions and to communicate only in English or French, consequently losing their traditional languages. Residential schools operated for over 100 years and were established in all Canadian provinces and territories except Newfoundland, Prince Edward Island, and New Brunswick. In total, there were approximately 130 residential schools, with the last school closing its doors in 1996.

A landmark Truth and Reconciliation Commission (TRC), which delivered its final report in 2015, found that, tragically, sexual and physical abuse at residential schools was widespread. It also estimated that at least 4,000 Indigenous children died in those schools, mainly from disease or malnourishment. Over 150,000 Indigenous children attended residential schools and, notably, the bodies of Indigenous children continue to be unearthed today from unmarked graves at residential school sites across Canada—more than 1,000 were discovered in 2020–2021 alone.

The harm inflicted by residential school policies continues to impact Indigenous children and families today. The disproportionate removal of Indigenous children by welfare agencies is part of the legacy of residential schools, which deprived their pupils of positive parenting, self-worth, and a sense of identity, contributing to high rates of poverty, substance use and addictions, and domestic and sexual violence (Truth and Reconciliation Commission of Canada [TRC], 2015). Indeed, Indigenous children 14 years and under comprise 52.2 percent of the population of children in care despite making up just over 7 percent of the kids in this country. These policies have also resulted in the overrepresentation of Indigenous persons in prison. While Indigenous adults accounted for 31 percent of Canada's incarcerated population in 2018–2019, they make up just 4.9 percent of the Canadian adult population (Government of Canada, 2021).

There have been a few apologies for the residential schools over the past three decades. In 1998, the Minister of Indian Affairs, Jane Stewart, delivered a "statement of reconciliation," apologizing to Indigenous peoples for the Canadian government's historical policies and practices. At the turn of the 20th century, the Moravian Mission and the International Grenfell Association established schools with dormitory residences for Indigenous children, with the support of the province of Newfoundland and Labrador. The last school closed in 1980. On June 11, 2008, on behalf of the

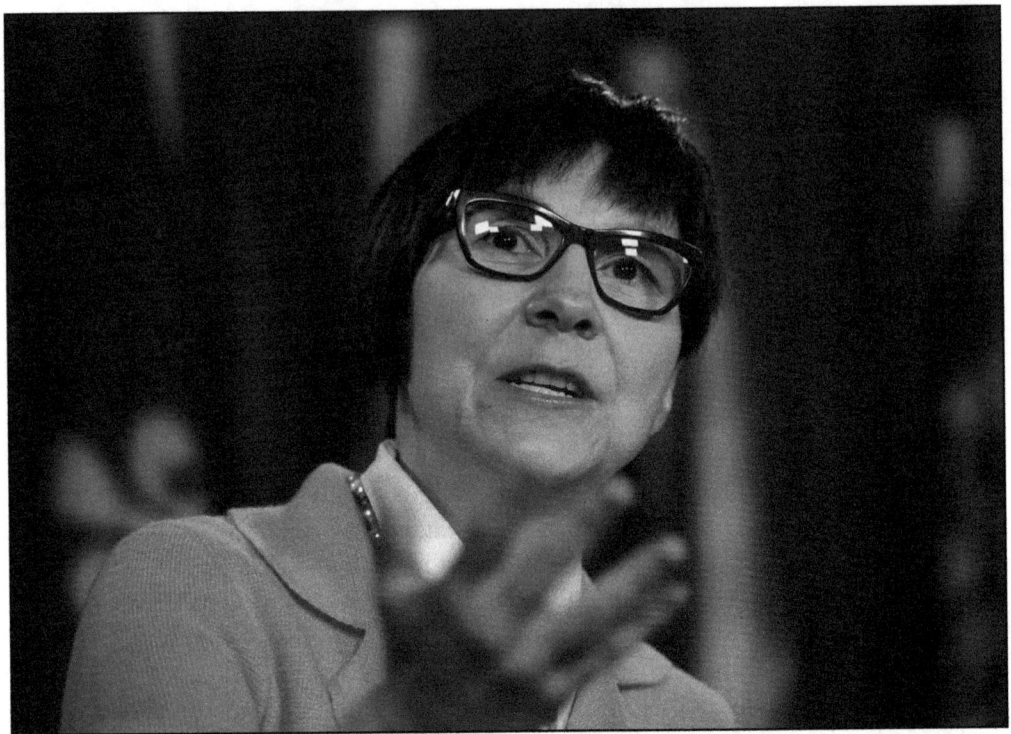

Figure 8.4: Cindy Blackstock, a renowned Indigenous scholar and activist on equality for Indigenous children, has worked on several successful human rights challenges, including a 13-year challenge that resulted in the landmark legal finding by the Canadian Human Rights Tribunal in September 2019. This finding stated that Canada wilfully and recklessly discriminated against Indigenous children on reserves by failing to provide funding for child and family services. She also has challenged the new Act (then Bill C-92), *respecting First Nations, Inuit and Métis children, youth and families*, because of the lack of accountability mechanisms and the unclear definition of what constitutes "the best interest of a child." This language allows a lot of discretion and has been problematically interpreted by non-Indigenous decision makers.

Source: Sean Kilpatrick/Canadian Press.

Government of Canada and all Canadians, then-Prime Minister Stephen Harper stood in the House of Commons to deliver an apology to students of Indian residential schools, their families, and communities. This apology did not include students from provincially run residential schools in Newfoundland and Labrador. On September 28, 2016, the Supreme Court of Newfoundland and Labrador approved a negotiated settlement to provide compensation to those who attended residential schools in Newfoundland and Labrador and those who may have suffered abuse. The settlement also includes provisions for healing and commemoration activities identified by former students. This apology also addresses Call to Action #29 outlined in the *Final Report of the Truth and Reconciliation Commission* (TRC, 2015), which implores the federal government "to work collaboratively with plaintiffs not included in the Indian Residential Schools Settlement Agreement." In the latest apology, which took place in 2017, Prime Minister Justin Trudeau apologized to the Residential School Survivors and their families:

> For every Innu, Inuit, and NunatuKavut child in Newfoundland and Labrador who suffered discrimination, mistreatment, abuse, and neglect in residential schools—we are sorry. While this long overdue apology will not undo the harm done, we offer it as a sign that we as a government and as a country accept responsibility for our failings. It is our shared hope that we can learn from this past and continue to advance our journey of reconciliation and healing. We have the power to be better and to do better.

Although important, apologies of this nature will never be enough. Great harm has been done.

Mental Health Consequences of Colonial Policies and Racism

The mental health inequities affecting Indigenous peoples in Canada are well documented and are directly attributable to the country's history of colonization, ongoing neocolonial policies, and racism. Despite this history, it is important to note that many Indigenous peoples are living well. For example, as noted in the "First Nations Mental Wellness Continuum" report (Health Canada, 2015), "First Nations have maintained their cultural knowledge in their ways of living (with the land and with each other) and in their language. These foundations have ensured First Nations people have strength, laughter, and resilience." In addition, statistics related to Indigenous mental health need to be understood as variable; the impact of colonialism, neocolonialism, racism, and so on, has not been the same for all Indigenous peoples or communities. Rather, mental health and wellness are associated with variation in access to education, housing, food security, employment, and health care and protective features such as connectedness to culture—to name several (Allan & Smylie, 2015; Auger, 2016).

However, higher rates of illicit drug and other substance use have been reported for Indigenous people as compared to non-Indigenous people and, although a smaller proportion of Indigenous persons consume alcohol than in the general population, the rate of problematic drinking is higher in the Indigenous population. In addition, depression has been found to occur more often than in the general population as well as PTSD.

Despite the fact that many Indigenous individuals are experiencing wellness, suicide rates also have consistently been shown to be higher among First Nations, Inuit, and Métis people in Canada as compared to rates among non-Indigenous

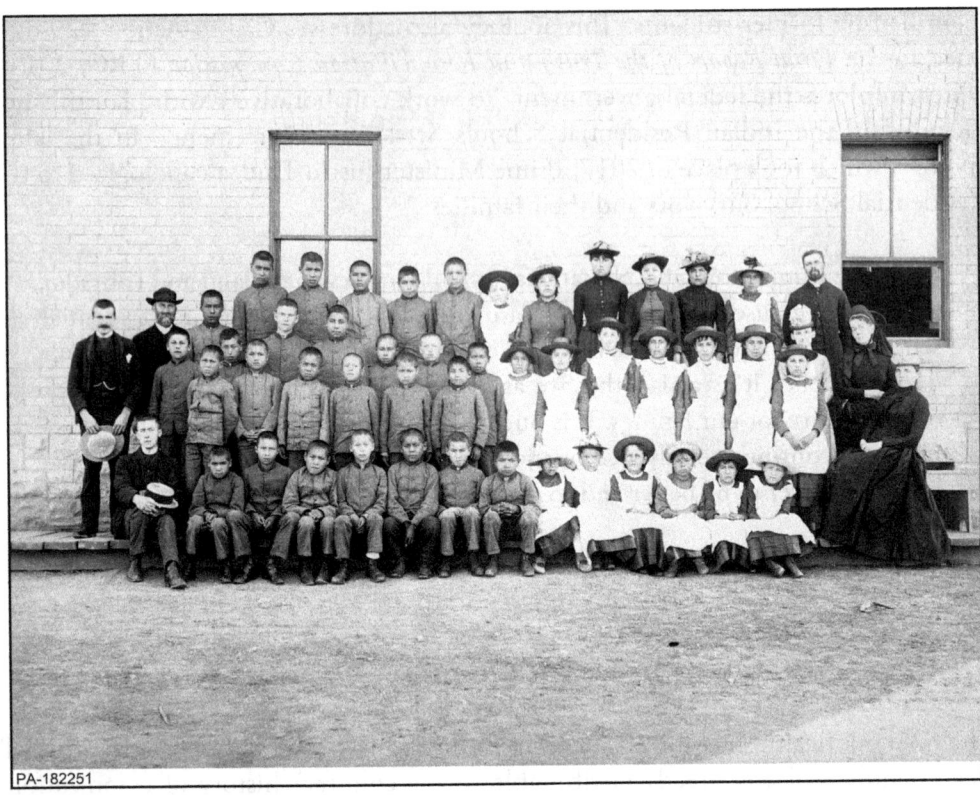

Figure 8.5: St. Paul's residential school in Middlechurch, Manitoba.

Source: Library and Archives Canada.

people. However, again, suicide rates vary by community, Indigenous group, age, and sex. For example, according to recent research, the suicide rate among First Nations people is three times higher than the rate among non-Indigenous people. Among First Nations people living on reserve, the rate is about twice as high as that among those living off reserve. Suicide rates have also been found to vary by First Nations band, with just over 60 percent of bands having a zero-suicide rate. The rate among the Métis is approximately twice as high as the rate among non-Indigenous people. Among Inuit people, the rate is approximately nine times higher than the non-Indigenous rate. Suicide rates and disparities are highest in youth and young adults (15 to 24 years), among First Nations males and among Inuit males and females (Kumar & Tjepkema, 2019).

The historical and ongoing impacts of colonization, forced placement of Indigenous children in residential schools in the 19th and 20th centuries, removal of Indigenous children from their families and communities during the "Sixties Scoop," and continuation of this practice today through the child welfare system and the forced relocation of communities have been well documented. These policies

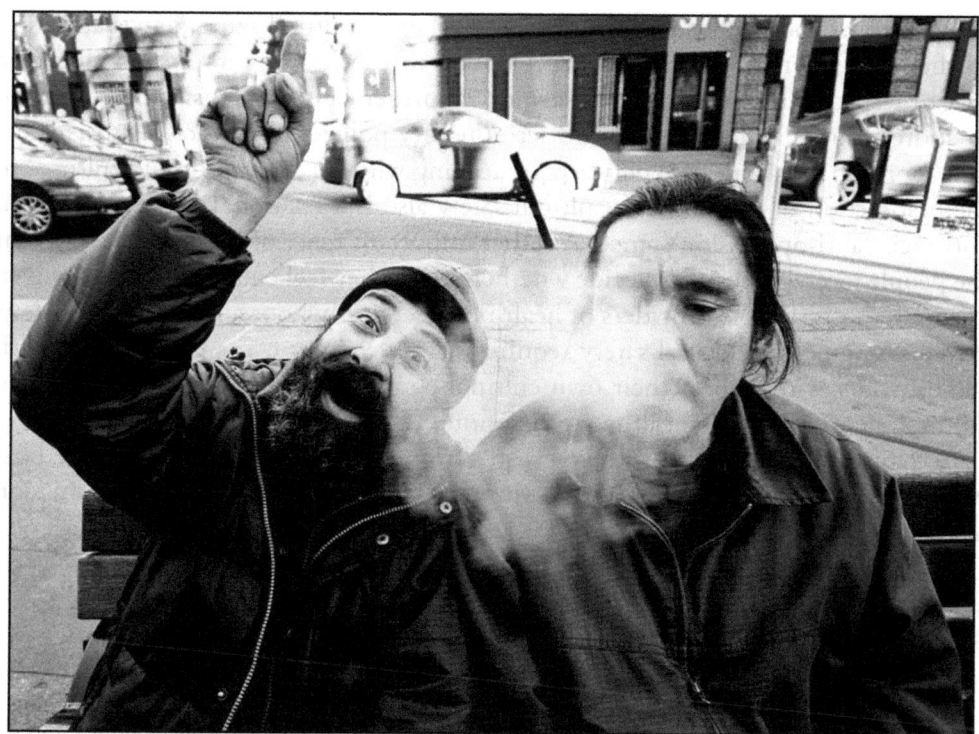

Figure 8.6: Colonization, discrimination, and loss of language and culture have led to intergenerational transmission of trauma and considerable mental health impacts among Indigenous peoples in Canada. For many Indigenous people, connecting with Indigenous friends and family, Elders, and communities can foster resilience and wellness.

Source: Chris Sang Yeob Park, Photographer.

and practices have resulted in the breakdown of families, communities, and political and economic structures. Loss of language, culture, and traditions; exposure to abuse; intergenerational transmission of trauma; and marginalization are suggested to be associated with the high rates of suicide (Kumar & Tjepkema, 2019). It is remarkable that First Nations, Inuit, and Métis people have survived the centuries of subjugation and colonization. Nevertheless, although many Indigenous peoples have demonstrated resilience to these multiple assaults, Indigenous peoples continue to carry the burden of history.

Cultural Safety and Decolonization

There has been growing recognition of the importance of ensuring that Canadian health care workers are culturally responsive, respectful, and safe in their interactions with First Nations, Inuit, and Métis people. The concept of **cultural safety** was developed in Aotearoa/New Zealand in response to health inequalities experienced by Māori, the Indigenous peoples of New Zealand. Cultural safety draws attention to the fact that many individuals feel unsafe in the health care system due to a lack of respect for their cultural identities. It further calls for transformative action to address power differentials and discriminatory policies and practices to create a safe approach to health care delivery. In keeping with our definition of "culture" in the first section of this chapter, cultural safety also is a relational concept—it is an anti-racist/anti-oppression stance. Another important tenet of cultural safety is that the people receiving services decide whether or not they feel culturally safe in a given encounter; it is not the providers of health care services who evaluate cultural safety. As a starting point, cultural safety requires self-reflection on the part of the health care provider with respect their own cultural context and the impact of their own cultural identities on the health care encounter (Browne et al., 2009).

We conclude this section with an excerpt from Bill Mussell, who chaired the First Nations, Inuit, and Métis Advisory Committee of the Mental Health Commission of Canada:

> *Decolonization* refers to a process where a colonized people reclaim their traditional culture, redefine themselves as a people and reassert their distinct identity.
>
> As a professional educator, mental health practitioner and consultant to First Nations, I see decolonization as the way to healing and restoring family and community health. The process requires:
>
> - learning how to learn and undertaking a journey to wellness that involves self-care
> - understanding forces of history that have shaped present day lifestyles
> - discovering, naming, and transmitting indigenous knowledge, values, and ways of knowing, together with understanding selected Western ways
> - applying and adapting both indigenous and Western knowledge, values, and ways of knowing to address present-day challenges effectively
>
> First Nations people must take positive control over their lives as individuals, families, and communities. They must build on who they are culturally and understand history from an Indigenous perspective. Reclaiming and building on cultural strengths contributes to a secure personal and cultural identity for all First Nations and other aboriginal groups. Grieving and healing of the losses suffered through colonization is a further step toward collective wellness and self-determination. More and more First Nations leaders and workers are calling for healing, family restoration and strengthened communities of care. These people promote a renewal of cultural practices and teaching history from an indigenous perspective. They call for education and training that combines the best of mainstream and indigenous knowledge, and for building the capacity of workers to improve the quality of life in their villages. A parallel process

of consciousness raising must occur within Canadian society, so stigma and discrimination against aboriginal Canadians can be eliminated, both on the personal and the structural levels of society. (Mussell, 2010)

Conclusion

Cultural and ethnic identities play important roles in shaping experiences of mental health and illness. Racism (and racialization) can cause substantial mental distress, and immigrants and refugees often experience challenges in adjusting to the changes and stresses they encounter. First Nations, Inuit, and Métis peoples have survived profound difficulties as a result of colonization, practices of forced assimilation, and separation of families through residential school systems. Activities to build cultural safety and support decolonization are means to bring about the healing and restoration of family and community life.

Glossary

acculturation: The gradual adoption of elements of the dominant culture and society by minority groups.
acculturative stress: This term refers to the difficulties immigrants face in relation to the process of adapting to the host society.
colonialization: The invasion, dispossession, forced assimilation, and subjugation of peoples by the dominant force/power for the political and economic benefit of the colonizing country—processes that remain active today.
cultural safety: A term developed in Aotearoa/New Zealand to bring awareness to and address health inequalities experienced by Māori, the Indigenous peoples of New Zealand. Cultural safety moves us beyond cultural awareness and cultural sensitivity to explicitly address inequitable power relations, racism, discrimination, and ongoing impacts of historical and current inequities in health care encounters.
culture: A complex network of meanings shaped by social, political, and historical processes—it is dynamic and ever-changing; it is relational.
ethnicity: A common history, language, and set of rituals that create a form of common identity and are shared by a group of people.
intersectionality: Refers to the complex intersection of social categorizations that create overlapping systems of discrimination and oppression. Basically, intersectionality is a lens for seeing the way in which various forms of inequality often operate together and exacerbate each other to create inequity.
racialization: A process of social differentiation or racial categorization by which people are labelled based on particular physical characteristics or arbitrary

ethnocultural or racial categories, and then dealt with in accordance with beliefs related to those labels.

racism: A set of attitudes and behaviours that can been found among a population in which social groups are identified, separated, treated as inferior or superior, and given differential access to power and other valued resources.

structural violence: Refers to the existence of unequal power, restricted access to resources, and systematic oppression resulting in the denial of basic needs. Closely aligned with social injustice, the arrangements are *structural* because they are embedded in the political and economic organization (institutional inequality) of our social world, and they are *violent* because they cause, influence, and govern individual experience.

Critical Thinking Questions

1. What is the difference between culture, race, and ethnicity?
2. What mental health challenges can be experienced as a result of acculturation?
3. Why are immigrants and people belonging to ethnic minority groups less likely to receive mental health services?
4. How has colonization impacted the mental health of Indigenous peoples?
5. What are some ways to build cultural safety and support decolonization of First Nations, Inuit, and Métis peoples?

Recommended Readings

Greenwood, M., de Leeuw, S., Lindsay, N. M., & Reading, C. (Eds.). (2018). *Determinants of Indigenous peoples' health in Canada: Beyond the social* (2nd ed). Canadian Scholars.

Kirmayer, L. J., & Valaskasis, G. G. (2008). *Healing traditions: The mental health of Aboriginal peoples in Canada*. UBC Press.

Nelson, S. E., & Wilson, K. (2017). The mental health of Indigenous peoples in Canada: A critical review of research. *Social Science & Medicine, 176*, 93–112. http://dx.doi.org/10.1016/j.socscimed.2017.01.021

Talaga, T. (2018). *All our relations: Finding the path forward*. Anansi.

Turpel-Lafond, M. E. (2020). *In plain sight: Addressing Indigenous-specific racism and discrimination in B.C. health care*. Government of British Columbia. https://engage.gov.bc.ca/app/uploads/sites/613/2020/11/In-Plain-Sight-Full-Report.pdf

Recommended Websites

Public Health Agency of Canada—Aboriginal Ways Tried and True. https://cbpp-pcpe.phac-aspc.gc.ca/aboriginalwtt

San'yas Indigenous Cultural Safety Training. www.sanyas.ca

Truth and Reconciliation Commission of Canada—Calls to Action. https://ehprnh2mwo3.exactdn.com/wp content/uploads/2021/01/Calls_to_Action_English2.pdf

University of Alberta, Faculty of Native Studies—Indigenous Canada, Massive Open Online Course. www.ualberta.ca/admissions-programs/online-courses/indigenous-canada/index.html

References

Agic, B., McKenzie, K., Tuck, A., & Antwi, M. (2016). *Supporting the mental health of refugees to Canada*. Mental Health Commission of Canada. https://www.mentalhealthcommission.ca/sites/default/files/2016-01-25_refugee_mental_health_backgrounder_0.pdf

Allan, B., & Smylie, J. (2015). *First Peoples, second class treatment: The role of racism in the health and well-being of Indigenous peoples in Canada*. The Wellesley Institute. https://www.wellesleyinstitute.com/wp-content/uploads/2015/02/Summary-First-Peoples-Second-Class-Treatment-Final.pdf

Auger, M. D. (2016). Cultural continuity as a determinant of Indigenous peoples' health: A metasynthesis of qualitative research in Canada and the United States. *The International Indigenous Policy Journal, 7*(4). https://doi.org/10.18584/iipj.2016.7.4.3

Azpiri, J. (2020, June 20). Allegations of B.C. health staff guessing alcohol levels prompt calls to address systemic racism. *Global News*. https://globalnews.ca/news/7089480/bc-health-racist-allegations/

Basok, T., & George, G. (2020, April 26). Migrant workers face further social isolation and mental health challenges during coronavirus pandemic. *The Conversation*. https://theconversation.com/migrant-workers-face-further-social-isolation-and-mental-health-challenges-during-coronavirus-pandemic-134324

Brant Castellano, M., Archibald, L., & DeGagne, M. (2008). *From truth to reconciliation: Transforming the legacy of residential schools*. Aboriginal Healing Foundation. https://www.ahf.ca/downloads/from-truth-to-reconciliation-transforming-the-legacy-of-residential-schools.pdf

Brian Sinclair Working Group. (2017). *Out of sight*. https://www.dropbox.com/s/wxf3v5uh2pun0pf/Out%20of%20Sight%20Final.pdf?dl=0

Browne, A. J., Varcoe, C., Smye, V., Reimer Kirkham, S., Lynam, J. M., & Wong, S. (2009). Cultural safety and the challenges of translating critically-oriented knowledge in practice. *Nursing Philosophy, 10*, 167–179. https://doi.org/10.1111/j.1466-769X.2009.00406.x

Browne, A. J., Varcoe, C. M., Wong, S. T., Smye, V. L., & Khan, K. B. (2014). Can ethnicity data collected at an organizational level be useful in addressing health and healthcare inequities? *Ethnicity and Health, 19*(2), 240–254. https://doi.org/10.1080/13557858.2013.814766.

Browne, A., Varcoe, C., Ford-Gilboe, M., Wathen, N. C., Smye, V., Jackson, B., Wallace, B., Pauly, B., Herbert, C., Wong, S., & Blanchet-Garneau, A. (2018). Disruption as opportunity: Impacts of an organizational-level health equity intervention in primary care clinics. *International Journal for Equity in Health, 17*, Article 154. https://doi.org/10.1186/s12939-018-0820-2

Caxaj, S., Cohen, A., Buffam, B., & Oudshoorn, A. (2020). Borders and boundaries in the lives of migrant agricultural workers: Towards a more equitable health services approach. *Witness: The Canadian Journal of Critical Nursing Discourse, 2*(2), 92–103. https://doi.org/10.25071/2291-5796.69

Cook, D. N. (1998). *Born to die: Disease and new world conquest, 1492–1650*. Cambridge University Press.

Corrigan, P. W., Bink, A. B., Schmidt, A., Jones, N., & Rüsch, N. (2016). What is the impact of self-stigma? Loss of self-respect and the "why try" effect. *Journal of Mental Health, 25*(1), 10–15. https://doi.org/10.3109/09638237.2015.1021902

Crenshaw, K. W. (2017). *On intersectionality: Essential writings*. The New Press.

Darwin, C. (1871). *The descent of man* (2nd ed.). John Murray.

Daschuk, J. W. (2013). *Clearing the plains: Disease, politics of starvation, and the loss of Aboriginal life* (Vol. 65). University of Regina Press.

Downey, B. (2020). Completing the circle: Towards the achievement of IND-equity—A culturally relevant health equity model by/for Indigenous populations. *Witness: The Canadian Journal of Critical Nursing Discourse, 2*(1), 97–110. https://doi.org/10.25071/2291-5796.59

Farmer, P. (2003). *Pathologies of power: Health, human rights, and the new war on the poor*. University of California Press.

First Nations Health Authority. (2021). *First Nations perspective on health and wellness*. https://www.fnha.ca/wellness/wellness-for-first-nations/first-nations-perspective-on-health-and-wellness

Ford-Gilboe, M., Wathen, N., Varcoe, C., Herbert, C., Jackson, B., Lavoie, J. G., Pauly, B., Perrin, N. A., Smye, V., Wallace, B., Wong, S. T., & Browne, A. J. (2018). How equity-oriented health care affects health: Key mechanisms and implications for primary health care practice and policy. *The Milbank Quarterly, 96*(4), 635–671. https://doi.org/ 10.1111/1468-0009.12349

George, U., Thomson, M. S., Chaze, F., & Guruge, S. (2015). Immigrant mental health, a public health issue: Looking back and moving forward. *International Journal of Environmental Research and Public Health, 12*, 13624–13648. https://doi.org/10.3390/ijerph121013624

Gerlach, A. J., Browne, A. J., Sinha, V., & Elliott, D. (2017). Navigating structural violence with Indigenous families: The contested terrain of early childhood intervention and the child welfare system in Canada. *The International Indigenous Policy Journal, 8*(3). https://doi.org/10.18584/iipj.2017.8.3.6

Government of Canada. (2021). *Reducing the numbers of Indigenous children in care*. https://www.sac-isc.gc.ca/eng/1541187352297/1541187392851

Graves, Jr., J. L. (2015). Why the nonexistence of biological races does not mean the nonexistence of racism. *American Behavioural Scientist, 59*(11), 1474–1495. https://doi.org/10.1177/0002764215588810

Health Canada. (2015). *First Nations Mental Wellness Continuum Framework—Full report.* https://thunderbirdpf.org/wp-content/uploads/2015/01/24-14-1273-FN-Mental-Wellness-Framework-EN05_low.pdf

Indian Act (R.S.C., 1985, c. I-5). https://laws-lois.justice.gc.ca/eng/acts/i-5/

Kumar, M. B., & Tjepkema, M. (2019). *Suicide among First Nations people, Métis and Inuit (2011–2016): Findings from the 2011 Canadian Census Health and Environment Cohort* (CanCHEC). Statistics Canada. https://www150.statcan.gc.ca/n1/en/catalogue/99-011-X2019001

Lowrie, M., & Malone, K. G. (2020, October 4). Joyce Echaquan's death highlights systemic racism in health care, experts say. *CTV News.* https://www.ctvnews.ca/health/joyce-echaquan-s-death-highlights-systemic-racism-in-health-care-experts-say-1.5132146

McConaghy, C. (2000). *Rethinking Indigenous education: Culturalism, colonialism and the politics of knowing.* Post Pressed.

McKenzie, K. (2019). Improving mental health services for immigrant, racialized, ethno-cultural and refugee groups. *Healthcare Papers, 8*(2), 4–9. https://doi.org/10.12927/hcpap.2019.25926

Mussell, B. (2010). Cultural pathways for decolonization. *Here to help.* www.heretohelp.bc.ca/publications/aboriginal-people/bck/2

Reimer Kirkham, S., & Anderson, J. M. (2002). Postcolonial nursing scholarship: From epistemology to method. *Advances in Nursing Science, 25*(1), 1–17.

Slack, J. D., & Grossberg, L. (2016). *Stuart Hall cultural studies 1983: A theoretical history.* Duke University Press.

Smye, V., & Browne, A. J. (2002). "Cultural safety" and the analysis of health policy affecting Aboriginal people. *Nurse Researcher: The International Journal of Research Methodology in Nursing and Health Care, 9*(3), 42–56.

Smye, V. L., & Oudshoorn A. (under review). Cultural implications for psychiatric mental health nursing. In C. Pollard & S. Jakubec (Eds.), *Varcarolis's Canadian Psychiatric Mental Health Nursing* (3rd ed., Chapter 8). Elsevier.

Souto, R. Q., Guruge, S. W., Merighi, M. A. B., & de Jesus, M. C. P. (2019). Immigrant partner violence among older Portuguese immigrant women in Canada. *Journal of Interpersonal Violence, 34*(5), 961–979. https://doi.org/10.1177/0886260516646101

Stackhouse, J. (2013, December 2). The 2013 Ismaili Centre Lecture. *The Globe and Mail.* https://www.theglobeandmail.com/community/editors-letter/the-2013-ismaili-centre-lecture/article15717835/

Statistics Canada. (2017). Immigration and ethnocultural diversity: Key results from the 2016 Census. https://www150.statcan.gc.ca/n1/daily-quotidien/171025/dq171025b-eng.htm

Truth and Reconciliation Commission of Canada [TRC]. (2015). *Honouring the truth, reconciling for the future: Summary of the final report of the Truth and Reconciliation Commission of Canada.* http://www.trc.ca/websites/trcinstitution/index.php?p=890

Turpel-Lafond, M. E. (2020). *In plain sight: Addressing Indigenous-specific racism and discrimination in B.C. health care.* Government of British Columbia. https://engage.gov.bc.ca/app/uploads/sites/613/2020/11/In-Plain-Sight-Full-Report.pdf

United Nations Refugee Agency. (1951). The Geneva Convention relating to the status of refugees. https://treaties.un.org/doc/Publication/MTDSG/Volume%20I/Chapter%20V/V-2.en.pdf

Vang, Z., Sigouin, J., Flenon, A., & Gagnon, A. (2015). The healthy immigrant effect in Canada: A systematic review. *Population change and lifecourse: Strategic knowledge cluster: Discussion paper series/Un Réseau stratégique de connaissances: Changement de population et parcours de vie: Documents de travail, 3*(1), 4. https://ir.lib.uwo.ca/pclc/vol3/iss1/4

Varcoe, C., Browne, A. J., Wong, S., & Smye, V. (2009). Harms and benefits: Collecting ethnicity in a clinical context. *Social Science & Medicine, 68*, 1659–1666. https://doi.org/10.1016/j.socscimed.2009.02.034

Chapter 9

Mental Health and Illness in Children and Youth

Skye Barbic, adapted from original chapter by
Elliot M. Goldner, Emily Jenkins, and Dan Bilsker

Our greatest natural resource is the minds of our children.
—Walt Disney (American film producer and director)

Introduction

Among the many species of the animal kingdom, it is humans, *homo sapiens*, that require the longest amount of time to reach maturity. Chimpanzees and gorillas take approximately 10 years to mature, while we require approximately twice as many years to do so. Anthropologists have found evidence indicating that our species first emerged approximately 200,000 years ago and that previous hominids, such as *homo neanderthalensis*, did not share the lengthy period of maturation that we require. Evolutionary psychologists contend that we require this lengthy period in order for our brains to develop and reach full intellectual capacity, particularly to achieve social intelligence.

This advanced brain development, including social and emotional intelligence, has supported young people growing up in Canada today to flourish in many ways. Indeed, this generation is among the most educated, connected, culturally safe, and diverse that our country has ever seen. They want to be engaged, challenge the status quo, and take the lead on building a sustainable future. They are also a generation with unprecedented issues to resolve, including climate crises, multiple pandemics, and other pressing issues, such as racial inequality, that have led to recent social justice movements. In this chapter, we examine the important periods of development and maturation occurring from the prenatal stage through transition to adulthood. A number of the social determinants of health that were listed in Chapter 3 are of particular relevance during this period, and we address these here. We also examine common mental illnesses that arise during this period and consider factors that may diminish the incidence of such challenges.

Social Determinants of Children's Mental Health

In order for children to grow and develop the capacity for good and enduring mental health, they require a safe and stable physical and social environment. It may be surprising to learn that in Canada, a relatively wealthy country, many children live in poverty and lack stable housing and other necessities of life. In fact, out of 36 Organisation for Economic Co-operation and Development (OECD) member countries, Canada ranks 17th in terms of its child poverty rates (Thévenon, 2018). According to a recent report, child poverty in Canada is on the rise, with 11.8 percent of Canadian children living in poverty (National Advisory Council on Poverty, 2021). Children under the age of 18 who live in families led by single women are more likely to live in poverty than children in families headed by a couple (National Advisory Council on Poverty, 2021). Moreover, many Canadian children experience homelessness, and recent studies indicate that the fastest growing segments among the homeless population are families with children under the age of 18 (Gaetz et al., 2016). As noted by the Homeless Hub (2021), the number of young people who become homeless in Canada each year is at least 40,000, and there may be as many as

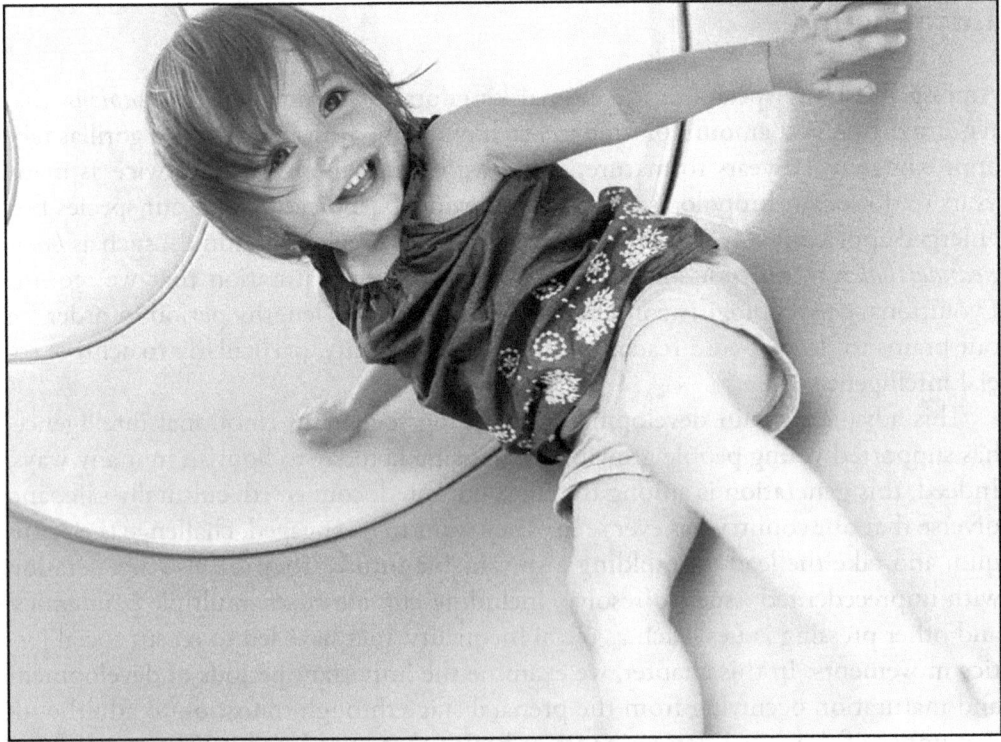

Figure 9.1: This little girl named Melina is having fun playing on the slide at the park. Children who are living in poverty often live in communities with less access to parks and recreational activities, which has an impact on their development and quality of life.

Source: Feryal Almazni, Photographer

7,000 homeless youth on any given night. Among homeless youth, there is a significant overrepresentation of those who identify as LGBTQ2+, Indigenous, and Black.

Two of the social determinants of health listed in Chapter 3 are directly pertinent to children and to the development of good mental health among Canada's populations—early life and education. As stated in a World Health Organization (WHO) document on social determinants of health, "What happens to the child in the early years is critical for the child's developmental trajectory and lifecourse" (2019). As a social determinant of health, "early life" comprises the period from prenatal development (i.e., before birth), through infancy (i.e., the first year after birth), and into early childhood. This period is of particular importance because of the high level of neural plasticity (i.e., the capacity for the brain to undergo development and build interconnections between brain cells) and because of the potential long-lasting effects of conditions and events experienced during this period. Healthy prenatal development requires proper nutrition, good maternal health, and an environment that is free from toxins or exposures that could interfere with the rapid growth and development that takes place during this period. Similarly, infancy and early childhood are crucial periods for the development of physical and mental health (WHO, 2012). We will discuss these periods in human development more thoroughly later in this chapter.

Education is an important social determinant of health, and it can exert significant influence on one's life trajectory over many years (Hahn & Truman, 2015). Early childhood education includes preschool and daycare, as well as the educational experiences a child receives at home and in the community. Significant emphasis has been placed on facilitating access to early childhood education for young children in order to promote cognitive and emotional development during this critical period. This is particularly important for children who experience risks to healthy development, such as those that arise due to poverty or parental mental illness or substance use challenges.

In a review of early childhood education programs in which program start, duration, and intensity were accounted for, Burger (2010) found that the majority of programs have substantial short-term benefits and more modest long-term effects on cognitive development. While these programs were especially advantageous for children from socioeconomically deprived backgrounds, they could not, in and of themselves, make up for the developmental deficits experienced by children from marginalized environments (Burger, 2010). In Canada, efforts are underway to identify children within early education programs who may need more support. Additionally, strategies have been developed to recognize and respond to gaps at a community-level. For example, the Early Development Instrument (EDI) is a Canadian-designed questionnaire that is completed by kindergarten teachers. It captures children's abilities to meet age-appropriate expectations including: (1) Physical Health and Well-being, (2) Social Competence, (3) Emotional Maturity, (4) Learning and Cognitive Development, and (5) Communication Skills and General Knowledge. Data from the EDI are used to inform policies and programs to best support child development. Recent EDI results indicate that 28 percent of children in Canada are vulnerable in one or more areas of development (Canadian Institute for Health Information, 2021), suggesting the ongoing need for early childhood education programming and community-level supports to decrease barriers to the social determinants of good health.

Beyond early childhood education programming, access to education in childhood and adolescence (in fact, throughout the entire lifetime) confers lasting benefits to both physical and mental health (Duncan et al., 2020; Goldfeld et al., 2018; Silva et al., 2016; Webb et al, 2016). In part, the benefits of education operate by opening up better opportunities for meaningful and rewarding employment, which in turn is linked to higher income, job security, and better housing options. In addition, education leads to heightened social skills and self-esteem.

In general, people with low education levels tend to have the worst health status (Borgonovi & Pokropek, 2016). Illiteracy is strongly associated with poverty, malnutrition, ill health, and increased rates of infant and child mortality (Lunze & Paasche-Orlow, 2014). This is further exacerbated in situations of low *health literacy*, which makes it more difficult to obtain and understand health information and to use it to make informed health decisions. In recent years, a lack of digital health literacy has been identified as an emerging challenge that is linked to poor health outcomes (Crawford & Serhal, 2020).

Research has found that children and young people who experience safe and supportive educational environments have an increased sense of connectedness to their schools and communities. School connectedness has been described as the belief by students that adults and peers in the school setting care about them both as learners and as individuals (Centers for Disease Control and Prevention, 2009; García-Moya et al., 2019). The important role that school connectedness plays in young peoples' mental health was illuminated during the COVID-19 pandemic, during which many school-aged children were transitioned to online learning due to school closures (Singh et al., 2020). In a systematic review of 15 studies describing nearly 23,000 children and youth, Panda and colleagues (2021) found that 79 percent were negatively affected by the pandemic, while 35 percent experienced boredom and 21 percent had sleep disturbances. Not surprisingly, the concept of school connectedness as an important determinant of health has gained substantial traction among researchers, educators, and public health professionals in recent years. Before the COVID-19 pandemic, this sense of connectedness was shown to be protective against a range of health challenges, including depression, violence, unsafe sexual activity, and harmful substance use (Arango et al., 2019; Weatherson et al., 2018). With this in mind, significant work must go into understanding how to best support children and youth in resuming their meaningful school-based connections and routines. This must include a sustained investment in mental health promotion programs to support children's well-being in school settings and timely access to early interventions.

Given the importance of education to the health of Canadians, it follows that great expectations and responsibilities are placed on our educational system. How well is it responding to this considerable challenge? Overall, Canada's educational institutions have been found to perform strongly when compared with those of other nations (OECD, 2018). Of course, there is always room for improvement; there are children in Canada whose needs are not adequately met. One substantial challenge is the ability of our school systems to address the diverse needs of our children,

> **Box 9.1: DAREarts: A Promising Community-Based Leadership Program Focused on Child and Youth Mental Health**
>
> While much of the health promotion programming that exists for children and youth takes place in school settings, there are also some innovative community-based programs that are showing great results. DAREarts is a program operating across Canada that aims to promote mental health among young people through leadership development and educational experiences in the arts. Participants in the program live with many barriers to well-being, including poverty and food insecurity, domestic violence in the home, bullying, and struggles in school. While typical leadership programs select students who are already demonstrating leadership capabilities, DAREarts believes that any young person can grow into a leader. The program further explains: "we see our programs as a critical intervention for children and youth who, for many reasons, may never consider themselves as leaders without support. We create a learning environment where participants can develop the skills, behaviors and confidence they need to see themselves as vital and capable change-makers." Building leadership capacity through the arts—including music, visual arts, and theatre—additionally helps young people express their creativity and confidence. Fun and engaging health promotion and prevention programs that are responsive to youths' needs, and the issues they face are an important component of a holistic approach to supporting the development of mentally healthy young people.

including their mental health needs. Howard Gardner, a psychologist, proposed the idea that there are many different components of intelligence, and consequently, education must be able to recognize and respond to these different strengths and capacities (Gardner & Hatch, 1989). Although Gardner's theory has been debated and disputed within the field of psychology, it has been embraced by many educators. The list provided in Table 9.1 will give you an idea of the different types of capacities being referred to in this theory.

Historically, our educational systems have emphasized the development of linguistic and logical-mathematical competence. Many educators feel that more diversity in school curricula is warranted to match different strengths and types of intelligence. Moreover, many policy makers believe that advancements can be made in supporting young peoples' well-being through cross-sector collaboration between schools and integrated youth services. **Integrated Youth Services** (IYS) represent a pan-Canadian and international movement towards building effective and cohesive services to better support children and youth. Many IYS projects in Canada focus on delivering integrated mental health and substance use services, youth and family support, primary care, educational opportunities, employment, and social services (i.e., housing). Organizations such as Youth Wellness Hubs Ontario, Foundry (in British Columbia), and Access Open Minds (with sites across Canada) are working with school communities in rural/remote, suburban, and urban settings, to identify "at risk" children and youth early, and to connect them to developmentally appropriate services and care.

Table 9.1: Different types of intelligence

Intelligence Type	End-States	Core Components
Logical-mathematical	Scientist Mathematician	Sensitivity to, and capacity to discern, logical or numerical patterns; ability to handle long chains of reasoning.
Linguistic	Poet Journalist	Sensitivity to the sounds, rhythms, and meanings of words; sensitivity to the different functions of language.
Musical	Composer Violinist	Abilities to produce and appreciate rhythm, pitch, and timbre; appreciation of the forms of musical expressiveness.
Spatial	Navigator Sculptor	Capacities to perceive the visual-spatial world accurately and to perform transformations on one's initial perceptions.
Bodily-kinesthetic	Dancer Athlete	Abilities to control one's body movements and to handle objects skillfully.
Interpersonal	Therapist Salesman	Capacities to discern and respond appropriately to the moods, temperaments, motivations, and desires of other people.
Intrapersonal	Person with detailed, accurate self-knowledge	Access to one's own feelings and the ability to discriminate among them and draw upon them to guide behaviour; knowledge of one's own strengths, weaknesses, desires, and intelligences.

Source: Gardner, H., & Hatch, T. (1989). Multiple intelligences go to school: Educational implications of the theory of multiple intelligences. *Educational Researcher, 18*(8), 4–10.

Box 9.2: Integrated Youth Services in Canada

In January 2020, at the World Economic Forum, an urgent call was made to invest in programs that expand access to care for young people. In response, Canada has been re-conceiving how services are delivered, specifically in the form of Integrated Youth Services (IYS). The emerging field of IYS seeks to guide system transformation to meet the needs of young people and their families. Programs such as Foundry in British Columbia and Youth Wellness Hubs Ontario are developing novel ways to engage children and youth to improve health outcomes. Countries such as Australia (headspace), Ireland (Jigsaw), and the United States (allcove) are also working towards the concept of timely access to IYS, including co-design of solutions with community leaders from schools alongside integration with health and academic plans. The evidence for these models continues to evolve (Mathias et al, 2021; Hetrick et al, 2017), with the shared vision of health and wellness for all young people, and the scaling of evidence to other jurisdictions nationally and internationally.

Development and Mental Health

Prenatal Development

Ensconced within the womb and dependent on the maternal physical environment during development, embryos (from conception to the 8th week of pregnancy) and fetuses (from the end of the 8th week until birth) are subject to various biological factors that may influence mental health. Healthy fetal development requires proper nutrition and good maternal health.

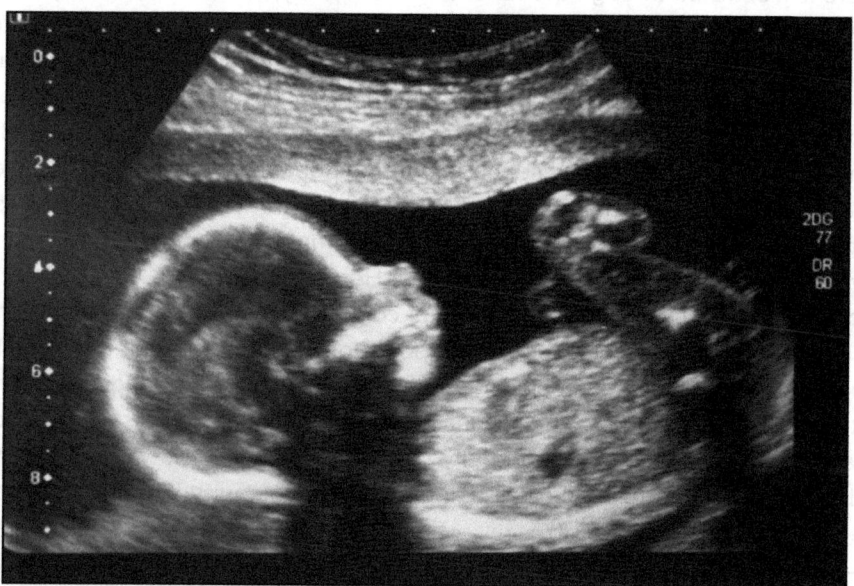

Figure 9.2: While still in the womb, the building blocks of mental health and well-being are already developing. While good maternal health and nutrition are known contributors to children's mental health throughout life, there is still much that is not known about fetal development and mental health and illness.

Source: iStockphoto/YsaL

Maternal malnutrition can have deleterious effects; for example, protein (essential amino acids) deprivation or glucose deprivation can result in an underdeveloped fetal brain. A tragic "natural experiment" in the 20th century allowed for study of the effects of malnutrition on mental health. From 1945 to 1946, the urban population in the Netherlands was exposed to acute starvation under Nazi occupation. A long-term follow-up study of children born to women who

> **Box 9.3: Biological Embedding**
>
> Depending on your disciplinary background and life experiences, some of you may find yourselves more closely relating to either the biological or social explanations for the development of mental health or illness. However, the two paradigms are not as separate as they may first appear. Through a process termed "biological embedding," the social factors that we are exposed to beginning in utero manage to "enter" our bodies and influence the development of our brains and central nervous system (Hertzman & Frank, 2006). A nice example of how this process occurs is illustrated through the functioning of the hypothalamic-pituitary-adrenal (HPA) axis. The HPA axis comprises of a set of brain and endocrine structures that influence the release of cortisol, a hormone secreted in response to experiences of stress. Cortisol serves an important function in our bodies and is involved in the "fight or flight" response to stress, providing a boost in energy and immune function, and lower pain sensitivity during periods of acute stress. However, prolonged exposure to the hormone (which is common with the chronic stresses encountered in today's society) can result in damage to various organ systems, leaving us vulnerable to illness and disease (Hertzman & Frank, 2006). Of particular concern is the fact that the HPA axis is conditioned, or "programmed," early in life, altering the way that our bodies respond to stress throughout the remainder of our lives! Thus, adverse social conditions or events (e.g., inadequate nutrition, limited parental bonding, poor access to early education, exposure to noxious substances, etc.), which are unequally distributed within society, have long-term implications for our health and well-being and influence our vulnerability to mental illnesses (Berens et al., 2017).

were pregnant during the famine found that they were significantly more likely to develop mental illnesses such as schizophrenia, mood disorder, and anti-social personality disorder when compared with children born at other times (Susser et al., 1998).

Some infectious illnesses that occur during pregnancy can adversely affect brain development, and various chemicals, toxins, and drugs that enter the maternal-fetal environment can also cause problems in mental development. The degree of impact of these factors ranges across a wide spectrum, from minimal effects that are difficult to detect to profound, permanent deficits in other instances.

> **Box 9.4: Fetal Alcohol Spectrum Disorder**
>
> Fetal Alcohol Spectrum Disorder (FASD) occurs as a result of damage to brain development caused by alcohol use during pregnancy. Infants with FASD display irritability, jitteriness, tremors, weak sucking reflexes, problems with sleeping and eating, failure to thrive, delayed development, poor motor control, and poor habituation. In childhood, challenges such as hyperactivity, attention difficulties, perceptual issues, cognitive deficits, language problems, and poor motor coordination are common. In adolescence and adulthood, the primary difficulties are memory impairments, problems with judgment and abstract reasoning, and poor adaptive functioning. How common is alcohol consumption during pregnancy? Research indicates that, in countries such as Canada and the US, the prevalence of alcohol consumption during pregnancy ranges from 10 to 15 percent (Popova et al., 2017).
>
> Some common secondary challenges characteristic of adolescents and adults with FASD include being unfocused and distractible. A diagnosis of FASD has also been found to be associated with difficulties with learning from experience, trouble understanding consequences and perceiving social cues, poor frustration tolerance, inappropriate sexual behaviours, problematic substance use, and difficulties with the law (Tsang et al., 2016). The exact amount of alcohol that can cause FASD is unknown and may vary between individuals (Roozen et al., 2018).

Infancy

Newborns interact with their environment quite differently than do adults. Their vision is relatively undeveloped, and they respond primarily to tactile (i.e., touch) and interoceptive stimuli (i.e., responses to internal stimuli such as hunger and thirst). Infants frequently let us know when something is amiss by crying, a powerful form of communication that few adults can ignore. Most of us have strong responses to crying infants and desperately want the crying to stop.

For the most part, infants are soothed when their basic needs are met (e.g., feeding them when they are hungry and changing their diapers when wet or soiled) and by touching, holding, rocking, cuddling, interacting with them, and stimulating their natural curiosity and interest in the world around them. Infants whose cries for food or comfort are ignored or produce angry and inconsistent responses by caregivers may have a difficult time trusting others and developing emotional bonds for the rest of their lives. This is reflected in Erik Erikson's theory (discussed in Chapter 3), in which he describes the first developmental stage (Trust vs. Mistrust) as the period during which infants must form loving, trusting relationships with caregivers or risk developing a sense of mistrust.

Unless supports are in place, a parent who struggles with a mental illness or substance use challenge may experience great difficulty in providing the consistent and ongoing nurturing, stimulation, and physical care that an infant or young child needs for optimal mental development. In some tragic circumstances, infants can suffer neglect and abandonment. Studies of both human and non-human primate infants have found that when infants are separated from their parents, three stages of emotional reactions follow. First is protest, in which infants cry and refuse to be consoled by others. Second is despair, in which infants are sad and passive. Third is detachment, in which infants actively disregard and avoid the parents if they return (Robertson & Bowlby, 1952).

Attachment theory was developed by psychologist John Bowlby, who theorized that a newborn child is biologically programmed to seek closeness with caregivers. Bowlby was intrigued by experimental studies of infant monkeys who had been removed from their mother's care. These studies found the young monkeys preferred to spend time with soft mother-like dummies that offered no food than with dummies that provided a food source but were less pleasant to touch (Harlow & Zimmerman, 1959). A central assumption in attachment theory, as applied to human children, is that sensitive responding by the parent or caregiver to infants' needs results in infants who demonstrate secure attachment, while lack of such sensitive or "attuned" responding results in insecure attachment.

Infant psychiatry or infant mental health represents a multidisciplinary field in which specialists seek to foster the mental health and well-being of infants, toddlers, preschoolers, and their families. Often, infant mental health specialists work with families identified as "high risk" to diminish the impact of social and economic risk factors. The intervention approach may include "treatments" that are informed by the biological, psychological, or social science perspectives; however, the primary focus is typically on supporting optimal infant-caregiver relationships.

In the Canadian context, researchers at the Children's Health Policy Centre led by Dr. Charlotte Waddell at Simon Fraser University have evaluated an infant mental health program called the "Nurse-Family Partnership," which was originally developed in the US over 40 years ago. The Nurse-Family Partnership program aims to provide young, first-time mothers who experience risk factors such as low income with intensive at-home supports from the prenatal period though to the child's second birthday. Over the course of the program, these moms and their babies will meet approximately 64 times with a public health nurse who will help to facilitate a sense of empowerment among these mothers through education and supports required to manage parental challenges. Studies of the Nurse-Family Partnership program conducted in the US have found the intervention to be associated with such outcomes as enhanced prenatal and early childhood mental health outcomes and decreased child and maternal mortality.

> **Box 9.5: Infant Psychiatry**
>
> Although a relatively new discipline, in the past few decades infant psychiatry has gained recognition as an important field. Many people tend to believe that infancy is a carefree period; however, young children can experience significant mental health challenges, particularly in the contexts of early developmental processes and the parent-child relationship. Mental health challenges in infants can manifest as prolonged crying, problems with sleeping or feeding, difficulties regulating emotions or attention, and aggressive behaviour. It is important that these issues are identified early so that there is an opportunity to improve developmental outcomes and promote positive parent-child relationships. One approach to treating infant mental health challenges is infant-parent psychotherapy, which is an attachment-based approach that focuses on reflective play, guidance, and aims to help parents process their emotions and caregiving experiences in relation to their interactions with their children.

Childhood

In early childhood, children are developing physical skills, including walking, grasping, and rectal sphincter control. According to Erikson (1963), in the Autonomy vs. Shame and Doubt development stage, young children from approximately 18 months to 3 years aim to learn autonomy (i.e., the ability to do certain things independently) and control. If these developments are not handled well by caregivers, the child may internalize persistent feelings of shame and doubt. This is the period when children learn to say "no," and it is common for parents to feel frustrated and exhausted by the frequent assertions of will and the temper tantrums that occur. In the subsequent stage of development identified by Erikson as Initiative vs. Guilt, which occurs from approximately 3 to 6 years of age, the child continues to become more assertive and to take more initiative. However, sometimes they may be too forceful, leading to feelings of guilt. According to Erikson's theory, in the next stage, Industry vs. Inferiority, lasting from about 6 to 12 years of age, the child must deal with demands to learn new skills or risk a sense of inferiority, failure, and incompetence.

For most children, family members will exert the greatest influence over a child's emotional and intellectual development. Children fortunate enough to have loving, nurturing family members who invest time and effort will usually flourish. Sometimes the most important bond and primary support to a child will be someone other than a parent—possibly an older sibling or another relative or family friend. Many grandparents play a special role in this regard, and we will return to a discussion of this important intergenerational bond in Chapter 10.

While cases of child maltreatment, such as abuse or neglect, are unsettling to hear about, it is well recognized that the impact of abuse, particularly in childhood, can greatly affect the mental health of the individual in later years. As discussed in

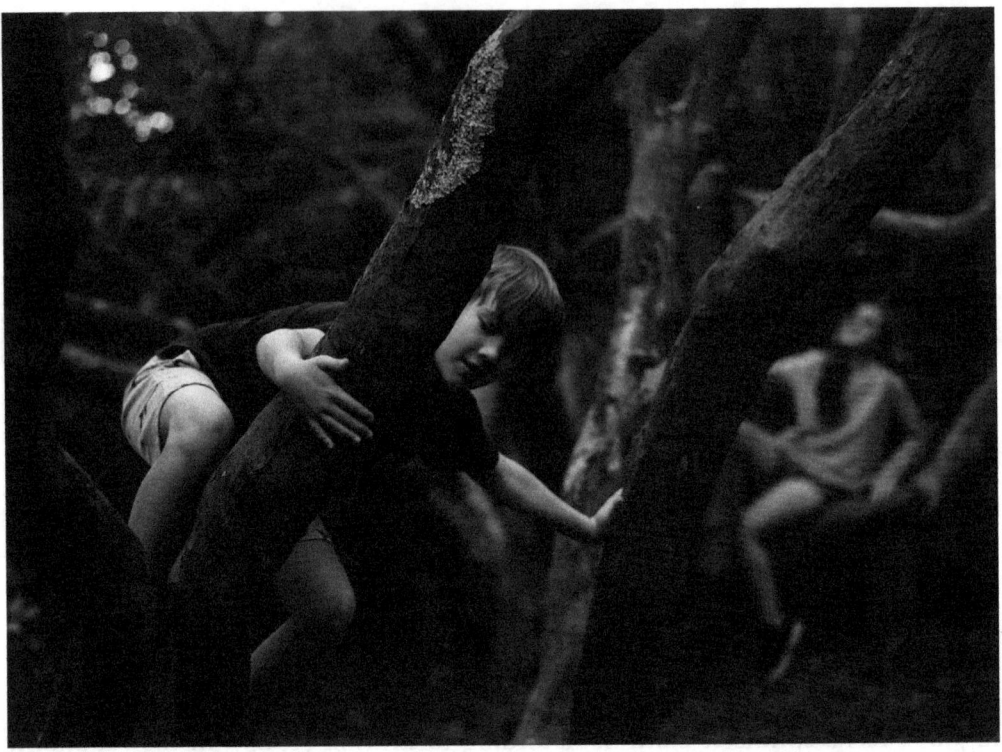

Figure 9.3: Healthy emotional growth in childhood includes the development of a sense of autonomy, comfort in social circumstances, self-generated initiative, and capacity for industrious activity. Play is the mechanism through which many of these competencies are derived. In recent years, "risky play" has emerged as a concept of interest among Canadian and international experts in childhood health and well-being. Risky play involves a focus on outdoor and informal play spaces with proximity to dangerous elements, such as water or the potential for getting lost. Risky play is responsive to concerns regarding the health effects of sedentary lifestyles as well as worries about the consequences of diminishing opportunities for children to partake in unstructured, unsupervised, and diverse outdoor play experiences as a result of "urbanization, the commercialization of play, risk-averse styles of parenting, the lure of indoor play technologies, and the pressures of academic achievement at increasingly younger ages" (Gerlach et al., 2019).

Source: Unsplash/Annie Spratt

Chapter 6, there is evidence to suggest that childhood maltreatment and early stressful experiences are associated with numerous physiological changes (Campbell et al., 2016; Kalmakis & Chandler, 2015). Furthermore, research has identified a possible causal relationship between childhood abuse and psychosis, as well as increased risk for major depressive disorder in young adulthood (Boyda et al., 2018; Selous et al., 2019). Child sexual abuse is associated with increased rates of childhood and adult mental illnesses (Kamiya et al., 2016). While it was once believed that children who are abused become abusers as adults, research has since demonstrated that this notion of a "cycle of abuse" is largely untrue (Michl-Petzing et al., 2019).

As we have discussed above, early education and schools play an important role in fostering the development of social and intellectual skills, and they are important environments for the emotional growth of our children. Whether at school, home, or elsewhere, adult oversight of children's behaviour is necessary to protect them from hurting themselves or others. In Chapter 3, we introduced Kohlberg's theory of moral development that was based, in part, on observations of children's interactions and their approach to moral dilemmas. Kohlberg noted that children tend to apply quite primitive rules of behaviour in which they do not consider whether their actions are hurtful or damaging to others, often being cruel. **Bullying** is usually defined as repeated negative acts, such as hitting, kicking, teasing, or taunting, committed by one or more children against others. A real or perceived power imbalance exists between the bully and victim. Bullying has been found to be common among children in school settings. In fact, in Canada, one in three young people report having experienced bullying (Molcho et al., 2009). Tragically, the long-term harms and consequences to the mental health of victims are often severe, and recent research indicates that those who have been bullied as children have an increased risk of depression, self-harm, and suicidality (Holt et al., 2015; Lereya et al., 2015).

Box 9.6: Roots of Empathy

Roots of Empathy is an evidence-based classroom initiative that has shown great success in reducing aggression among schoolchildren by enhancing social and emotional competence and increasing empathy. The Roots of Empathy initiative fosters the development of "emotional literacy" by bringing infants into the classroom to help young children learn to understand their own and others' emotions. The program is designed around visitation by a local infant and parent who come to the classroom every few weeks over the school year. A trained Roots of Empathy instructor guides students to observe the baby's development and to label the baby's feelings. In this experiential learning process, the baby is the "teacher" and helps children to identify and reflect on their own feelings and the feelings of others. Emotional literacy provides the foundation for safer and more caring classrooms. Children build their capacity for understanding their own and others' feelings (empathy), and as a result, they are less likely to physically, psychologically, or emotionally hurt each other through bullying and other cruelties. In the Roots of Empathy initiative, children also develop skills to challenge cruelty and injustice. Messages of social inclusion and activities that are consensus building contribute to a culture of caring that shifts the tone of the classroom. Research results from national and international evaluations of the initiative indicate significant reductions in aggression and increases in pro-social behaviour (Santos et al., 2011).

Source: Adapted from Roots of Empathy. (2021). *About our program*. https://rootsofempathy.org

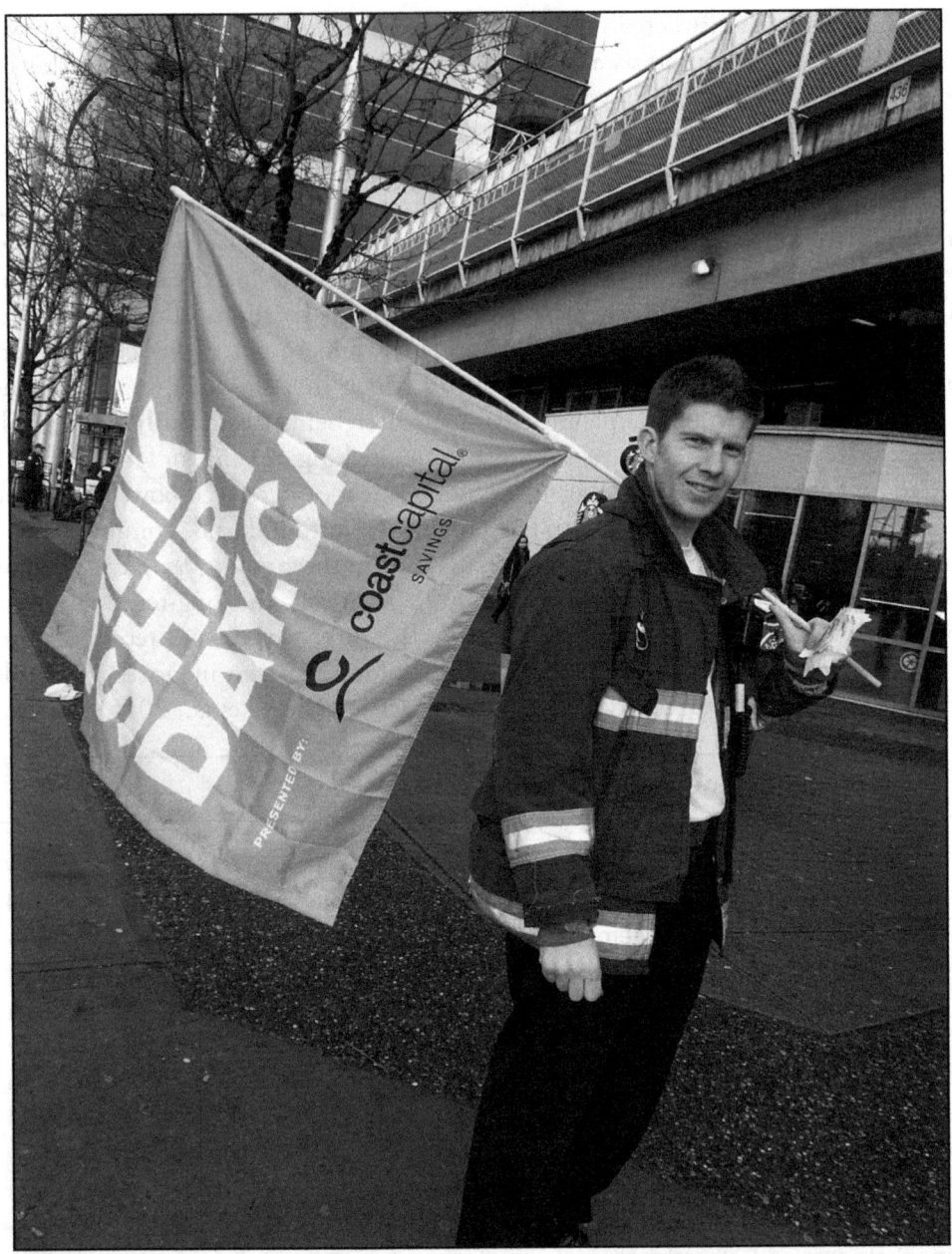

Figure 9.4: In recent years, there have been a number of community efforts to bring awareness to bullying, such as the annual Canada-wide Pink Shirt Day.

Source: Cassidy Jones, Photographer

Adolescence

According to Erikson (1963), an adolescent's challenge is Identity vs. Role Confusion (ages 12 to 18), during which time the youth must form a sense of identity in relation to such things as gender roles, occupational endeavours, and religious beliefs. Typically, a teenager's world is no longer centred within the family, but in the more exciting realm of peers and youth culture. Not all young people will go through a period of intense adolescent rebellion, but almost all will identify ways to differentiate themselves from previous generations, often by their dress, preferences in music, and political or social values.

Adolescence is often a time of many firsts: first date, first love, first sexual encounter, first job, and first experimentation with substances such as alcohol or other drugs. Academic stress, peer pressure, and learning to establish health routines are all part of this phase. However, today's teens face unique challenges that older generations might not have encountered. This includes navigating the digital world, responding to climate change, engaging in efforts to promote social justice, and dealing with unprecedented economic uncertainty. The risks and negative consequences encountered by young people during adolescence can be very serious, including

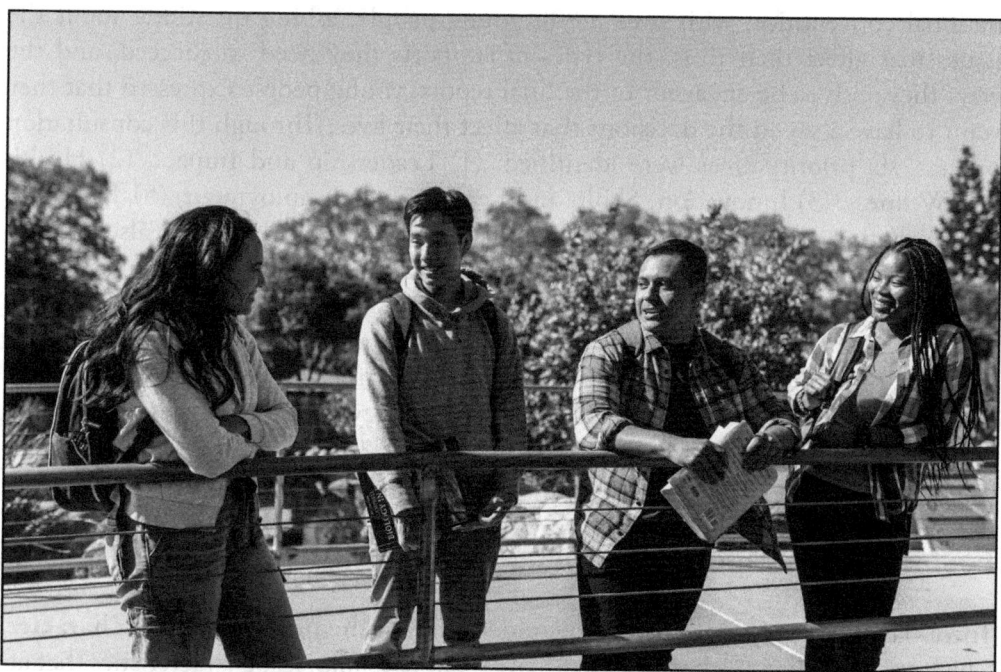

Figure 9.5: Adolescence is a period during which one establishes a distinctive identity and is exposed to a host of new experiences and challenges.

Source: Pexels/RODNAE Productions

problematic substance use (i.e., associated with harms). Maintaining and building strong and supportive relationships, as well as early intervention for those youth experiencing struggles, is critical to supporting this stage of development as needs emerge and change.

Transition to Adulthood

It is difficult to delineate where adolescence ends and adulthood begins. Often, young (and older) adults continue to work on challenges that emerged during earlier stages of development. Studies have found that young adults in Canada are making so-called key life transitions (i.e., beginning full-time jobs, working towards financial independence, finding their partner, starting a family) later and later (Statistics Canada, 2018). Some sociologists have dubbed this as a "failure to launch" and consider it the result of recent social and economic changes, such as increased housing costs and fewer career opportunities. The COVID-19 pandemic presented additional risks to this sub-group, with many young people accumulating debt, being socially isolated, delaying their studies, or returning home to live with their parents.

Regardless of the specific challenges being faced, prioritizing the voices of young people is crucial in developing relevant and impactful supports for the transition from adolescence to adulthood. In 2018, the Government of Canada launched a national conversation with over 5,000 young people, asking questions about the issues that affect their lives, the types of supports they need to succeed, and the ways they wish to be engaged. In the final report, young people expressed that they want to have a say in the decisions that affect their lives. Through this consultation process, six priority areas were identified: (1) Leadership and Impact, (2) Health and Wellness, (3) Innovation, Skills, and Learning, (4) Employment, (5) Truth and Reconciliation, and (6) Environment and Climate Action. The report also emphasizes that social participation and leadership are an integral part of young people's lives, and that they need to have their perspectives and voices heard. Further, a collective effort is required to eliminate discrimination and structural racism, advance a culture of equity, and promote full participation of all young people in Canada. The consultation resulted in Canada's first Youth Policy focusing on these six priority areas (Government of Canada, 2020).

Fostering Character and Social Responsibility

There has been a growing interest in understanding the development of **character**, which has been described as an individual's set of psychological characteristics that affect their ability and inclination to function morally (Berkowitz, 2002). Christopher Peterson and Martin Seligman (2004) have aimed to describe the core virtues that are consistently valued across cultures and time. The main virtues identified are wisdom, courage, humanity, justice, temperance, and transcendence (see Table 9.2).

Table 9.2: Character virtues and strengths

Character Virtues	Strengths
Wisdom and Knowledge	1. Curiosity/Interest in the world
	2. Love of learning
	3. Judgment/Critical thinking/Open-mindedness
	4. Ingenuity/Originality/Practical intelligence/Street smarts
	5. Social intelligence/Personal intelligence/Emotional intelligence
	6. Perspective
Courage	7. Valour and bravery
	8. Perseverance/Industry/Diligence
	9. Integrity/Genuineness/Honesty
Humanity and Love	10. Kindness and generosity
	11. Loving and allowing oneself to be loved
Justice	12. Citizenship/Duty/Teamwork/Loyalty
	13. Fairness and equity
	14. Leadership
Temperance	15. Self-control
	16. Prudence/Discretion/Caution
	17. Humility and Modesty
Transcendence	18. Appreciation of beauty and excellence
	19. Gratitude
	20. Hope/Optimism/Future-mindedness
	21. Spirituality/Sense of purpose/Faith/Religiousness
	22. Forgiveness and mercy
	23. Playfulness and humour
	24. Zest/Passion/Enthusiasm

Source: Peterson, C., & Seligman, M. (2004). *Character strengths and virtues: A handbook and classification*. Oxford University Press.

There is hope that an increased understanding of how these virtues can be fostered during childhood will lead to a more socially responsible and caring society. It appears that childhood is a critical period during which it is essential for these virtues to be relayed and incorporated into a life pattern. We will return to this topic in Chapter 17.

Mental Disorders in Children and Youth

Although some mental health challenges emerge for the first time later in life, the majority of mental disorders begin either in childhood or adolescence (Lee et al.,

2014). Indeed, 75 percent of all mental health challenges first occur between the ages of 12 and 24 years (Patel et al., 2016). For example, depressive disorders, anxiety disorders, and anorexia nervosa all typically emerge before the age of 18. The most prevalent mental disorders among children and youth are depression and anxiety disorders, and their features are similar to those seen in adults and described in Chapter 4. Across Canada, studies have been conducted on children between the ages of 6 to 18, and it has been estimated that nearly 13 percent of young people in this age group experience mental disorders that cause clinically significant symptoms (Waddell et al., 2014). At this point in time, prevalence estimates of mental disorders in younger children are not known. In the remainder of this chapter, we provide a brief description of the mental disorders that commonly begin during this developmental period. At the end of the chapter, we recommend additional reading for those who wish to obtain a more detailed and comprehensive understanding of mental disorders that affect children and youth.

Childhood mental disorders are sometimes distinguished as being either externalizing or internalizing. **Externalizing disorders** are those in which distress is turned outwards and directed towards others in a disruptive manner. In contrast, distress is turned inward in **internalizing disorders**. However, many conditions affecting children cannot be placed sensibly within this simplistic dichotomy.

One group of disorders that fits well under the category of externalizing disorders are **disruptive behaviour or dissocial disorders**. These disorders are "characterized by behaviours [that] range from those described as disruptive—that is, markedly and persistently defiant, disobedient, provocative or spiteful—to behaviours that are considered dissocial because they persistently violate the basic rights of others or major age-appropriate societal norms, rules, or laws" (WHO, 2020). The ICD further specifies that this pattern of conduct must persist for more than 12 months and constitute severe behavioural disturbance that is well beyond ordinary mischief. The following examples are listed in the ICD: "aggression towards people or animals; destruction of property; deceitfulness or theft; and serious violations of rules" (WHO, 2018).

Another group of disorders includes what is widely referred to as **attention deficit hyperactivity disorder** or ADHD. Children with this disorder have difficulty focusing their attention and are easily distracted. Often they experience compulsive behaviours and are hyperactive; that is, they have marked difficulty remaining still for any period. Attentional deficits associated with these disorders may persist throughout childhood and adolescence into adulthood, whereas the symptoms of hyperactivity and impulsivity tend to diminish with age. Even though many children with ADHD ultimately adjust, they are more likely to drop out of school and fare more poorly in their later careers than others.

While both disruptive behaviour or dissocial disorders and ADHD are considered externalizing in their behavioural manifestations, anxiety and fear-related disorders tend to be internalizing in nature. Most young children display some degree of distress upon separation from their primary caregivers (usually their mothers), between the ages of 8 and 14 months. Separation anxiety disorder is diagnosed when the fear of separation is unusually intense or interferes with social functioning and persists beyond the typical age period. Another fear-related disorder is selective mutism, which involves a lack of speech that is believed to be volitional (i.e., willed) on the part of the child. Selective mutism may be a reaction to a traumatic event or a symptom of extreme shyness.

Another group of mental disorders affecting children are **tic disorders**. According to the ICD,

> Primary tics or tic disorders are characterized by the presence of chronic motor and/or vocal (phonic) tics. Motor and vocal tics are defined as sudden, rapid, non-rhythmic, and recurrent movements or vocalizations, respectively. In order to be diagnosed, tics must have been present for at least one year, although they may not manifest consistently. (WHO, 2018)

Autism spectrum disorder, categorized as a pervasive developmental disorder in the ICD-11, is a complex condition that results in deficits in social interaction, communication, and behaviour. While the severity of symptoms can vary tremendously, children with autism typically also display various repetitive behaviours and routines and obsessions with particular objects. Some children with autism have quite severe impairment of language and may be completely non-verbal. Autism can be diagnosed between the ages of one and three, as symptoms are apparent even in young children. Individuals with autism are often unable to respond appropriately in social exchanges and struggle in forming relationships, which can be disheartening for parents, whose children may not reciprocate affection. Although the cause of autism remains unknown, it is thought to be a developmental disorder that involves an interaction of genetic and environmental factors. No medication is currently available to treat the primary symptoms of autism, but there are a variety of behavioural interventions that are helpful and are most beneficial if they begin as soon as a child is diagnosed; early intervention of autism ensures the best possible prognosis. One behavioural treatment that is widely utilized is Applied Behaviour Analysis (ABA). The underlying theory promotes "positive" behaviour and discourages "negative" behaviour. Despite its widespread use, ABA has been critiqued by many autistic people and advocates as attempting "to make children with autism 'normal'" by enforcing particular behaviours, rather providing teaching and support for self-identified needs and challenges (DeVita-Raeburn & Spectrum, 2016). As each individual with autism is unique, outcomes of treatment vary drastically.

Conclusion

A lengthy period of human maturation is required for the development of complex brain function and achievement of social and emotional intelligence. Social determinants that are particularly germane to the development of children's mental health are early life and education.

Many factors influence human development from the prenatal period through adulthood. Erik Erikson produced a theoretical framework that delineates specific developmental tasks considered to be central to various stages of development in infancy, childhood, adolescence, and adulthood. Currently, efforts are underway to understand the development of and specific virtues and strengths of character. Work is also underway in Canada to remove the structural barriers to health and wellness for children and young people to enhance equity.

The majority of mental disorders first begin during childhood or adolescence and the most prevalent mental conditions in young people are depressive and anxiety disorders. A wide range of disorders first seen in childhood are described in the ICD system.

Glossary

attachment theory: Developed by John Bowlby, this theory suggests that newborn children are biologically programmed to seek closeness with caregivers.
attention deficit hyperactivity disorder: A disorder in which individuals have great difficulty focusing attention and are easily distracted. People with ADHD can find it hard to remain still and can struggle with impulsivity.
bullying: Repeated negative acts, such as hitting, kicking, teasing, or taunting, committed by one or more people towards another.
character: An individual's set of psychological characteristics or virtues that affect that person's ability and inclination to function morally.
disruptive behaviour or dissocial disorders: Disorders characterized by a repetitive and persistent pattern of behaviour in which the basic rights of others or major age-appropriate societal norms, rules, or laws are violated.
externalizing disorders: Disorders in which distress is turned outward and directed towards others in a disruptive manner.
integrated youth services: A community-based program that provides youth-focused and integrated services to improve the health and well-being of young people and their families.
internalizing disorders: Disorders in which distress is turned inward, as is common in those with depression or anxiety disorders.
tic disorders: Disorders involving involuntary, rapid, non-rhythmic, recurrent movements, or vocalizations.

Critical Thinking Questions

1. Describe the relationship between education and mental health. How can educational systems respond to the diverse needs of young people?

2. Select one of the stages of development discussed in this chapter and describe its key features.
3. What are some of the challenges facing adolescents as they transition to adulthood?
4. What are the differences between internalizing and externalizing disorders? Provide examples of specific disorders.
5. Select a childhood/adolescent mental disorder and describe its characteristics.

Recommended Readings

Crain, W. (2015). *Theories of development: Concepts and applications* (6th ed.). Psychology Press.

Kostouros, P., & Thompson, B. (2018). *Child and youth mental health in Canada: Cases from front-line settings*. Canadian Scholars.

Szatmari, P., & Bryden, P. (2020). *Start here: A parent's guide to helping children through mental health challenges*. Simon & Schuster.

Yung, A. R., Cotter, J., & McGorry, P. D. (2020). *Youth mental health: Approaches to emerging mental ill-health in young people*. Routledge.

Recommended Websites

Children's Health Policy Centre—Simon Fraser University. https://childhealthpolicy.ca
Children's Mental Health Ontario. www.cmho.org
DAREarts. www.darearts.com
Frayme. https://frayme.ca
Kids Help Phone. https://kidshelpphone.ca
Teen Mental Health. www.teenmentalhealth.org

References

Arango, A., Cole-Lewis, Y., Lindsay, R., Yeguez, C. E., Clark, M., & King, C. (2019). The protective role of connectedness on depression and suicidal ideation among bully victimized youth. *Journal of Clinical Child & Adolescent Psychology, 48*(5), 728–739. https://doi.org/10.1080/15374416.2018.1443456

Berens, A. E., Jensen, S. K. G., & Nelson III, C. A. (2017). Biological embedding of childhood adversity: From physiological mechanisms to clinical implications. *BMC Medicine, 15*, Article 135. https://doi.org/10.1186/s12916-017-0895-4

Berkowitz, M. W. (2002). The science of character education. In D. Damon (Ed.), *Bringing in a new era in character education* (pp. 43–64). Hoover Institution Press.

Borgonovi, F., & Pokropek, A. (2016). Education and self-reported health: Evidence from 23 countries on the role of years of schooling, cognitive skills and social capital. *PloS One, 11*(2), e0149716. https://doi.org/10.1371/journal.pone.0149716

Boyda, D., McFeeters, D., Dhingra, K., & Rhoden, L. (2018). Childhood maltreatment and psychotic experiences: Exploring the specificity of early maladaptive schemas. *Journal of Clinical Psychology, 74*(12), 2287–2301. https://doi.org/10.1002/jclp.22690

Burger, K. (2010). How does early childhood care and education affect cognitive development? An international review of the effects of early interventions for children from different social backgrounds. *Early Childhood Research Quarterly, 25*(2), 140–165. https://doi.org/10.1016/j.ecresq.2009.11.001

Campbell, J. A., Walker, R. J., & Egede, L. E. (2016). Associations between adverse childhood experiences, high-risk behaviors, and morbidity in adulthood. *American Journal of Preventive Medicine, 50*(3), 344–352. https://doi.org/10.1016/j.amepre.2015.07.022

Canadian Institute for Health Information. (2021). *Children are vulnerable in areas of early development*. https://yourhealthsystem.cihi.ca/hsp/inbrief#!/indicators/013/children-vulnerable-in-areas-of-early-development/;mapC1;mapLevel2;/

Centers for Disease Control and Prevention. (2009). *School connectedness: Strategies for increasing protective factors among youth*. US Department of Health and Human Services.

Crawford, A., & Serhal, E. (2020). Digital health equity and COVID-19: The innovation curve cannot reinforce the social gradient of health. *Journal of Medical Internet Research, 22*(6), e19361. https://doi.org/10.2196/19361

DeVita-Raeburn, E., & Spectrum. (2016, August 11). Is the most common therapy for autism cruel? *The Atlantic*. https://www.theatlantic.com/health/archive/2016/08/aba-autism-controversy/495272/

Duncan, R. J., Duncan, G. J., Stanley, L., Aguilar, E., & Halfon, N. (2020). The kindergarten Early Development Instrument predicts third grade academic proficiency. *Early Childhood Research Quarterly, 53*, 287–300. https://doi.org/10.1016/j.ecresq.2020.05.009

Erikson, E. H. (1963). *Childhood and society* (2nd ed.). W.W. Norton.

Gaetz, S., Dej, E., Richter, T., & Redman, M. (2016). *The state of homelessness in Canada 2016*. Canadian Observatory on Homelessness Press. https://homelesshub.ca/sites/default/files/SOHC16_final_20Oct2016.pdf

García-Moya, I., Bunn, F., Jiménez-Iglesias, A., Paniagua, C., & Brooks, F. M. (2019). The conceptualisation of school and teacher connectedness in adolescent research: A scoping review of literature. *Educational Review, 71*(4), 423–444. https://doi.org/10.1080/00131911.2018.1424117

Gardner, H., & Hatch, T. (1989). Educational implications of the theory of multiple intelligences. *Educational Researcher, 18*(8), 4–10. https://doi.org/10.3102/0013189X018008004

Gerlach, A. J., Jenkins, E., & Hodgson, E. (2019). Disrupting assumptions of risky play in the context of structural marginalization: A community engagement project in a Canadian inner-city neighbourhood. *Health & Place, 55*, 80–86. https://doi.org/10.1016/j.healthplace.2018.11.008

Goldfeld, S., O'Connor, M., Cloney, D., Gray, S., Redmond, G., Badland, H., Williams, K., Mensah, F., Woolfenden, S., Kvalsig, A., & Kochanoff, A. T. (2018). Understanding child disadvantage from a social determinants perspective. *Journal of Epidemiology & Community Health, 72*(3), 223–229. http://dx.doi.org/10.1136/jech-2017-209036

Government of Canada. (2020). *Canada's Youth Policy.* https://www.canada.ca/content/dam/y-j/documents/YP-ENG.pdf

Hahn, R. A., & Truman, B. I. (2015). Education improves public health and promotes health equity. *International Journal of Health Services, 45*(4), 657–678. https://doi.org/10.1177/0020731415585986

Harlow, H. F., & Zimmerman, R. R. (1959). Affectional responses in the infant monkey. *Science, 130*(3373), 421–432.

Hertzman, C., & Frank, J. (2006). Biological pathways linking the social environment, development, and health. In J. Heymann, C. Hertzman, M. L. Barer, & R. G. Evans (Eds.), *Healthier societies: From analysis to action* (pp. 35–57). Oxford University Press.

Hetrick, S. E., Bailey, A. P., Smith, K. E., Malla, A., Mathias, S., Singh, S. P., O'Reilly, A., Verma, S. K., Benoit, L., Fleming, T. M., Moro, M. R., Rickwood, D. J., Duffy, J., Eriksen, T., Illback, R., Fisher, C. A., & McGorry, P. D. (2017). Integrated (one-stop shop) youth health care: Best available evidence and future directions. *Medical Journal of Australia, 207*(S10), S5–S18. https://doi.org/10.5694/mja17.00694

Holt, M. K., Vivolo-Kantor, A. M., Polanin, J. R., Holland, K. M., DeGue, S., Matjasko, J. L., Wolfe, M., & Reid, G. (2015). Bullying and suicidal ideation and behaviors: A meta-analysis. *Pediatrics, 135*(2), e496–e509. https://doi.org/10.1542/peds.2014-1864

Homeless Hub. (2021). *Youth homelessness overview.* https://www.homelesshub.ca/toolkit/youth-homelessness-overview

Kalmakis, K. A., & Chandler, G. E. (2015). Health consequences of adverse childhood experiences: A systematic review. *Journal of the American Association of Nurse Practitioners, 27*(8), 457–465. https://doi.org/10.1002/2327-6924.12215

Kamiya, Y., Timonen, V., & Kenny, R. A. (2016). The impact of childhood sexual abuse on the mental and physical health, and healthcare utilization of older adults. *International Psychogeriatrics, 28*(3), 415–422. https://doi.org/10.1017/S1041610215001672

Lee, F. S., Heimer, H., Giedd, J. N., Lein, E. S., Šestan, N., Weinberger, D. R., & Casey, B. J. (2014). Adolescent mental health—Opportunity and obligation. *Science, 346*(6209), 547–549. https://doi.org/10.1126/science.1260497

Lereya, S. T., Copeland, W. E., Costello, E. J., & Wolke, D. (2015). Adult mental health consequences of peer bullying and maltreatment in childhood: Two cohorts in two countries. *The Lancet Psychiatry, 2*(6), 524–531. https://doi.org/10.1016/S2215-0366(15)00165-0

Lunze, K., & Paasche-Orlow, M. K. (2014). Limited literacy and poor health: The role of social mobility in Germany and the United States. *Journal of Health Communication, 19*(Suppl 2), 15–18. https://doi.org/10.1080/10810730.2014.946115

Mathias, S., Tee, K., Helfrich, W., Gerty, K., Chan, G., & Barbic, S. P. (2021). Foundry: Early learnings from the implementation of an integrated youth service network. *Early Intervention in Psychiatry.* https://doi.org/10.1111/eip.13181

Michl-Petzing, L. C., Handley, E. D., Sturge-Apple, M., Cicchetti, D., & Toth, S. L. (2019). Re-examining the "cycle of abuse": Parenting determinants among previously maltreated, low-income mothers. *Journal of Family Psychology, 33*(6), 742–752. https://doi.org/10.1037/fam0000534

Molcho, M., Craig, W., Due, P., Pickett, W., Harel-Fisch, Y., & Overpeck, M. (2009). Cross-national time trends in bullying behaviour 1994–2006: Findings from Europe and North America. *International Journal of Public Health, 54*(2), 225–234. https://doi.org/10.1007/s00038-009-5414-8

National Advisory Council on Poverty. (2021). *Building understanding: The first report of the National Advisory Council on Poverty.* https://www.canada.ca/content/dam/esdc-edsc/documents/programs/poverty-reduction/national-advisory-council/reports/2020-annual/Building_understanding_FINAL_Jan_15.pdf

Organisation for Economic Co-operation and Development [OECD]. (2018). *PISA 2015: Results in focus.* https://www.oecd.org/pisa/pisa-2015-results-in-focus.pdf

Panda, P. K., Gupta, J., Chowdhury, S. R., Kumar, R., Meena, A. K., Madaan, P., Sharawat, I. K., & Gulati, S. (2021). Psychological and behavioral impact of lockdown and quarantine measures for COVID-19 pandemic on children, adolescents and caregivers: A systematic review and meta-analysis. *Journal of Tropical Pediatrics, 67*(1), fmaaa122. https://doi.org/10.1093/tropej/fmaa122

Patel, V., Chisholm, D., Parikh, R., Charlson, F. J., Degenhardt, L., Dua, T., Ferrari, A. J., Hyman, S., Laxminarayan, R., Levin, C., Lund, C., Mora, M. E. M., Petersen, I., Scott, J., Shidhaye, R., Vijayakumar, L., Thornicroft, G., Whiteford, H., & DCP MNS Author Group. (2016). Addressing the burden of mental, neurological, and substance use disorders: Key messages from Disease Control Priorities. *The Lancet, 387*(10028), 1672–1685. https://doi.org/10.1016/S0140-6736(15)00390-6

Peterson, C., & Seligman, M. (2004). *Character strengths and virtues: A handbook and classification.* Oxford University Press.

Popova, S., Lange, S., Probst, C., Parunashvili, N., & Rehm, J. (2017). Prevalence of alcohol consumption during pregnancy and Fetal Alcohol Spectrum Disorders among the general and Aboriginal populations in Canada and the United States.

European Journal of Medical Genetics, 60(1), 32–48. https://doi.org/10.1016/j.ejmg.2016.09.010

Robertson, J., & Bowlby, J. (1952). Responses of young children to separation from their mothers. *Courrier du Centre International de l'Enfance, 2*, 131–142.

Roots of Empathy. (2021). *About our program.* https://rootsofempathy.org/roots-of-empathy/

Roozen, S., Peters, G. J. Y., Kok, G., Townend, D., Nijhuis, J., Koek, G., & Curfs, L. (2018). Systematic literature review on which maternal alcohol behaviours are related to fetal alcohol spectrum disorders (FASD). *BMJ Open, 8*(12), e022578. https://doi.org/10.1136/bmjopen-2018-022578

Santos, R. G., Chartier, M. J., Whalen, J. C., Chateau, D., & Boyd, L. (2011). Effectiveness of school-based violence prevention for children and youth: A research report. *Healthcare Quarterly, 14*, 80–91. https://doi.org/10.12927/hcq.2011.22367

Selous, C., Kelly-Irving, M., Maughan, B., Eyre, O., Rice, F., & Collishaw, S. (2019). Adverse childhood experiences and adult mood problems: Evidence from a five-decade prospective birth cohort. *Psychological Medicine, 50*(14), 2444–2451. https://doi.org/10.1017/S003329171900271X

Silva, M., Loureiro, A., & Cardoso, G. (2016). Social determinants of mental health: A review of the evidence. *The European Journal of Psychiatry, 30*(4), 259–292.

Singh, S., Roy, D., Sinha, K., Parveen, S., Sharma, G., & Joshi, G. (2020). Impact of COVID-19 and lockdown on mental health of children and adolescents: A narrative review with recommendations. *Psychiatry Research, 293*, 113429. https://doi.org/10.1016/j.psychres.2020.113429

Statistics Canada. (2018). *Canadian youth and full-time work: A slower transition.* https://www150.statcan.gc.ca/n1/pub/11-630-x/11-630-x2017004-eng.htm

Susser, E., Hoek, H. W., & Brown, A. (1998). Neurodevelopmental disorders after prenatal famine: The story of the Dutch Famine Study. *American Journal of Epidemiology, 47*(3), 213–216.

Thévenon, O. (2018). *Tackling child poverty in Canada: OECD social, employment and migration working papers, no. 220.* OECD iLibrary. https://www.oecd-ilibrary.org/employment/tackling-child-poverty-in-canada_dd4dcfa6-en

Tsang, T. W., Lucas, B. R., Olson, H. C., Pinto, R. Z., & Elliott, E. J. (2016). Prenatal alcohol exposure, FASD, and child behavior: A meta-analysis. *Pediatrics, 137*(3), e20152542. https://doi.org/10.1542/peds.2015-2542

Waddell, C., Shepherd, C., Schwartz, C., & Barican, J. (2014). *Child and youth mental disorders: Prevalence and evidence-based interventions.* Children's Health Policy Centre, Simon Fraser University.

Weatherson, K. A., O'Neill, M., Lau, E. Y., Qian, W., Leatherdale, S. T., & Faulkner, G. E. (2018). The protective effects of school connectedness on substance use and physical activity. *Journal of Adolescent Health, 63*(6), 724–731. https://doi.org/10.1016/j.jadohealth.2018.07.002

Webb, S., Janus, M., Duku, E., Raos, R., Brownell, M., Forer, B., Guhn, M., & Muhajarine, N. (2016). Neighbourhood socioeconomic status indices and early childhood development. *SSM Population Health, 3*, 48–56. https://doi.org/10.1016/j.ssmph.2016.11.006

World Health Organization. (2012). *Social determinants of health and well-being among young people.* https://www.euro.who.int/__data/assets/pdf_file/0003/163857/Social-determinants-of-health-and-well-being-among-young-people.pdf

World Health Organization. (2018). *ICD-11 for mortality and morbidity statistics (ICD-11 MMS): 2018 version.*

World Health Organization. (2019). *Social determinants of health—Early child development.* https://www.who.int/social_determinants/themes/earlychilddevelopment/en/

World Health Organization. (2020). *ICD-11 diagnostic guidelines: Disruptive behaviour or dissocial disorders.*

Chapter 10

Mental Health and Illness in Older Adults

That's what an elder is. He's one who knows the teachings, who knows them so well that he's able to live by them. And he's lived through all those stages of life, and he's held onto them and now he can give people those teachings and not only can he give them those teachings, he can help them to understand them because he's lived it. That's what an elder is.
—Ojibway Traditional Teacher on "What is a 'real' Elder?"

Introduction

Life expectancy in Canada is relatively high, though the drug poisoning crisis and COVID-19 have led to a slight decline in recent years. In 2019, the average life expectancy in Canada was 82 years (84 years for females and 80 years for males)—one of the longest life expectancies of all countries (The World Bank, 2021). Worldwide, the average life expectancy is 73 years and Figure 10.1 shows the shockingly wide range of life expectancies across different regions of the world (World Health Organization [WHO], 2021).

The proportion of older adults in Canada has been increasing progressively and is anticipated to continue to rise over the coming decades. In the 1930s, about 5 percent of the population was 65 years of age or older, and in 2019 this had grown to approximately 17.5 percent (Statistics Canada, 2019b). Statistics Canada has projected that by 2068, this proportion will rise to between 21.4 and 29.5 percent (Statistics Canada, 2019c).

It is not uncommon for people in their seventies, eighties, and nineties to be living active and rewarding lives. Nevertheless, there are unique mental health challenges that affect older adults. In this chapter, we examine both the strengths and challenges that are common in this phase of life. We will discuss efforts that are used

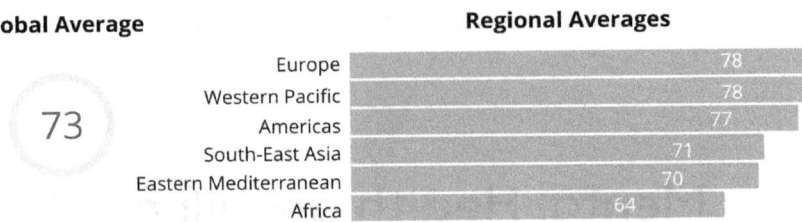

Figure 10.1: This graph shows the wide range of life expectancies that exist in various regions around the world.

Source: Adapted from the World Health Organization. (2021). Life expectancy at birth (years). https://www.who.int/data/gho/data/indicators/indicator-details/GHO/life-expectancy-at-birth-(years)

to promote good mental health among older Canadians, while signalling important issues that are being addressed in the treatment of mental health challenges within this section of our population.

Age, Experience, and Wisdom

One of the great benefits of advanced age is having had the opportunity to gain knowledge and experience that can produce wisdom. Many spiritual and cultural traditions describe historical or mythical figures who have transmitted insights gained through long lives or immortality, such as King Solomon, Confucius, the Norse god Odin, or the wizards and enchantresses found in fantasy tales such as *The Lord of the Rings*. Various cultures, including those of Indigenous peoples, have long traditions of honouring and valuing the wisdom of elders.

There are many well-known examples of profound contributions to society made by individuals of advanced age. At 79 years old, Sir Winston Churchill, the famous British leader who steered his country through the challenges of the Second World War, was in his second term as prime minister when he was awarded the Nobel Prize for literature for his historical and biographical writing and for his oratory. Pierre Berton, one of Canada's best-known journalists who published 50 books on Canadiana, continued to write and publish during his eighties. Since they have great experience and knowledge, older adults often play key roles in our organizations and societies; younger colleagues often obtain mentorship and guidance from their older counterparts.

Within families, the role of grandparent is one of particular importance. Grandparents are often able to provide children with non-judgmental love and acceptance, thus supporting a child's developmental and emotional needs. A child is often comforted by grandparents and obtains important feelings of safety, security, and self-esteem as a result of being loved and attended to by caring elders. Grandparents can also help to support busy or stressed parents through providing emotional, financial, or physical support and by taking on some child care responsibilities. A relationship with a grandchild gives grandparents a second opportunity to connect with children. Sometimes, accumulated wisdom and a less harried and frenetic lifestyle allows them an opportunity to improve on the parenting they were able to provide the first time around. An old Welsh proverb states: "Perfect love sometimes does not come until the first grandchild."

When parents experience extreme challenges caring for children, grandparents may end up becoming primary providers of child care and support. This often happens when parents encounter difficulties due to physical or mental illnesses or substance use challenges. Grandparents may be asked by parents to step in when children are proving too difficult for parents to manage or when parents become overwhelmed by circumstances or responsibilities.

Of course, an important connection between the old and young is not exclusive to grandparents and their grandchildren. Wisdom, life experience, and love can be passed along the generations by other family members too and by those who have no biological or familial relationship with a child. Many communities have developed programs that match older adults with children and youth who are in need of some additional support, encouragement, and love.

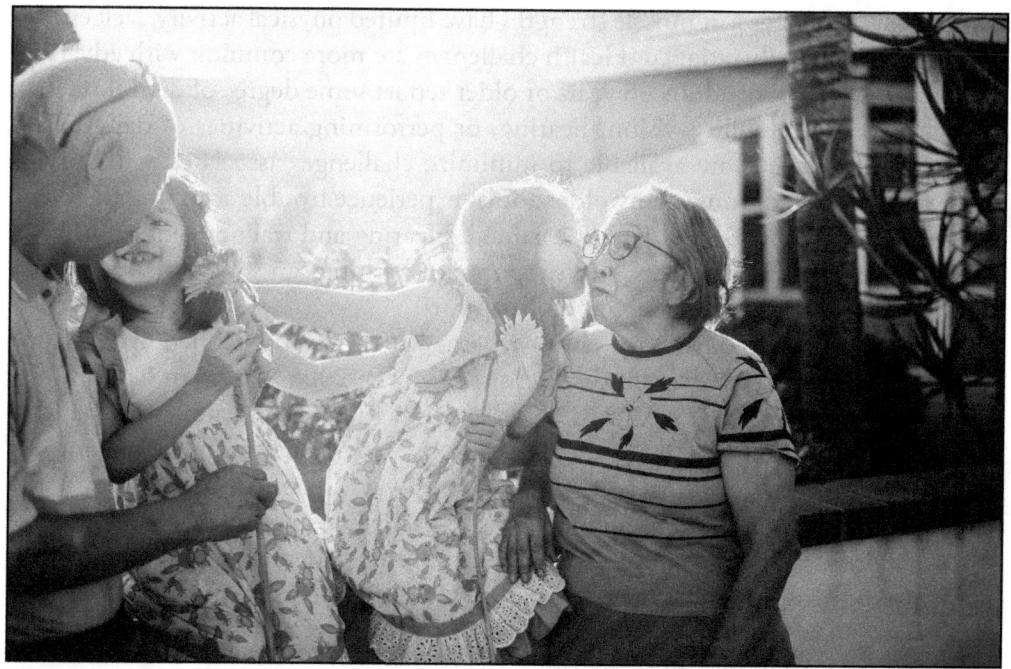

Figure 10.2: Grandparents and grandchildren enjoying each other's company. Research conducted by Fuller-Thomson and colleagues (2014) in Canada suggests that time spent with grandchildren provides older adults with a sense of purpose—and confirms that "grandchildren are fun!"

Source: Pexels/RODNAE Productions

Health, Illness, and Frailty among Older Adults

A large national longitudinal research study, the Canadian Study of Health and Aging, examined more than 10,000 people aged 65 or older across Canada, repeatedly obtaining information from the same group of individuals every 5 years over a 15-year period. The study found that three-quarters of these Canadians described their health as being "very good" or "pretty good" (Ebly et al., 1996). Even those who indicated having significant disability due to heart disease, limited physical mobility, or decreased vision often rated their health to be very good. This may be because they have adjusted to such changes over time, or it could be due to a tendency of older people to minimize complaints about poor health. Many older Canadians, however, experience substantial difficulties with their physical or mental health or both.

Although it is an oversimplification, older adults are often characterized as either "fit" or "frail." Those who are fit are considered to enjoy good overall health and to have the capacity to live full and independent lives. Those considered **frail** have significant physical or mental health challenges that interfere with their independence and require them to depend on others for aspects of care and daily function. Commonly, they have lost muscle strength, have limited physical activity, lack endurance, and/or are easily fatigued. Health challenges are more common with advanced age and close to half of adults 65 years or older report some degree of disability, such as difficulty with mobility, vision, hearing, or performing activities of daily living. Although various aids are available to minimize challenges associated with a wide range of health conditions, many older adults experience trouble accessing these and miss out on the benefits that could be gained. Hearing and walking aids, motorized wheelchairs, seat lifts for toilets, and supports for bathing can substantially improve quality of life and minimize pain and discomfort.

Some older adults experience chronic pain, which can be defined as pain that persists for more than a few months. Results from the 2005 Canadian Community Health Survey show that 27 percent of older adults living in private homes, and 38 percent living in long-term health care institutions, experience chronic pain. Chronic pain can impact an individual's life in numerous ways, including day-to-day activities, sleep and eating patterns, and mood. Research has shown that irrespective of other comorbidities, older adults experiencing chronic pain are more likely to be unhappy. Additionally, chronic pain can induce feelings of irritability, make it difficult to concentrate or remember things, and can contribute to anxiety and depression.

Loss, Loneliness, and Isolation

As people reach advanced age, it is inevitable that they will lose friends, family members, and colleagues to illness and death. Such loss takes a large toll. When one partner in a couple dies, the surviving individual often describes their experience as "losing a part of oneself." This may be a terribly difficult adjustment for couples who have spent much of their lives together or who have formed close intellectual or emotional bonds and joint senses of identity. When couples have divided various responsibilities over many years, such as managing finances, preparing food, or organizing social activities, the surviving spouse may find it difficult to take on unfamiliar tasks that were previously done by the deceased.

Some older adults are fortunate to have adult children, other family members, or friends who rally around them and help to ensure that their needs are being well looked after. However, many older people are estranged from family members and may not have a network of social support. In this case, they are at risk of being isolated and disconnected. Marginalized older adults often have few resources, and those who have no income, retirement savings, or other material goods may be forced to rely on shelters, social housing supports, or charitable agencies to survive.

Modern societies have been criticized as being **ageist**, that is, characterized by prejudice and discrimination on the basis of people's age. Intensified by advertising and mass marketing activities, the vibrancy and beauty of youth often becomes a preoccupation reinforced by frequent exposure to images of young models, actors, athletes, and celebrities. In societies like ours, which are sometimes described as being "youth obsessed," older adults are often considered irrelevant. This can be observed in the employment setting, where older adults frequently face discrimination during hiring processes, being passed over in favour of younger applicants. Even in their social and family relationships, they are often treated as unimportant and obsolete. For many aging individuals, the entrenched ageist attitudes and behaviours that exist in our society contribute to feelings of worthlessness (Ravary et al., 2019). These feelings may contribute, in part, to the higher rates of suicide observed among older adults, where men are at particularly high risk, especially those who are single or living alone (Statistics Canada, 2019a). Poor physical health, social isolation, changing social roles, and loss of independence are other factors that are associated with suicide among older adults.

Erik Erikson, the psychologist known for describing developmental phases that occur sequentially through the course of human life (see the discussion of his framework in Chapter 3), considered the final developmental phase to be one that juxtaposes Ego Integrity vs. Despair. Erikson proposed that, towards the end of one's life, the inevitability of mortality must be faced, and we are impelled to review the meaningfulness of our lives, knowing that we have limited time left. Erikson's theory proposes that there is a spectrum of experience. At one end are those who feel positively about their lives, seeing themselves as being fortunate to have experienced happiness and satisfaction, a condition Erikson described as "ego integrity." The other extreme is despair over the lack of meaning or satisfaction that one construes when reviewing the course of their life. Although most people end up feeling positive towards the end of their lives, many will also experience a mixture of feelings that include both satisfaction and regrets.

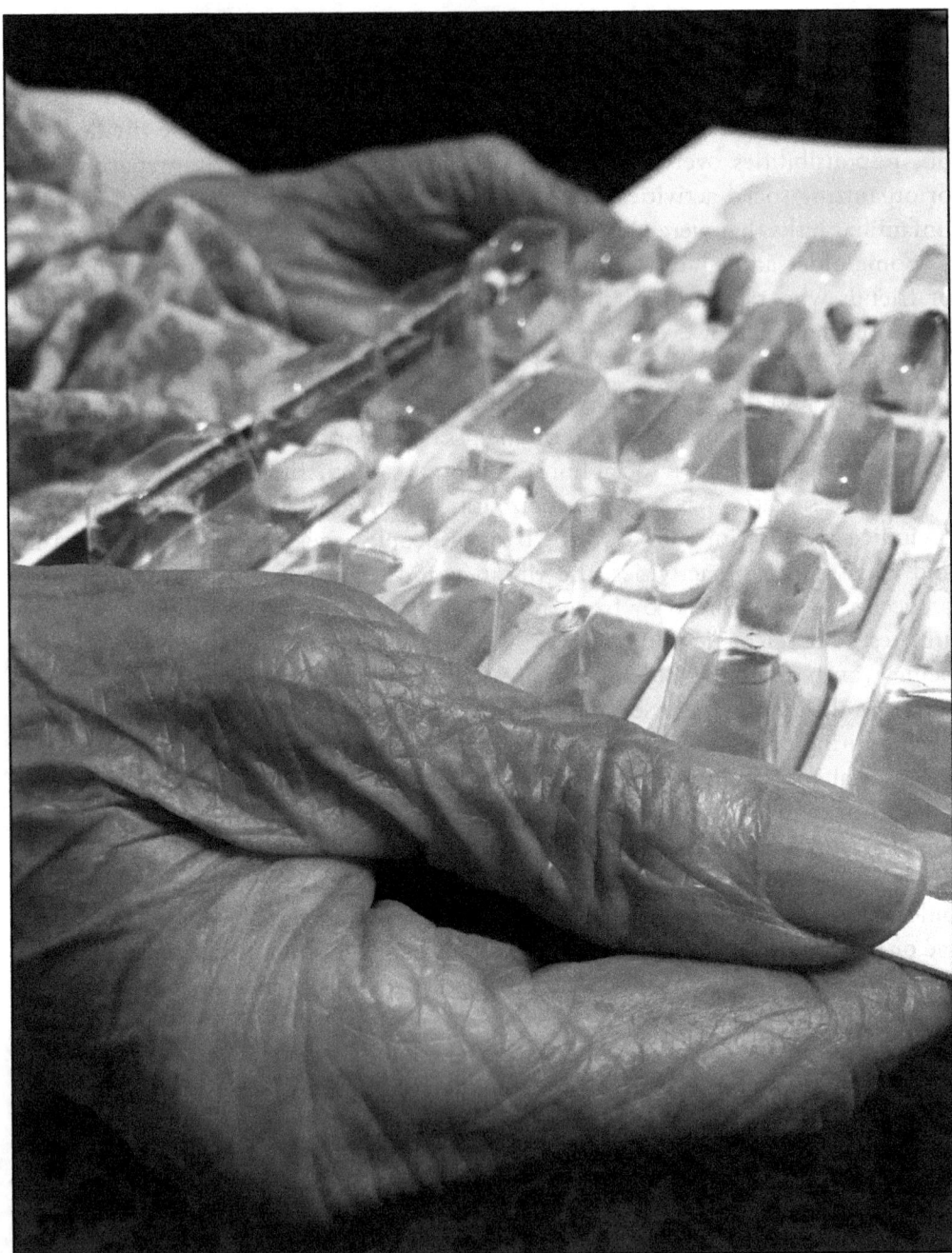

Figure 10.3: Older adults experiencing depression are at greater risk for *polypharmacy*, the regular use of multiple medications that may lead to adverse side effects or reactions. While pharmaceutical approaches may be beneficial for treating depression, health care providers should regularly evaluate medications to ensure that they are continuing to meet the client's needs.

Source: Daman Pabla, Photographer

Depression in older adults is seen much more often among those who feel regretful about their lives and in those who are experiencing substantial physical health challenges or who are isolated. We will discuss approaches to prevent and treat depression and other mental health challenges later in this chapter.

Death and Dying

Existential philosophers and anthropologists have brought attention to the weight carried by humans in being so aware of our own mortality. They point out that, along with the many advantages that humans have over the rest of the animal kingdom as a result of our highly developed brains, we are cursed with a serious drawback: we foresee and imagine our own deaths (Becker, 1973). Although in Canada most of us are fortunate enough to survive to a ripe old age, ultimately, we all face death. As Erikson indicated, this will be easier for those who have come to terms with their lives than those who feel a nagging sense of dissatisfaction or who hold many regrets.

Box 10.1: The Five Stages of Grief

The model developed by psychiatrist Elisabeth Kübler-Ross for understanding how we respond to the knowledge of impending death is widely known and used in caring and supporting those who are terminally ill (Kübler-Ross, 1973). She described five stages that humans commonly experience. However, these do not necessarily follow in the order that they are typically listed, nor do all people experience each stage. Responses are highly personal and individual, although Kübler-Ross did state that all people will experience at least two. The five stages are listed below and are accompanied by a representative statement that characterizes the thoughts and feelings that predominate in each stage:

Denial—*"This can't be happening to me."*
Anger—*"Why me? It's not fair!"*
Bargaining—*"I'll do anything for more time."*
Depression—*"I'm so sad, why bother with anything? I'm going to die."*
Acceptance—*"It's going to happen. I may as well prepare for it."*

In recent years, efforts have been made to help people die in comfortable surroundings. Where possible, most people would prefer to be in their homes or usual residences rather than in hospital. This can be supported by physicians, nurses, and other health care professionals, sometimes working together as a team and delivering care to dying people in their homes. However, in some circumstances, hospital or institutional care is preferred or necessary. Palliative care units and hospices are designed to be responsive to the emotional and spiritual needs of people who are dying and allow individuals to avoid unnecessary medical procedures. When cure is not possible, and often it is not, then a primary goal of health care should be to relieve suffering. Thankfully, advances in pharmacotherapy and new anaesthetic techniques, such as nerve blocks and spinal anaesthetics, often provide highly effective methods to remove or diminish pain. Consequently, most people with advanced or invasive disease can be helped to live their final days without profound physical suffering or discomfort. In June 2016, the Criminal Code of Canada was amended to allow for **Medical Assistance in Dying** (also referred to as MAID) for those deemed eligible. Since this time, there have been over 13,000 medically assisted deaths in the country, most of which were for people who experienced advanced illness and whose natural death was foreseeable. In 2021, following a thorough review of the regulations, additional provisions were added to the laws that govern MAID. Still in process, however, are guidelines and safeguards to inform how MAID may be used in cases where the sole condition is a mental illness (Government of Canada, 2021).

Cognitive Impairment and Memory Loss in Older Adults

The degree to which older people experience or exhibit problems with cognitive functions or memory loss varies widely. Many people maintain very sharp mental faculties well into their eighties and nineties. Some continue to engage in complex and challenging computational or linguistic activities, demonstrate formidable debating skills, and show little, if any, signs of limitations when compared to young whippersnappers. However, some older people observe that certain memory functions are not as sharp as they once were. The evidence for structural changes in the brain causing difficulties in memory associated with aging is still being studied and analyzed by researchers. Changes in structure of the grey or white matter of the brain have been associated with memory loss in some studies (Nyberg, 2017), and it is found that conditions such as hypertension (high blood pressure) may put some people at risk for repeated vascular and structural damage that impairs brain function over time (Tadic et al., 2016). Excessive use of alcohol or other psychoactive substances may lead to profound memory problems and other cognitive disturbances in older age as a result of physiological changes that occur in the brain.

Although older people sometimes worry when they notice themselves being forgetful or misplacing keys, studies have found that mild memory loss symptoms such as these are not a sign of impending dementia for most individuals (Eshkoor et al., 2015). Many of the memory challenges that older people experience have been found to have a psychological basis and may be a consequence of stress, mild depression, or being overtired. More serious memory challenges affect the ability to carry out everyday life activities. When older people are getting lost in familiar places; becoming confused about time, dates, people, or places; or forgetting to eat

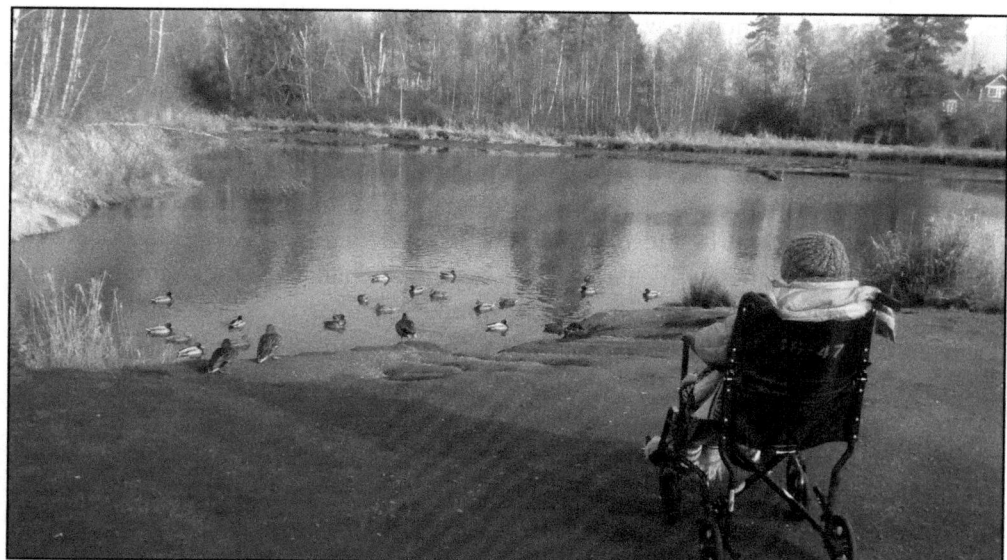

Figure 10.4: When a person is facing death, it is a very important time for family members. This photograph was taken by a student whose grandmother was facing death. Her comments about this photograph are as follows: "This is a picture of my grandma a couple of days before she died of leukemia. She was 90 years old and a healthy and strong woman who lived as a widow for 20+ years. She used to wear black almost every day to show her mourning and grief of my grandpa being gone. When she knew she was passing away she decided that she wanted to be removed from the hospital setting and just come home because she would rather die there than in a hospital bed. In this picture, I wanted to take her out and show her my favourite park that she had never seen before. I wanted to spend some time with her because I knew she didn't have much time left to live. I remember she said, 'Oh my, look at all those ducks, this is so lovely Jeanelle, thank you so much.' I will always remember this day and never forget it."

Source: Jeanelle Aldaba, Photographer

regularly, a careful determination of their cognitive and memory functions is needed and measures to ensure their safety are essential. Progressive memory challenges and other cognitive deficits in older adults may be caused by various medical conditions, such as hypothyroidism, HIV illness, or Parkinson's disease, but are commonly associated with the development of dementia.

Dementia in Older Adults

Dementia is a clinical syndrome that is characterized by general and irreversible loss of mental capabilities, such as memory, reasoning, judgment, and the ability to communicate. Most older adults do not have any signs of dementia; in 2013–2014, the prevalence of dementia was only 7.1 percent among those 65 years or older (Public Health Agency of Canada, 2017). However, the likelihood of having dementia increases progressively with advancing age. For example, while the prevalence of dementia is less than 1 percent among individuals 65–69 years, it rises to approximately 25 percent in individuals over 85 years.

There are many potential causes of dementia, with pathophysiological mechanisms that vary considerably. The most common cause of dementia is **Alzheimer's disease**. This disease is associated with characteristic structural changes to the brain, including **plaques** (i.e., small, dense deposits that accumulate in the spaces between brain cells, scattered throughout the brain) and **tangles**, (i.e., twisted strands of protein that are found within brain cells). As brain cells degenerate and die, the brain shrinks markedly in some regions. Researchers are working to understand the mechanisms that underlie Alzheimer's disease and their relationship to the structural changes.

Other types of dementia include those that are caused by vascular problems, infections, brain injury, excessive use of alcohol or other psychoactive substances, and nutritional deficiencies. Vascular dementias develop as a result of repeated loss of brain cells when blood vessels in the brain are damaged as a result of stroke, hypertension (high blood pressure), or other problems that interfere with the supply of oxygen to the brain.

Stages and Progression of Dementia

Irrespective of cause, dementia is sometimes classified into a series of stages according to the severity of cognitive disturbance that is present. The rate of progression

---

Box 10.2: Music Therapy

In recent years, there has been growing recognition of the therapeutic and healing nature of music for individuals with Alzheimer's or other forms of dementia. Rhythmic responses while listening to music require little cognitive processing, as they are controlled by the motor centre of the brain. This means that a person with dementia can actively engage in music even during late stages of the disease. Music is used to create positive moods and emotions, initiate social interaction, manage stress and agitation, and, perhaps most profoundly, stimulate memory recall. Many individuals tend to associate music with life events, memories, and emotions—whether they be good or bad. Music therapists will play music that is familiar to the individual from an era that is previous to their dementia, to which there has been an overwhelmingly positive response. Some people will recall memories that they associate with the music, others will sing or dance, and some have even remembered how to play instruments and can accompany the performer. For those who are able to dance, music therapy has increased physical activity, which can have tremendous health benefits for those who are generally otherwise sedentary. Worldwide, there has been an increase in non-profit organizations and music students volunteering to perform in long-term residential care facilities, as evidence grows for this non-pharmaceutical alternative approach to managing dementia.

varies substantially from one person to the next, though, on average, it will take about 10 years for progression from early, mild symptoms through to the development of severe dementia and profound disability.

The appearance of symptoms of dementia is often very gradual, and early symptoms may only be apparent in hindsight. In early stages, people may become apathetic and unable to adapt to changes. Memory problems may become evident through frequent repetition of questions, misplaced items, or confusion about events. Some people may appear to become more self-centred and less concerned with the feelings of others or become more irritable or upset when things do not go smoothly.

In moderate stages of dementia, symptoms are more disabling. Memory problems generally become significant with more frequent and extensive forgetfulness and confusion about time, people, or events. If away from familiar surroundings, an individual may become lost. In this stage, it is not unusual for people to wander out of their residences, walking aimlessly and unable to find their way home. Irritability and difficulties in behaviour may increase, and it is not uncommon for people to neglect their food intake and hygiene.

With severe dementia, disability becomes profound. Memory loss often becomes so severe that individuals can no longer recognize close family members or friends. Some individuals may become aggressive or combative, and many become incontinent and unable to feed or dress themselves.

It is essential to carry out careful assessments of the ability of people with dementia to perform activities of daily living to ensure their safety and proper care. Structured assessments have been developed to determine one's capacity to undertake activities such as meal preparation, shopping, telephone use, handling personal finances, travelling alone by car or public transportation, dressing, grooming, bathing, and toileting. Such assessments are carried out by occupational therapists (OTs) or other health care workers and are used to determine the level of care and support needed.

Box 10.3: A New Alzheimer's Treatment?

Although there is currently no cure for Alzheimer's disease, recent studies performed on mice have rendered promising results. It is currently believed that Alzheimer's is a result of a buildup of amyloid plaque that interferes with the function of neurons and causes brain cells to die. Researchers in the study injected microbubbles into the brains of the mice; they disturb the blood-brain barrier when activated by ultrasound. This then allows molecules to enter the brain and stimulate cells that reduce amyloid plaque. In mice, this resulted in an elimination of amyloid plaque in 75 percent of treated mice. After treatment, mice responded better on memory tests and object recognition. Studies in human subjects are currently underway, including out of labs located in Toronto, Canada. Early findings suggest the safety and feasibility of this intervention, providing interesting insight into possible future treatments for this degenerative disease (Lipsman et al., 2018).

Health Promotion, Illness Prevention, and Treatment

In this section, we will discuss treatments and interventions that can be put into place to help people with dementia and other mental health challenges. Before doing so, however, we will describe some of the population and public health approaches that can help to promote good mental health and prevent mental health challenges among older adults.

Mental Health Promotion and Illness Prevention Strategies

The development of healthy practices and patterns of behaviour early in life may prove to be important in promoting one's mental health in later years. For example, healthy nutritional intake, moderation in the use of alcohol, physical exercise patterns, and social skills that are developed when someone is young, may contribute to good mental health as we age. Wearing helmets when cycling or participating in sports that involve a risk of head injury is a good practice that can prevent mental challenges later in life.

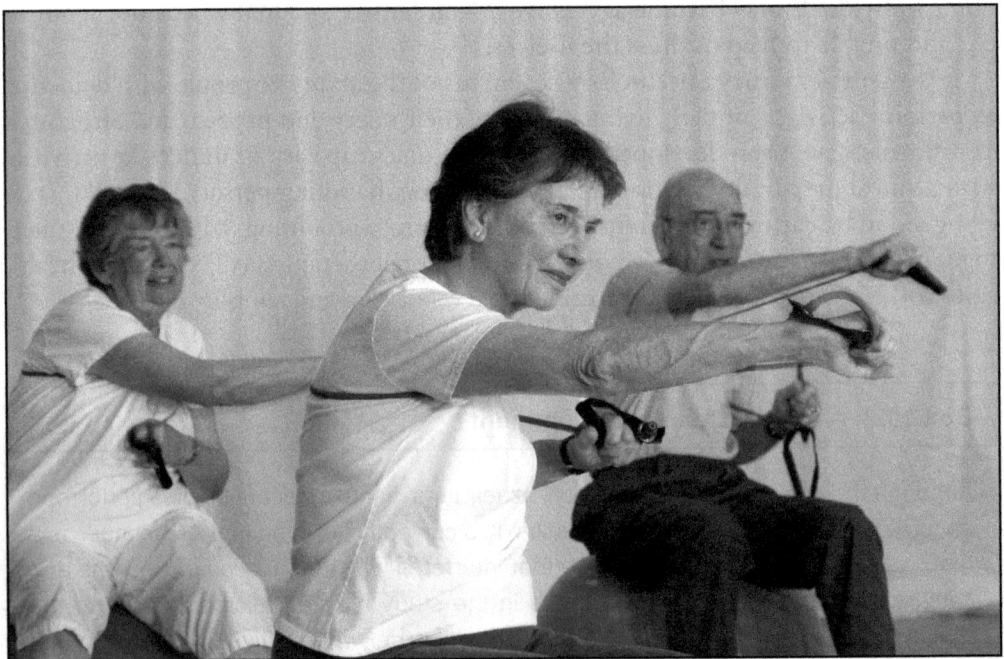

Figure 10.5: The development of healthy practices and patterns of behaviour early in life may prove to be important in promoting mental health in later years. Exercise promotes both mental and physical health, and there are many creative adaptations for older adults such as the chair exercises shown here.

Source: iStockphoto/alwekelo

There are also valuable health promotion and illness prevention strategies that can be put in place later in life. Programs that keep older adults physically and mentally active will help them to maintain cognitive abilities and social function and enjoy a higher quality of life. Work has also been done to help people who must cope with chronic physical health conditions by providing them with effective strategies to prevent depression and other negative consequences. Relief of pain, improvement of mobility, and social connectedness can have a strong impact on preventing depression and despair. Another beneficial strategy is to target preventive interventions to help older adults who are at particular risk of experiencing mental health challenges because of recent circumstances, such as the loss of a job or death of a spouse. Group programs and activities that connect people who have had similar experiences provide an excellent means of preventing illness through mutual support and other benefits of social networks.

Independence, Support, and Residential Care

Support services, home care workers, and various aids can be put in place to help older adults continue to live at home, even when they require regular care. These may be available through the health care system, social services, or community agencies such as the Alzheimer Society Canada. Often, however, much of the care of older adults falls to a spouse, adult children, friends, or other family members. If the person who needs care has severe physical or mental health challenges, then the burden on the caregiver can become great. It is not uncommon for one member of an older couple to become exhausted and overwhelmed by the continuous burden of providing care to a spouse. Since family members so often play a key role in looking after and supporting the care of older adults, health care providers must work closely and collaboratively with family members. Frequently, educational sessions or materials are made available to help family members gain the best possible knowledge about how to provide good quality support.

As described earlier, many older adults are left without family members or friends to help them. Such individuals are at high risk for adverse outcomes and can easily "fall through the cracks" unless there is a dedicated effort by health care workers to address their needs. It is not uncommon to discover that an older adult is experiencing such significant challenges that residential care is required in order to manage health concerns and protect physical safety. Such care is provided in what are referred to as "**long-term care facilities**" or "nursing homes." These facilities provide 24-hour personal care, nursing care, and medical attention, and they generally include social and recreational opportunities for residents.

Caring for People with Dementia

Individuals with dementia are often unable to recognize their own cognitive difficulties. This can lead to conflict or disputes with family members, friends, or caregivers who perceive them as requiring additional care or institutional treatment. In the early stages of dementia, people will frequently struggle with memory problems. Some forms of dementia, such as Alzheimer's disease, can sometimes be slowed in the early-to-intermediate stages with cholinesterase inhibitor medications. Although medical and physical intervention are important components of care for people with more advanced dementia, the quality of interpersonal and environmental support that is made available is a critical factor in determining how well or poorly individuals manage. At times, facilities and services for people with dementia may find it difficult to recruit skilled staff and financial cutbacks may result in staffing levels that are insufficient to provide quality time to residents (Boscart et al., 2019). Indeed, the troubling conditions of these care settings have been highlighted within the context of the COVID-19 pandemic, during which Canada had "the worst record among wealthy nations for COVID-19–related deaths in long-term care facilities" (Webster, 2021), which many considered a "national disgrace." Ideally, frequent human contact and caring interactions will form a substantial component of treatment provided to older adults, including people with dementia.

Box 10.4: Managing Memory Difficulties

The following approaches are useful in helping individuals with dementia to manage memory difficulties that might otherwise create problems and cause them to feel excessive distress:

1. *Diminish stress and distraction*. Memory problems are intensified with stress and in distracting situations where there is a lot of noise or activity. It helps to provide quieter and more relaxed surroundings where it is easier to concentrate on one thing at a time.
2. *Provide orienting information and avoid challenging questions*. It helps to provide cues and assistance to help people remember and orient themselves to people and places. For example, it is helpful to say "Look, your niece, Susan, has come to visit you" rather than "Do you remember who this is?"
3. *Instill a regular routine*. A regular routine around meals, bathing, exercise, and other activities often helps people to feel more secure and makes it easier to remember daily activities.
4. *Use memory aids*. Lists and clearly written instructions can help stimulate an individual's memory and support them in carrying out daily activities.

Treatment of Depression and Grief in Older Adults

As discussed in Chapter 4, depressive illnesses are among the most prevalent mental illnesses experienced throughout the lifespan. Among older adults, depression can be a substantial problem that requires careful attention and treatment. Depression is more common among older adults who are facing substantial physical health challenges, are socially isolated, or who have experienced substantial loss, such as the death of loved ones or the loss of employment or housing.

As in other phases of life, the treatment of depression is often multi-modal and may require intervention to help solve specific challenges that are contributing to one's depression (such as social isolation or physical disability) as well as counselling, psychotherapy, and use of medications or other physical treatments.

Antidepressant medications may be an effective treatment for depression among older adults. However, caution is required with their use in this age group due to potential side effects, interactions with other medications, or other difficulties that older people may have in metabolizing or tolerating antidepressant medications. In Chapter 14, we discuss the treatment known as "electroconvulsive therapy" (ECT), in which electrical current is passed through electrodes placed on an individual's head, resulting in a seizure of electrical activity throughout the brain. Although this sounds dangerous and odd, ECT appears to be a relatively safe and effective treatment for severe depression (Dong et al., 2018). Whereas the use of antidepressants is associated with substantial risks of medical complications, ECT can often be used safely, and consequently it is quite frequently used as a treatment for depression in older adults.

Responding to the Growing Older Adult Population

As mentioned at the beginning of this chapter, the proportion of older adults in Canada is increasing. Relatedly, recent research predicts that there will be doubling in the rate of dementia over the next decade (Alzheimer Society Canada, 2019). How will our health and social service systems respond to the needs of older adults as they grow in numbers? Efforts are being put in place to develop innovative approaches to health-promoting, preventive, and early intervention activities that will help keep older people healthier and more independent in the future. There is also increased training of health care and social service staff to develop the skills and knowledge needed to provide good care to older adults, including thoughtful attention to their mental health needs. Nevertheless, the challenges faced by our "greying population" are significant, and we must continue to ensure that we pay attention to the needs of our elders' mental health.

Conclusion

Older age often brings wisdom and experience, and most older Canadians enjoy good mental health, despite the inevitable aches and pains and the increased likelihood of various physical health challenges. Many older adults experience loss of loved ones, and some will end up lonely and socially isolated. This age cohort is at risk of suffering economic hardships and often end up marginalized in our communities, dependent on social services and supports. Various resources have been developed to help older adults live fuller, more active lives. Treatments to address depression and improve care of those with dementia are available. Additionally, palliative care offers an approach to help people at the end of their lives to experience more comfort and dignity, and changes to laws governing Medical Assistance in Dying (MAID) now mean that individuals who are experiencing significant health challenges can seek medical help to support their death. Increased attention to health promotion and illness prevention across the life course appears to foster good mental health in the later years.

Glossary

ageist: Prejudice and discrimination on the basis of people's age.
Alzheimer's disease: The most common cause of dementia; associated with characteristic structural changes to the brain.
dementia: A clinical syndrome characterized by general and irreversible loss of mental capabilities such as memory, reasoning, judgment, and the ability to communicate.
frail: The presence of significant physical or mental health challenges that interfere with older adults' independence and require them to depend on others for aspects of care and daily function.
long-term care facilities: Institutions that provide 24-hour personal care, nursing care, and medical attention and generally include social and recreational opportunities for residents.
Medical Assistance in Dying (MAID): The provision of medical help to support death for people who experience advanced illness and whose natural death is foreseeable.
plaques: Small, dense deposits that accumulate in the spaces between brain cells, scattered throughout the brain.
tangles: Twisted strands of protein that are found within brain cells.

Critical Thinking Questions

1. What are some of the unique mental health challenges that affect older adults?
2. Is modern society an ageist society? Explain.
3. Describe the stages of dementia.
4. Select a mental health promotion or mental illness prevention strategy. Briefly describe the approach and explain how it can benefit the mental health of older adults.
5. What are key factors to consider when caring for older adults with dementia or other mental health challenges?

Recommended Readings

Hartt, M., Biglieri, S., Rosenberg, M. W., & Nelson, S. E. (Eds.). (2021). *Aging people, aging places: Experiences, opportunities, and challenges of growing older in Canada*. Bristol University Press.

Picard, A. (2021). *Neglected no more: The urgent need to improve the lives of Canada's elders in the wake of a pandemic*. Random House Canada.

Prohaska, T. R., Anderson, L. A., & Binstock, R. H. (2012). *Public health for an aging society* (3rd ed.). Johns Hopkins University Press.

Zarit, S. H., & Zarit, J. M. (2012). *Mental disorders in older adults: Fundamentals of assessment and treatment* (2nd ed.). Guilford Press.

Recommended Websites

Alzheimer Society Canada. www.alzheimer.ca

Canadian Coalition for Seniors' Mental Health. www.ccsmh.ca

Public Health Agency of Canada—Healthy Aging in Canada: A New Vision, A Vital Investment—A Discussion Brief. www.phac-aspc.gc.ca/seniors-aines/alt-formats/pdf/publications/public/healthy-sante/vision/vision-eng.pdf

World Health Organization—Mental Health of Older Adults. www.who.int/news-room/fact-sheets/detail/mental-health-of-older-adults

References

Alzheimer Society Canada. (2019). Latest information and statistics. https://alzheimer.ca/en/Home/Get-involved/Advocacy/Latest-info-stats

Becker, E. (1973). *The denial of death*. Free Press.

Boscart, V. M., McNeill, S., & Grinspun, D. (2019). Dementia care in Canada: Nursing recommendations. *Canadian Journal on Aging/La Revue Canadienne du Vieillissement, 38*(3), 407–418. https://doi.org/10.1017/S071498081800065X

Dong, M., Zhu, X. M., Zheng, W., Li, X. H., Ng, C. H., Ungvari, G. S., & Xiang, Y. T. (2018). Electroconvulsive therapy for older adult patients with major depressive disorder: A systematic review of randomized controlled trials. *Psychogeriatrics, 18*(6), 468–475. https://doi.org/10.1111/psyg.12359

Ebly, E. M., Hogan, D. B., & Fung, T. S. (1996). Correlates of self-rated health in persons aged 85 and over: Results from the Canadian Study of Health and Aging. *Canadian Journal of Public Health/Revue canadienne de Santé publique, 87*(1), 28–31.

Eshkoor, S. A., Hamid, T. A., Mun, C. Y., & Ng, C. K. (2015). Mild cognitive impairment and its management in older people. *Clinical Interventions in Aging, 10*, 687–693. https://doi.org/10.2147/CIA.S73922

Fuller-Thomson, E., Serbinski, S., & McCormack, L. (2014). The rewards of caring for grandchildren: Black Canadian grandmothers who are custodial parents, co-parents, and extensive babysitters. *GrandFamilies, 1*(1), 4–31.

Government of Canada. (2021). *New medical assistance in dying legislation becomes law.* https://www.canada.ca/en/department-justice/news/2021/03/new-medical-assistance-in-dying-legislation-becomes-law.html

Kübler-Ross, E. (1973). *On death and dying.* Routledge.

Lipsman, N., Meng, Y., Bethune, A. J., Huang, Y., Lam, B., Masellis, M., Herrmann, N., Heyn, C., Aubert, I., Boutet, A., Smith, G. S., Hynynen, K., & Black, S. E. (2018). Blood–brain barrier opening in Alzheimer's disease using MR-guided focused ultrasound. *Nature Communications, 9,* Article 2336. https://doi.org/10.1038/s41467-018-04529-6

Nyberg, L. (2017). Functional brain imaging of episodic memory decline in ageing. *Journal of Internal Medicine, 281*(1), 65–74.

Public Health Agency of Canada. (2017). *Dementia in Canada, including Alzheimer's disease: Highlights from the Canadian Chronic Disease Surveillance System.* https://www.canada.ca/en/public-health/services/publications/diseases-conditions/dementia-highlights-canadian-chronic-disease-surveillance.html

Ravary, A., Stewart, E. K., & Baldwin, M. W. (2019). Insecurity about getting old: Age-contingent self-worth, attentional bias, and well-being. *Aging & Mental Health, 24*(10), 1636–1644. https://doi.org/10.1080/13607863.2019.1636202

Statistics Canada. (2019a). *Deaths and age-specific mortality rates, by selected grouped causes.* https://www150.statcan.gc.ca/t1/tbl1/en/tv.action?pid=1310039201

Statistics Canada. (2019b). *Population estimates on July 1st, by age and sex.* https://www150.statcan.gc.ca/t1/tbl1/en/tv.action?pid=1710000501

Statistics Canada. (2019c). *Population projections: Canada, provinces and territories, 2018 to 2068.* https://www150.statcan.gc.ca/n1/daily-quotidien/190917/dq190917b-eng.htm

Tadic, M., Cuspidi, C., & Hering, D. (2016). Hypertension and cognitive dysfunction in elderly: Blood pressure management for this global burden. *BMC Cardiovascular Disorders, 16*(1), 208. https://doi.org/10.1186/s12872-016-0386-0

Webster, P. (2021). COVID-19 highlights Canada's care home crisis. *The Lancet, 397,* 183. https://doi.org/10.1016/S0140-6736(21)00083-0

The World Bank. (2021). *Life expectancy at birth—Canada.* https://data.worldbank.org/indicator/SP.DYN.LE00.IN?locations=CA

World Health Organization. (2021). *Global Health Observatory (GHO) data: Life expectancy.* https://www.who.int/data/gho/data/indicators/indicator-details/GHO/life-expectancy-at-birth-(years)

Chapter 11

Responding to Mental Health Crisis, Emergency, and Disaster

> I have left orders to be awakened at any time in case of national emergency, even if I'm in a cabinet meeting.
> —Ronald Reagan (40th US president)

Introduction

In this chapter, we discuss how various systems and services in Canada respond to mental health challenges. When mental distress increases to unmanageable levels or puts individuals at risk of harm, a mental health challenge can become a **crisis** or emergency. It is particularly important to respond well during such situations, both because risk of harm must be averted and because the handling of such incidents can have long-standing impacts on those who experience them. If a person feels that they were treated unfairly or inappropriately, this negative impression of treatment systems and services can be difficult to change. Consequently, a person who has had a bad experience during a mental health crisis or emergency may be reluctant to receive services in the future. In some circumstances, this can detract from opportunities to obtain meaningful support and recovery.

Coping

While there are numerous approaches to understanding human behaviour and the ways that people deal with life challenges and overcome obstacles to achieve their goals, coping plays a key role (Lazarus, 1993). **Coping** can be characterized as finding ways to accomplish goals despite barriers and challenges. Each of us has goals to accomplish, even from the very beginning of our lives. Infants cannot articulate their goals, and yet they must accomplish goals of considerable difficulty—learning to walk, acquiring language, and dealing with the frustrating and inconsistent behaviours of adults. These are formidable challenges! With maturation, goals change, as do the barriers to their attainment, and the person finds new ways to overcome obstacles and (mostly) attain goals. Over time, goals become increasingly individualized—one person may seek excellence in a sport, another might pursue financial success, and so forth.

For much of the world's population, coping is often focused on the need to remain adequately fed, clothed, and sheltered. For most of us living in higher-income countries, such as Canada, goals and needs mostly involve the struggle to be loved, esteemed, and successful. A useful way to think about these different levels of needs and goals is in terms of Abraham Maslow's Hierarchy of Needs (see Figure 11.1). Each of these needs, at each level, represents important goals that require a different set of cognitive and behavioural skills and approaches, that is, different **coping strategies** (Carver et al., 1989).

Individuals develop unique ways of accomplishing goals: habitual behaviours, modes of problem solving, forms of social interaction, and so on. These characteristic

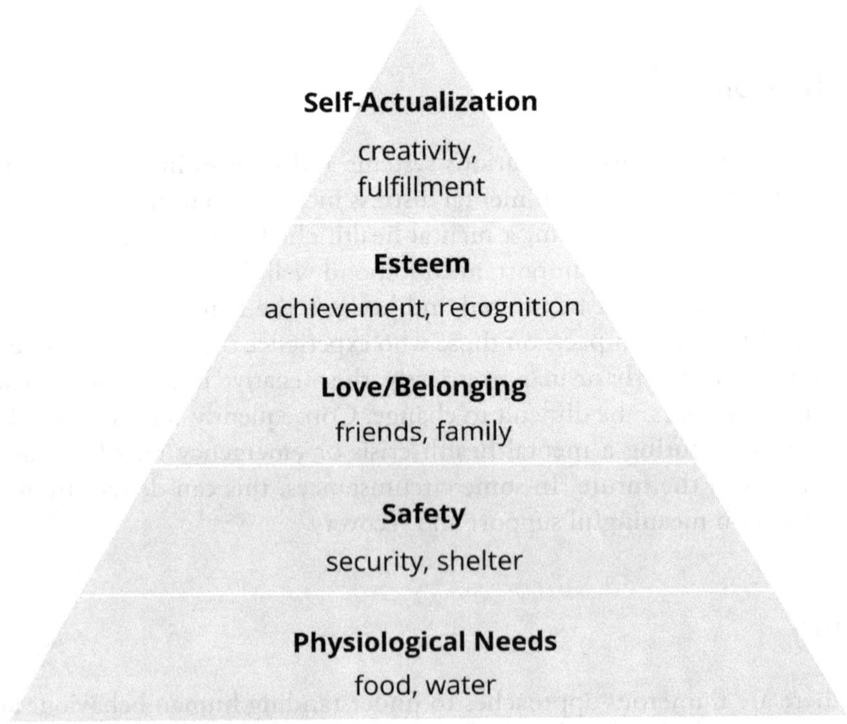

Self-Actualization
creativity, fulfillment

Esteem
achievement, recognition

Love/Belonging
friends, family

Safety
security, shelter

Physiological Needs
food, water

Figure 11.1: In Maslow's Hierarchy of Needs, the greatest and most fundamental needs occur at the bottom of the pyramid and must be achieved before the individual will be able to rise up the pyramid towards the ultimate goal of achieving their full potential, or *self-actualization*.

ways of thinking and acting in order to accomplish goals can be described as "coping styles." Each of us has a characteristic coping style, our own way of making a path through this difficult life to reach the goals important to us. For example, one person will approach a looming deadline for a term paper mainly through problem-focused coping, cancelling other activities to focus on the paper, or applying for an extension. Another person will respond with emotion-focused coping, seeking reassurance from friends or convincing oneself that the term paper doesn't really mean that much (Folkman & Lazarus, 1985). If you think about people you know, you can see how each has a characteristic coping style. When under stress, one person will increase exercise, another will increase social activities, another will spend more time alone, and another will drink more alcohol. They all have coping styles that typically work, most of the time, and only become problematic when exaggerated, self-destructive, or overly fixed.

Stress

When the demands and challenges of your life situation exceed your capacity to manage them you will experience **stress**. Stress can be defined as "the result of a relationship with the environment that the person appraises as significant for [their] well-being, and in which demands tax or exceed available coping resources" (Montero-Marin et al., 2014). There are many definitions of stress, but they all share this basic concept of an imbalance between demands and coping capacity. When challenges operate in this way, taxing or overtaxing an individual's coping ability, they are described as **stressors**. Note that a situation perceived by one person as highly stressful may be perceived by another as minimally stressful, depending on each person's particular coping style and goals. For example, if it is extremely important to be perceived as self-reliant, then asking for help may be a significant stressor; for someone who does not place such a high value on a self-reliant image, asking for help will not be stressful at all.

Most of us deal with a certain degree of stress as we grapple with problematic life situations and challenges. It's part of being human. Ideally, we will put our own internal resources into play effectively and, if needed, obtain assistance from friends, family members, health professionals, and others. But sometimes the level of stress becomes unmanageable, and our coping resources are exhausted. At those times, we may enter a state of crisis.

Crisis

In the crisis state, we feel overwhelmed by our life situation—we experience ourselves as unable to cope with important challenges and to achieve crucial goals. Our usual means of maintaining balance are unsuccessful and we feel a sense of disequilibrium or even chaos (Echterling et al., 2018). When we have difficulty coping, we tend to increase our efforts and shift to a mode of "urgent coping" in order to regain control—perhaps turning to family members for extra support or taking time away from work or school activities. It is when these attempts to regain equilibrium fail that we can find ourselves in a state of crisis.

Crisis states have been defined as

> limited time periods of upset in the psychosocial functioning of individuals, precipitated by current exposure to environmental stressors, which appear to be turning points in the development of mental disorder. (Caplan, 1989)

This brings us to one of the key elements of crisis states—someone may have a coping style that works quite well in their usual life situation, but then the situation changes. Perhaps the level of stress increases dramatically, or a different kind of stress emerges. Picture someone with a fairly rigid and emotion-focused style of coping. This person is comfortable with a high level of predictability in work and personal life but is suddenly given a new kind of work project that is unpredictable and quite novel. This person might find the new project to be exceedingly difficult. Their natural tendency would be to seek reassurance from friends and vent about the situation—but if this is unsuccessful, they may become increasingly anxious and unhappy, feeling inadequate. Furthermore, if this person receives negative feedback about their handling of the situation, they might begin to experience stress effects such as poor sleep, excessive worry, or anxiety. As this continues, this person might go into a state of crisis—this might include becoming depressed due to the feeling of helplessness and the failure of their usual coping style.

Another key element of crisis is that individuals may do "more of the same"—that is, show an exaggerated form of their usual coping style—and perhaps make the situation worse. This person who has an emotion-focused style of coping and who can be quite rigid might become even more rigid and emotion-focused. This may involve them desperately seeking out others' support and sympathy while trying to respond to the stressful situation and return to a more predictable set of tasks (which could elicit resentment from others and worsen the situation). Or consider individuals who tend to become indignant and slightly aggressive when others do not comply with their wishes—this behaviour may trigger resentment and resistance on the part of others, which in turn may lead to increased anger and indignation, creating more resistance, and so forth. If that spiral of ineffective coping continues long enough, they might find themselves in a state of crisis. It is common for individuals to enter a state of crisis through this kind of vicious spiral, with situational difficulties being handled by relatively ineffective coping mechanisms, leading to more frustration and an increase in the same ineffective coping, leading to a worsened situation (see Figure 11.2).

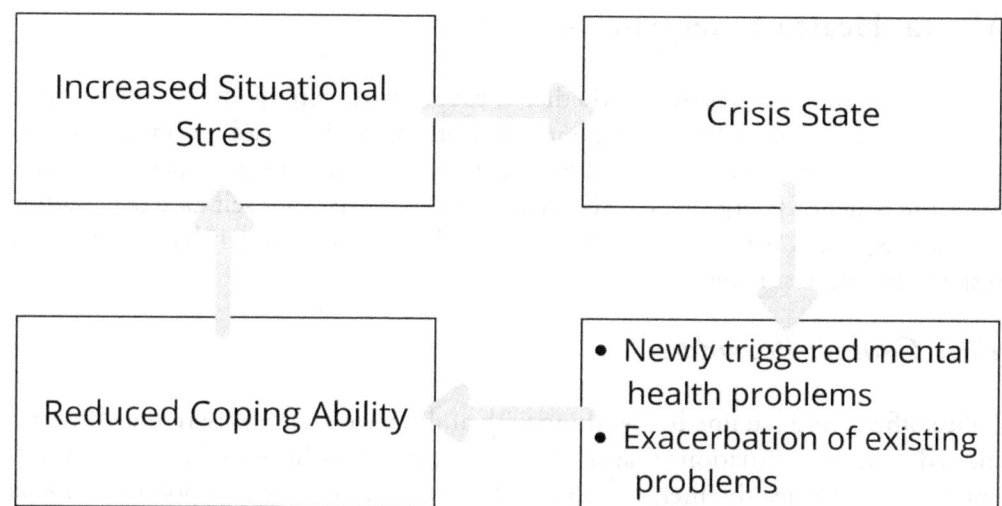

Figure 11.2: Crisis cycle.

Mental Health and Crisis

The state of crisis relates to mental health challenges in several ways. First, it may be that an individual has a long-standing mental health condition that reduces their ability to cope with life challenges and therefore makes this person more vulnerable to crisis. In this case, the mental health condition would represent a vulnerability to stress and a risk factor for crisis (Devylder et al., 2013). Second, a long-standing mental health condition may in itself represent a substantial source of stress—for example, if a chronic psychotic condition causes an individual to be evicted from housing and become homeless. Homelessness represents an extraordinarily stressful life situation, sufficient to overwhelm anyone's coping skills and cast them into crisis. Furthermore, a stressful situation may exacerbate a pre-existing mental health condition, making its symptoms acutely worse in the context of the crisis state. For example, an individual with bipolar disorder might find that a situation of unusual stress triggers the onset of manic symptoms—needless to say, the presence of manic symptoms will make it harder to cope with the stressful situation. This can feed into the kind of crisis spiral we described above. Third, high situational stress and loss of control associated with a crisis state may trigger mental health symptoms, especially depression or anxiety. It is not uncommon for people with depression to describe themselves as feeling helpless and unable to deal with life challenges, in effect, as feeling "defeated" by their lives. This state of feeling a lack of control and inability to change present circumstances has been described as "learned helplessness" (Seligman, 1972) and is viewed as a central feature of depression. Alternatively, the sense of overwhelming fear or apprehension often associated with crisis may give rise to anxiety symptoms, such as panic or obsessive worry.

Mental Health Emergencies

If a crisis state is not resolved (whether through extra coping efforts, lessening of situational stress, or additional support from others) and instead becomes more intense, it may transition to a mental health emergency. In the emergency state, there are acute issues of safety, whether because of dangerously poor self-care (e.g., failing to eat adequately, exposing oneself to physical risks, etc.) or self-harm behaviour (especially risk of suicide).

First-Contact Providers

Police officers and paramedics working with ambulance services are frequently summoned to address situations that involve unpredictable behaviour by people experiencing a mental health emergency. Indeed, they are often the first point of contact in such situations. It may be that police are called when an individual who is experiencing psychosis begins yelling on the street or when someone expresses suicidal intent. Police officers are often placed in difficult situations, where they have to work outside of their range of training and comfort. At times, this results in the use of physical aggression, which may have been avoided if a mental health care provider were involved. In the summer of 2020, concerns about police involvement in responding to mental health emergencies rose to prominence following several cases in which people with mental ill health were harmed or even lost their life during a police "wellness check" or other altercation. In response, some mental health advocates engaged in campaigns to "defund" the police and redirect resources to mental health services and response. Even prior to these events, however, there was a move towards including mental health workers in police response units to help defuse situations with the least possible violence. Further initiatives such as these are still very much needed

The Mental Health Act

When police or paramedics suspect that a person may be suffering with a mental health challenge, they are empowered to transport that individual to a hospital or other facility under the **Mental Health Act**, a piece of legislation that governs such circumstances. Each province and territory has a unique Mental Health Act, so there is variation across the country in regard to various details, such as the length of time that someone may be detained or hospitalized on an involuntary basis. Typically, an assessment by one or more physicians is required within a certain time period. If an individual is judged by these physicians to require hospitalization because of mental health reasons, the individual may be ordered to stay in a "designated mental health facility," typically a hospital, on an involuntary basis. When the Mental Health Act is applied in this way, the procedure is referred to as "committal."

One of the key issues that arises with hospitalizations due to mental health challenges is that of balancing the goal of ensuring safety (protecting the individual from causing harm to self or others) with the goal of ensuring that rights are respected (imposing the least possible restriction on the individual). In line with the first goal, hospitals will typically rely on legal certification or committal procedures, gaining the authority to hold the individual in hospital with or without their consent. This does not mean that hospitals now have a free hand in administering treatments—the legislation governing committal defines the sorts of treatment that may be administered against the patient's will and those that may not be administered without permission (given by the patient or by a designated representative of the patient). Typically, individuals who have been committed to a facility have the right to ask that this decision be reconsidered within a fixed period of time by a review board. These individuals must be clinically evaluated, and committal must be formally renewed at legally fixed intervals.

When a patient refuses prescribed treatment, such as antipsychotic medication, a number of complex procedures come into play. One is the evaluation of the patient's competence with regard to making treatment decisions. If the patient is judged by a physician to be incompetent to make treatment decisions, a "substitute decision-maker" may be appointed, either a person who has been selected by the patient, the nearest relative, the Public Guardian, or another individual identified by provincial legislation (Psychiatric Patient Advocate Office, 2016).

A fairly recent variation on committal is the community treatment order, which requires the individual to accept specific treatment or support in the community for a specified period of time. A supervisor will be designated to oversee this order and ensure that the individual is receiving the required care, for example, appearing for community clinic follow-up visits. The community treatment order can be enforced, that is, the supervising physician can authorize a police officer to apprehend the individual, who is then taken to a designated facility for examination.

When it comes to involuntary hospitalization, clinical and legal worlds meet in a way that causes much anxiety and potential conflict for health care providers, family members, and, of course, individuals experiencing mental health emergencies. The nature and details of these intersections between health care and law are often poorly understood, even by those working directly with the legislation (e.g., clinicians, police). Given this, we dedicate Chapter 13 entirely to this topic, covering the nuances of the Mental Health Act as well as patients' experiences with this legislation.

Hospital Emergency Departments

Hospitals have emergency departments to which individuals experiencing mental health emergencies can be brought for urgent care. Yet hospital emergency departments are hectic places; individuals with mental health emergencies often have a difficult time dealing with these environments. Furthermore, emergency departments are more geared towards managing physical emergencies, and staff in these settings often feel poorly equipped to effectively care for people experiencing mental health challenges. Consequently, mental health emergencies are ideally handled in hospital units specialized for this kind of work. Over the last 20 years, hospitals across North America have developed various kinds of intensive and brief stay units focused on rapid assessment and treatment of mental health emergencies.

Crisis Lines, Shelters, and Other Crisis Services

Not all mental health crises or emergencies are dealt with in hospital emergency departments or other health care settings. Some are averted and addressed through crisis lines, which generally provide quick access to advice, information, and referral over the telephone. Staff may respond by steering a person to appropriate resources or by helping to de-escalate crises. Crisis lines may be operated by volunteers or paid workers and are often run by non-profit organizations and societies. Similar services can also be provided face-to-face or through mobile services, delivered by individuals or small teams of mental health professionals who travel (usually by car) to meet with an individual in crisis and provide help (Guo et al., 2014). Mobile services provide a critical connection between people experiencing mental health emergencies and other elements of the system of mental health response (hospitals, community health care providers, family members, police, etc.). Some of the advantages of mobile services include the ability to assess a patient's support system in context, better grasp the perspective of the patient and other caregivers, and more effectively preserve the patient's sense of autonomy.

Shelters provide short-term accommodation for people who are homeless or who are experiencing crises that have interrupted their living arrangements. Shelters are often needed by individuals who have been the subject of domestic violence or who have encountered a dispute, including youth who have left home. Many of these types of crises are precipitated by mental health challenges. The Canadian government reported that in 2018 there were 15,859 shelter beds operating each night in Canada (Government of Canada, 2018). Nevertheless, shelter beds are often in short supply, leading some individuals to seek temporary refuge in tents in city parks. Many people who experience homelessness identify these encampments as a safer and more independent alternative to shelter beds; however, city bylaws often prohibit overnight camping and people living in these temporary shelters experience frequent evictions, which can be quite distressing to those also experiencing mental health crises.

Acute Hospitalization

Following an assessment in a hospital emergency department (or other care setting), health care professionals may conclude that a person requires inpatient hospital treatment for an acute mental health challenge. Typically, this is done to ensure a safe environment for stabilization and treatment, but it may also be recommended when it is

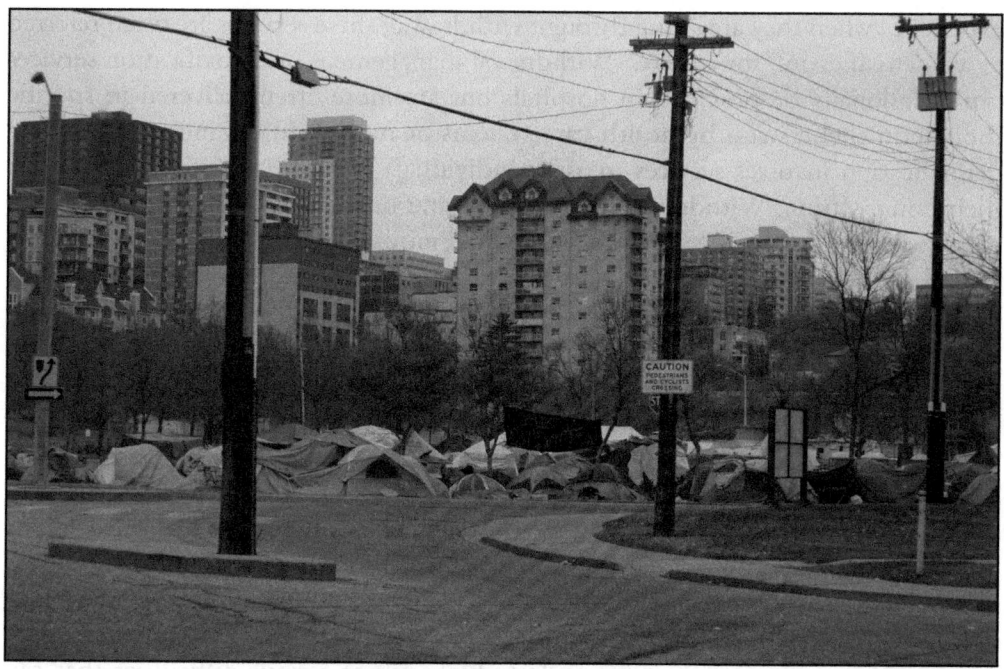

Figure 11.3: An encampment for people experiencing homelessness in Edmonton, Alberta. Tents provide temporary shelter, but challenging conditions such as evictions and extreme weather may further exacerbate mental health crises.

Source: Shutterstock/EdmontonMartin

judged that a person needs very intensive interventions that could not be administered on an outpatient basis. Hospital treatment for mental health conditions is generally provided in psychiatric inpatient units that are staffed and designed to address specific needs. These include the need for safety, which is commonly a concern among people who are acutely suicidal or experiencing intense psychotic symptoms. Treatment services often include medication, crisis management, and counselling or therapy, which may take place in individual and group settings. Inpatient psychiatric hospitalization tends to be relatively brief (averaging approximately two weeks), and efforts are made to make follow-up arrangements to continue treatment following discharge.

Acute Withdrawal Management and Detoxification Services

As discussed in Chapter 5, people who have become dependent on alcohol and/or other drugs often experience profound withdrawal symptoms when their use is stopped or interrupted. Withdrawal from such psychoactive substances can involve extreme physical illness and discomfort, and in some cases, death. **Withdrawal management** services primarily address the physical health challenges that people experience when they are going through withdrawal; these services are often referred to as "detoxification" or "detox." Withdrawal management or detoxification services can occasionally be provided in hospitals but are more often delivered in specific short-term shelters run by health care systems or non-profit organizations. Home detoxification involves services to assist individuals to undergo withdrawal within their home setting. Withdrawal management and detoxification may involve treatment with various medications to block or diminish physical symptoms of withdrawal, reduce adverse physical health complications and, ideally, include supportive care, counselling, or therapy.

Common Mental Health Emergencies

There are many mental health emergency situations, but the most frequent situations are the suicidal, psychotic, and substance use emergencies described in the following sections. These situations often overlap. Indeed, mental health emergencies frequently involve combinations of suicidality, acute psychosis, and substance use. Individuals with concurrent disorders (i.e., substance use in combination with another mental illness) are at particularly high risk of serious difficulties that can overwhelm coping mechanisms and lead to emergency situations.

Regardless of the type of precipitating factors at play, it is important that health care professionals and others who respond to crises do their utmost to minimize the distress that people experience when they are in the midst of a mental health emergency. Compassionate treatment that avoids the use of force or physical restraint and maintains a respectful approach will help to create a sense of trust that may have long-lasting benefits. As discussed in Chapter 6, a person who feels they have been treated inappropriately or violently by hospital staff, police, or others during a mental health crisis may experience trauma and develop an enduring mistrust and avoidance of health care, contributing to poor outcomes.

The Suicidal Emergency

When a person's coping abilities are overwhelmed, often triggered by increased stress or mental health challenges, suicidal thoughts and behaviours may develop. In such circumstances, health care providers will first aim to determine the level of suicide risk, which requires the assessment of a number of key factors. These include whether the person has made an active suicide plan, the dangerousness of any such plans, access to potentially lethal means of self-harm, previous self-harming behaviour, situational factors that could precipitate further crises, specific mental or substance use challenges that could influence suicidal behaviour, and the presence or absence of social supports.

The next major task is to help the person to lessen their suicidal feelings, that is, to address suicidality as a clinical problem. Various interventions can be used to help reduce suicide risk depending on the particular situation and circumstances being faced by the individual. Treatment of outstanding mental health and/or substance use challenges may assist in diminishing suicidal ideas and impulses. Often, it is beneficial to work with the individual experiencing suicidal thoughts to identify alternative ways of thinking about problems that may feel impossible to fix. A useful explanatory model helps people to recognize that serious suicidal thoughts often arise when they feel that their lives have the following three characteristics:

- *Intolerability* (their life situation is so painful that it seems unbearable)
- *Interminability* (it feels like the challenging circumstances will go on forever)
- *Inescapability* (it seems like nothing they've tried has changed or will change their experience)

The next task is to help strengthen coping mechanisms, including increased tolerance for distressing emotions, modification of unrealistic and discouraging thoughts, and systematic problem-solving activities. The individual is helped to implement positive coping skills used previously. This is done by examining strategies that have been used successfully to manage challenging situations in the past and then being encouraged to apply some of these same skills. Another common intervention is the co-development of a safety plan. This consists of a written plan to help the individual stay safe in the short term, for example, by removing means of self-harm and identifying strategies for self-regulation and for accessing help from others. The person is assisted in sharing the safety plan with their support network, including health care providers, family members, and friends, in an effort to strengthen feelings of connectedness and support.

The Psychotic Emergency

Individuals in this kind of emergency state are experiencing a severe disturbance to their capacity to distinguish reality and think in a rational manner. Often, they have confused and frightening thoughts that can sometimes lead to behaviours that place themselves or others at significant risk. For example, an individual who believes that people are conspiring against them may "protect" themselves by physically assaulting strangers or refusing to eat in case their food is poisoned. Psychotic emergencies can occur with mental illnesses such as schizophrenia or bipolar disorder if psychotic symptoms such as delusions or hallucinations are prominent.

The first priority of health care professionals and first-contact providers will be to calm the individual and provide a safe environment to reduce any risk of harm. This often involves a strategy known as "rapid tranquilization," in which medications with antipsychotic or sedating properties are used to help de-escalate or settle the individual (Hirsch & Steinert, 2019). Once this initial risk reduction phase has been completed, clinical attention will focus on pharmacological treatment to reduce delusions and hallucinations.

More recently, there has been a shift in the standard approach to the short-term management of aggressive behaviour associated with a psychotic emergency. This involves a transition from a reliance on restrictive interventions, such as physical restraint or seclusion, to the use of "skills, methods, and techniques to reduce or avert imminent violence and defuse aggression when it arises (for example, verbal de-escalation)" (National Institute for Health and Care Excellence, 2015). Under this new approach, restrictive interventions are implemented only after efforts to de-escalate have failed. Note that this approach requires considerable training to enhance staff skill in sophisticated behavioural management techniques. Should a mental health service impose an expectation of non-restrictive management without adequate staff training, an unintended consequence might be that of exposing staff—and people experiencing mental health emergencies—to increased risk of physical and psychological harm.

Once there has been a meaningful degree of improvement in symptoms and safety, clinical focus will ideally shift to ensuring that the individual has community resources in place (e.g., housing, financial support, clinical services and supports, and so on) to make a successful transition out of hospital and to prevent recurrence of the problems that led up to the emergency situation.

The Substance Use Emergency

Individuals dependent upon psychoactive substances such as alcohol, cocaine, and methamphetamine may develop significant mental health challenges. For example, an individual who is intoxicated on methamphetamine may become disorganized and agitated and be brought to hospital by police or paramedics. Measures to prevent harm may be required, such as providing a safe environment or administering medications to diminish agitation. As the drug-induced state subsides over one or several days, the individual typically returns to "baseline" (their typical level of functioning) and is discharged. As discussed earlier, individuals who are in withdrawal from substance use may develop acute physical problems involving damage or dysfunction of bodily organs and may require withdrawal management services. Depression, psychosis, or other symptoms of mental illness may also occur as part of the withdrawal process.

Those who have experienced a crisis or emergency due to substance use should be assisted in accessing treatment services or other supports aimed at reducing substance use harms once the crisis has passed. Tragically, this does not usually occur, in part, because of the extremely limited availability of treatment services for substance use disorders. Although some high-quality treatment programs exist in Canada, they are not widely available, and many are not covered by our public health insurance plans. Therefore, unless an individual or family is able to pay "out of pocket" for such a program or has special benefits through their employers that will cover such services, treatment may be inaccessible. Another contributor to the service gap is the poor integration and communication among various systems that respond to the needs of individuals with substance use challenges. A report on substance use treatment in Canada noted: "People who may have significant health challenges, at a time of great personal strain, must navigate a complex and ever-changing labyrinth of services and supports" (National Treatment Strategy Working Group, 2008).

Responding to Disasters and Public Health Emergencies

Disasters and public health emergencies may occur as a result of "natural" environmental events (e.g., floods, earthquakes, and tsunamis); large-scale accidents (e.g., industrial fires and explosions, plane crashes); terrorist and wartime attacks and violence; or "extraordinary events" that pose a significant public health risk (e.g., spread

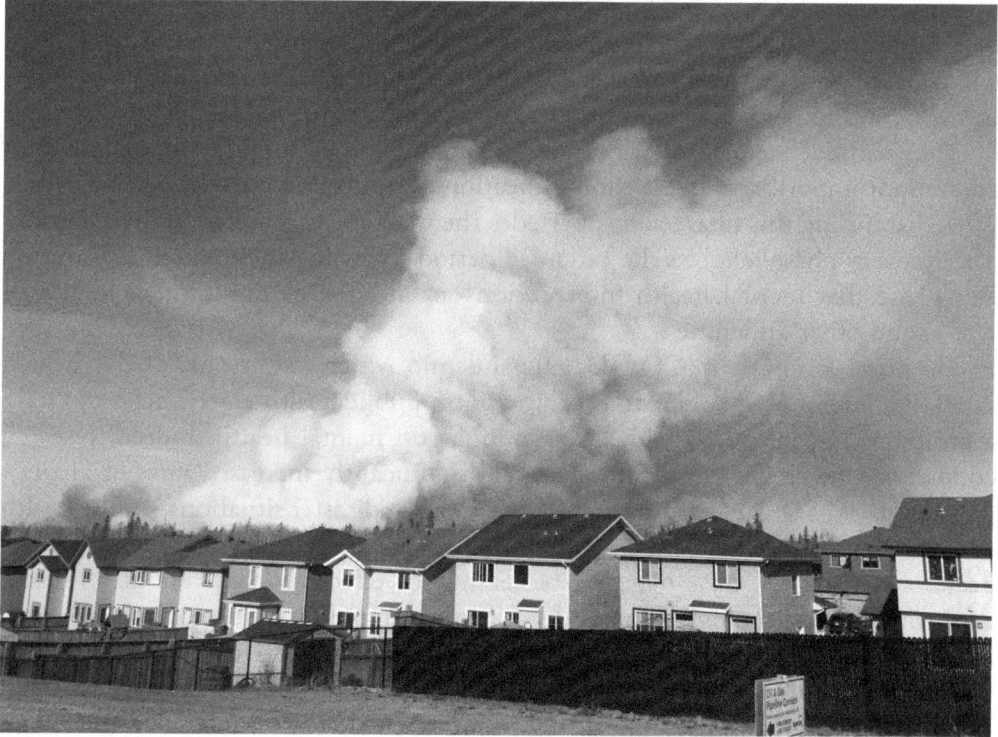

Figure 11.4: A wildfire burns behind a neighbourhood in Fort MacMurray, Alberta, in 2016. The day after this photo was taken, fire swept through the town, forcing over 88,000 people to evacuate. Thousands of buildings and homes were destroyed, and reconstruction efforts are still ongoing. Wildfires and other disasters have had significant impacts on the psychological health of Canadians.

Source: Shutterstock/CSDigitalMedia

of disease). In addition to the toll of death and injury, such disasters and emergencies may result in profound trauma that often affects the mental health of large groups of people simultaneously.

Since the 9/11 terrorist attack in the US in 2001, much has been learned about the nature of disaster response and approaches to enhance people's coping in the aftermath (Feder et al., 2016; Park et al., 2008). Fortunately, most individuals are able to recover from disasters with only transitory mental health symptoms that do not result in persistent psychological consequences or require formal intervention to restore mental health (Christodoulou et al., 2016). However, a portion will develop persistent post-traumatic stress disorder (PTSD; Beaglehole et al., 2018); it has been found that those who provide emergency response services are at particular risk.

Three phases have been described in relation to disaster response: the preparedness phase, the response phase, and the recovery phase (Laurendeau et al., 2007). The preparedness phase involves the advance planning and preparation of actions, communications, and leadership roles, including the training of individuals who will be responsible for various aspects of disaster response. The response phase refers to the period immediately following the disaster, when re-establishment of feelings of safety, confidence, competence, and social cohesion among the population is of paramount importance. Clear communication of information to the general public is needed during this phase and supersedes the need for psychological intervention. The recovery phase involves the extended period following the disaster. It is during this phase that mental health interventions are needed to diminish incidence of PTSD and other difficulties.

The novel coronavirus (COVID-19) pandemic, which was first declared in March 2020, has taught us that like disaster situations, public health emergencies can have a profound impact on individual and population mental health. Indeed, research conducted during the pandemic identified significantly increased rates of anxiety, depression, PTSD, and suicidality. However, unlike disaster situations, public health emergencies may not be contained to a discrete geographic region and certain aspects of disaster response may not be feasible or effective (e.g., central outreach, deployment of psychological responders). Moreover, public health emergencies such as pandemics are largely invisible—unlike a natural disaster—with limited observable indicators of safety or resolution of the threat. As Jacob Stern (2020) wrote in *The Atlantic* early on in the COVID-19 pandemic, "when a wildfire ends, the flames subside and the smoke clears. 'You have an event, and then you have the rebuild process that's really demarcated … It's not like a hurricane goes on for a year.' But pandemics do not respect neat boundaries: They come in waves, ebbing and flowing, blurring crisis into recovery." These and other elements of a public health emergency can contribute to heightened feelings of fear, uncertainty, and anxiety. If they persist for an extended period of time, they can overwhelm peoples' coping abilities and increase risk for prolonged or clinically significant mental health challenges. Indeed, some experts predict that the COVID-19 pandemic will result in a global mental health crisis of unprecedented magnitude—suggesting the need for substantial and coordinated recovery responses.

Conclusion

When usual coping mechanisms are overwhelmed, individuals may experience mental health crises or emergencies. An initial response to such situations may be carried out by police, paramedics, and other first responders; they will often transport people who are in crisis to hospital emergency departments for assessment. Crisis lines, emergency shelters, and other services can help to avert problems, provide temporary support, and assist people in obtaining additional help.

Common mental health emergencies include suicidal, psychotic, and substance use emergencies. Following assessment, people who are determined to require inpatient admission are hospitalized to receive treatment that usually includes medications and individual or group counselling or therapy. Withdrawal management, also known as "detoxification" services, may be provided to individuals who are experiencing substantial physical and mental health challenges during acute withdrawal from psychoactive substances.

Studies of the psychological outcomes of people who experience traumatic events, including disasters and public health emergencies, have found that most people have only transient problems, but some will experience persistent PTSD and other mental health challenges. Negative psychological outcomes can be minimized through good preparedness, well-organized responses immediately following disasters, and provision of appropriate interventions during the longer-term recovery phase.

Glossary

coping: Finding ways to accomplish goals despite obstacles and challenges.
coping strategies: A set of cognitive and behavioural skills and approaches used to meet goals and needs.
crisis: Limited time periods of upset in the psychological functioning of individuals, precipitated by current exposure to environmental stressors, which appear to be turning points in the development of mental illnesses.
Mental Health Act: A piece of legislation that regulates involuntary transportation and admission to psychiatric services for individuals suspected of experiencing mental illness.
stress: Occurs when the perceived pressure exceeds one's perceived ability to cope.
stressors: Environmental challenges that tax or overtax an individual's coping ability.
withdrawal management: Services that primarily address the physical health challenges that people experience when they are going through withdrawal from psychoactive substances.

Critical Thinking Questions

1. What are the key elements of a crisis?
2. What are the three ways in which a state of crisis relates to mental health?
3. What is the Mental Health Act and what issues arise with hospitalization due to mental health challenges?
4. Select one type of common mental health emergency and describe the tasks involved in addressing it.
5. What are the three stages in response to disaster? Briefly describe each stage.

Recommended Readings

Benas, N., & Hart, M. (2017). *Mental health emergencies: A guide to recognizing and handling mental health crises*. Hatherleigh Press.

Glick, R. L., Zeller, S. L., & Berlin, J. S. (Eds.). (2020). *Emergency psychiatry: Principles and practice*. Wolters Kluwer.

Halpern, J., & Vermeulen, K. (2017). *Disaster mental health interventions: Core principles and practices*. Routledge.

Lazarus, R. (2006). *Stress and emotion: A new synthesis*. Springer.

Taylor, C. (2019). *The psychology of pandemics: Preparing for the next global outbreak of infectious disease*. Cambridge Scholars Publishing.

Recommended Websites

Canadian Mental Health Association—Coping with Mental Health Crises and Emergencies. https://cmha.bc.ca/documents/coping-with-mental-health-crises-and-emergencies-2

Centres for Disease Control and Prevention—Emergency Preparedness and Response. https://emergency.cdc.gov

Crisis Services Canada. www.crisisservicescanada.ca/en

Mental Health First Aid Canada. www.mhfa.ca

References

Beaglehole, B., Mulder, R. T., Frampton, C. M., Boden, J. M., Newton-Howes, G., & Bell, C. J. (2018). Psychological distress and psychiatric disorder after natural disasters: Systematic review and meta-analysis. *The British Journal of Psychiatry, 213*(6), 716–722. https://doi.org/10.1192/bjp.2018.210

Caplan, G. (1989). Recent developments in crisis intervention and the promotion of support services. *Journal of Primary Prevention, 10*(1), 3–25.

Carver, C. S., Scheier, M. F., & Weintraub, J. K. (1989). Assessing coping strategies: A theoretically based approach. *Journal of Personality and Social Psychology, 56*(2), 267–283.

Christodoulou, G. N., Mezzich, J. E., Christodoulou, N. G., & Lecic-Tosevski, D. (Eds.). (2016). *Disasters: Mental health context and responses.* Cambridge Scholars Publishing.

Devylder, J. E., Ben-David, S., Schobel, S. A., Kimhy, D., Malaspina, D., & Corcoran, C. M. (2013). Temporal association of stress sensitivity and symptoms in individuals at clinical high risk for psychosis. *Psychological Medicine, 43*(2), 259–268. https://doi.org/10.1017/S0033291712001262

Echterling, L. G., Presbury, J. H., & Edson McKee, J. (2018). *Crisis intervention: Building resilience and resolution in troubled times.* Cognella Academic Publishing.

Feder, A., Mota, N., Salim, R., Rodriguez, J., Singh, R., Schaffer, J., Schechter, C. B., Cancelmo, L. M., Bromet, E. J., Katz, C. L., Reissman, D. B., Ozbay, F., Kotov, R., Crane, M., Harrison, D. J., Herbert, R., Levin, S. M., Luft, B. J., Moline, J. M., ... Reissman, D. B. (2016). Risk, coping and PTSD symptom trajectories in World Trade Center responders. *Journal of Psychiatric Research, 82*, 68–79. https://doi.org/10.1016/j.jpsychires.2016.07.003

Folkman, S., & Lazarus, R. S. (1985). If it changes it must be a process: Study of emotion and coping during three stages of a college examination. *Journal of Personality and Social Psychology, 48*(1), 150–170.

Government of Canada. (2018). *Shelter capacity report 2018.* https://www.canada.ca/en/employment-social-development/programs/homelessness/publications-bulletins/shelter-capacity-2018.html

Guo, S., Biegel, D. E., Johnsen, J. A., & Dyches, H. (2014). Assessing the impact of community-based mobile crisis services on preventing hospitalization. *Psychiatric Services, 52*(2), 223–228. https://doi.org/10.1176/appi.ps.52.2.223

Hirsch, S., & Steinert, T. (2019). The use of rapid tranquilization in aggressive behavior. *Deutsches Ärzteblatt International, 116*(26), 445–452. https://doi.org/10.3238/arztebl.2019.0445

Laurendeau, M. C., Labarre, L., & Senécal, G. (2007). The psychosocial dimension of health and social service interventions in emergency situations. *Open Medicine, 1*(2), 102–106.

Lazarus, R. S. (1993). Coping theory and research: Past, present, and future. *Psychosomatic Medicine, 55*(3), 234–247.

Montero-Marin, J., Prado-Abril, J., Demarzo, M. M. P., Gascon, S., & García-Campayo, J. (2014). Coping with stress and types of burnout: Explanatory power of different coping strategies. *PloS One, 9*(2), e89090. https://doi.org/10.1371/journal.pone.0089090

National Institute for Health and Care Excellence. (2015). *Violence and aggression: Short-term management in mental health, health and community settings.* https://nice.org.uk/guidance/ng10

National Treatment Strategy Working Group. (2008). *A systems approach to substance use in Canada: Recommendations for a national treatment strategy.* http://www.ccsa.ca/Resource%20Library/nts-systems-approach-substance-abuse-canada-2008-en.pdf

Park, C. L., Aldwin, C. M., Fenster, J. R., & Snyder, L. B. (2008). Pathways to posttraumatic growth versus posttraumatic stress: Coping and emotional reactions following the September 11, 2001, terrorist attacks. *American Journal of Orthopsychiatry, 78*(3), 300–312. https://doi.org/10.1037/a0014054

Psychiatric Patient Advocate Office. (2016). *Substitute decision makers (SDMs).* https://www.sse.gov.on.ca/mohltc/ppao/en/Pages/InfoGuides/2016_SDMs.aspx?openMenu=smenu_InfoGuides

Seligman, M. (1972). Learned helplessness. *Annual Review of Medicine, 23*(1), 407–412.

Stern, J. (2020, July 7). This is not a normal mental-health disaster. *The Atlantic.* https://www.theatlantic.com/health/archive/2020/07/coronavirus-special-mental-health-disaster/613510/

Chapter 12

Mental Health and the Criminal Justice System

Amanda Butler, Katherine Rossiter, and Tonia Nicholls

Injustice anywhere is a threat to justice everywhere.
—Martin Luther King, Jr. (American minister, activist, and civil rights leader)

Introduction

You might be asking: "What is the relevance of the criminal justice system to a book about the mental health system?" In fact, there are many important intersections between these two systems, including determining when it is appropriate to divert a person with a mental illness to an alternative system, as well as addressing their unique service needs from within the criminal justice system. Two common law principles provide the rationale for criminal justice officials to intervene in the lives of people with mental illnesses. Firstly, officials are granted power and authority to protect the safety of the community. Secondly, the *parens patriae* doctrine (Latin for "parent of the nation") is the authority of the government to intervene in the lives of people who are in need of protection (Lamb et al., 2002; Service, 2010). We begin this chapter with a brief overview of the criminal justice system in Canada. We then examine the characteristics and unique needs of people with mental illnesses who come into contact with the law, and the psychosocial circumstances that often result in the overrepresentation of people with mental illnesses in the criminal justice system. Finally, we discuss the relevance of mental illness at successive stages of the criminal justice process, including tribunals and programs developed specifically to respond to people with mental illnesses who come into contact with the criminal justice system.

The Criminal Justice System in Canada: A Brief Overview

Similar to the Canadian mental health system, the criminal justice system in Canada is comprised of a series of government agencies and institutions. The three main parts of this system include law enforcement (police), adjudication and dispositions (courts, Review Boards), and the agencies responsible for detaining and supervising sentenced offenders (correctional facilities and community corrections, forensic mental health services). Responsibility for the criminal justice system is shared between the federal, provincial, and municipal governments. The *Constitution Act of 1867* gave exclusive jurisdiction over matters of criminal law to the Parliament of Canada. Although the *Criminal Code* is federal law, provincial governments are responsible for forensic mental health services and for carrying out *Criminal Code* prosecutions. The provinces have the power to name quasi-criminal offences (also known as regulatory offences) within their jurisdictions. For example, provinces determine who can sell alcohol and under what conditions. Furthermore, the provinces are largely responsible for the administration of justice, and provincially established courts administer both civil and criminal law. Jurisdiction over correctional services is shared between the provincial and federal governments. People who are detained while waiting to be sentenced (i.e., remanded) or who are sentenced to custody for less than two years serve time in provincial facilities, whereas people sentenced to custody for two years or more serve time in federal facilities.

Most municipal governments in urban areas are given the authority to maintain their own local police forces. In 2019, there were 137 stand-alone municipal police services and 36 First Nations self-administered police services in Canada (Conor et al., 2020). Provincial police forces operating in Ontario (Ontario Provincial Police), Quebec (Sûreté du Québec), and Newfoundland (the Royal Newfoundland Constabulary) provide policing for communities without municipal police forces. The Royal Canadian Mounted Police (RCMP) is the Canadian national police agency, providing service at the federal level; they are also contracted to provide services in every province except Ontario and Québec. Because policing is largely a municipal and provincial responsibility, there is a great deal of variability in police structure, governance, and operations.

Part XX.1 of the federal Criminal Code concerns persons who were suffering from a mental disorder at the time they committed a criminal offence and/or at the time of their trial. A person may be found **Not Criminally Responsible on account of Mental Disorder** (NCRMD or "NCR") or Unfit to Stand Trial (UST) by a court if the *Criminal Code* criteria for the **disposition** (outcome of a charge) are met. An accused person who is found NCR or UST will come under the **Review Board** system, rather than the criminal court system. A Review Board is an administrative tribunal, established by the *Criminal Code*. Its purpose is to make decisions and orders concerning the liberty of individuals whom courts have found to be NCR for crimes committed while they were suffering from a mental illness, or whose mental illness makes them unfit to stand trial on criminal charges. The rationale for the Review

Board system is that special expertise is required to make appropriate decisions regarding individuals with mental illnesses.

If a person is arrested and convicted of a crime, depending on the severity of the crime and a range of individual and circumstantial factors, they may be sentenced to a term in custody or in the community. **Bail** is the procedure to determine if a person charged with a criminal offence will be released or detained while awaiting trial. **Probation**, which falls under provincial jurisdiction, is an option that allows a person to serve their sentence in the community, with conditions prescribed in a probation order. For those in federal custody, parole is a type of conditional release whereby an individual may serve a part of their sentence in the community under specified conditions.

A comprehensive discussion of the criminal justice system in Canada is beyond the scope of this chapter, but as is likely evident, the legislative framework is extremely complicated. The constitutional structure of Canada, with shared responsibility across all levels of government, poses many challenges to the efficiency and effectiveness of the system and the people who come into contact with it.

Figure 12.1: The courthouse in London, Ontario. Courts determine whether a person with a mental disorder is fit to stand trial within the court system, or whether they are deemed Not Criminally Responsible on account of Mental Disorder (NCRMD) or Unfit to Stand Trial (UST).

Source: Unsplash/Scott Webb

Overrepresentation of People with Mental Illnesses in the Criminal Justice System

People with mental illnesses are overrepresented at all levels of the criminal justice system, including interactions with police, courts, and corrections (Fazel & Danesh, 2002; Fazel & Seewald, 2012). Indeed, research suggests that as many as 1 in 20 police dispatches involves a person with a mental illness (Brink et al., 2011). A study of police interventions with people with mental illnesses in Montreal, Quebec, found that the most common intervention outcome was informal (e.g., counsel and release), followed by referral to hospital, and lastly, arrest (Charette et al., 2011). In the recent past, the number of and public profile of police encounters with persons with mental illnesses have increased significantly (Kouyoumdjian et al., 2019).

Once arrested, people with mental illnesses are more likely to be charged, are less likely to be released on bail, and are likely to spend considerably longer in custody before receiving bail (Council of State Governments Justice Centre, 2012; Charette et al., 2014). A Canadian study found that police interventions involving people with mental illnesses use 87 percent more resources than those involving individuals without mental illnesses (Charette et al., 2014). Importantly, the bail system disproportionately penalizes people who are living in poverty, who use substances, and/or who suffer from mental illnesses, by imposing strict conditions, including abstaining from using substances, housing conditions, treatment orders, check-in requirements, curfews, and no-contact conditions (i.e., orders to stay away from certain people or places). Symptoms of certain mental illnesses can impair one's ability to comply with bail conditions, adhere to treatment, and manage daily living. Although a person released on bail has not been found guilty of a crime, breaching a bail condition is a criminal offence in Canada (even if the breach does not involve criminal activity). Onerous bail conditions contribute to a revolving door cycle of rearrest, recharging, and reincarceration, especially among people with mental illnesses (John Howard Society of Ontario, 2015).

Given that we see disproportionate numbers of people with mental illnesses at all levels of the criminal justice system, it is not surprising that individuals with mental illnesses are also overrepresented within correctional institutions. A study conducted in British Columbia drew on intake screening data for every adult incarcerated over a nine-year period and found that the prevalence of any mental health need or substance use disorder among people admitted to provincial prison increased from 61 percent in 2009 to 75 percent in 2017. Furthermore, the proportion of people with co-occurring mental health needs *and* substance use disorders more than doubled during this time period (Butler et al., 2021). Similarly, between 1998 and 2007, the proportion of people in federal correctional facilities with significant mental health needs more than doubled in Canada (Sapers, 2011). Below, we consider explanations for this over-representation.

The Impact of Deinstitutionalization

Beginning in the 1960s, jurisdictions across Canada, and internationally, began to downsize and close major psychiatric institutions. Reasons for this transition included increasing awareness of inhumane conditions in some psychiatric hospitals, advances in psychotropic medications, changes in societal attitudes towards mental illnesses and civil liberties, and reduced government budgets (Kim, 2014). Psychiatric **deinstitutionalization** refers to a process of shifting mental health care from institutional care to community-based outpatient settings, as discussed in Chapter 1. Significant problems were produced by early reform efforts where the reduction in inpatient beds outpaced the expansion of community-based services and supports (Livingston et al., 2011). Previously, when people were institutionalized for severe and persistent mental illnesses, they were provided housing in large asylums. In this post-deinstitutionalization era, a place to live at the end of a hospital stay for psychiatric care is not guaranteed and people are regularly discharged to the street or shelters (Forchuk et al., 2006). This practice increases the risk of criminalization, homelessness, and unmet needs. **Transinstitutionalization** refers to deinstitutionalization policy reforms resulting in the movement of people with mental illnesses to institutions that are not designed for or equipped to provide quality mental health care (Livingston et al., 2011).

Risk Factors for Crime and Violence among People with Mental Illnesses

The relationship between mental illnesses and criminal offending and violence has been a hotly debated topic for several decades, and there are challenges to interpreting research evidence on this issue. For example, the use of very broad definitions, such as "any mental disorder," blur important distinctions between specific syndromes and violence; and there is great variability in the literature regarding what constitutes violence (Douglas et al., 2009). The pendulum has swung between a resolutely assumed link between mental illnesses and violence, to the view that any link between these experiences cannot be made due to a lack of sufficient evidence. Recent research has taken a more nuanced approach, abandoning the general question of whether mental illnesses cause violence for the more sophisticated question:

> What particular symptoms of psychosis, under which situational circumstances, and in combination with which personal or situational factors, are associated with increased or decreased risk of various kinds of violence? (Douglas et al., 2009).

Most people with mental illness never engage in violence. In rare cases, such as when someone is experiencing a psychotic illness (see Chapter 4) for the first time or engaging in problematic substance use, the risk of violence is elevated (Large & Nielssen,

2011). However, most mental illnesses, including psychotic disorders, are highly treatable and therefore, the risk of violence can be diminished by access to quality mental health services (Langeveld et al., 2014). When a mental illness and substance use disorder co-occur (referred to as concurrent disorders or dual diagnosis), the risk profile looks different from those with a mental illness alone. Among people released from prison, those with co-occurring disorders are more likely to be returned within one year of release compared to those with a mental illness alone (Messina et al., 2004; Wilson et al., 2014). Additionally, the risk of violence is significantly elevated (Douglas et al., 2009; Large & Nielssen, 2011). The relationship between concurrent disorders and violence is extremely complex. Some drugs may act on brain mechanisms that increase the risk of aggressive behaviour; drugs may also interact with or even cause psychotic symptoms, which increases the probability of violence. That said, there is no definitive evidence that most types of substances directly cause violent behaviour (White et al., 2019). Research evidence supports the conclusion that mental illnesses are an important consideration, but the proportion of societal violence that is attributable to mental illness is very low (Bonta et al., 2014; Skeem et al., 2014).

Social Determinants of Health and Criminal Behaviour

Research on the relationship between mental illnesses and crime often ignores the broader social and environmental context in which mental illnesses are embedded. Social determinants of health (discussed in detail in Chapter 3) are the conditions in which people are born, grow, live, work, and age. These conditions are shaped by money, power, resources, policy, and prevailing political ideologies. The social determinants of criminal behaviour are similar to the social determinants of health, which suggest that a public health approach to crime prevention can reduce crime and improve public safety. Considerable research demonstrates that efforts to reduce poverty, homelessness, and stigma could have a very positive effect on reducing mental illnesses and the risk of criminal offending.

Poverty explains part of the relationship between mental illnesses and other social problems through factors such as lower educational attainment, under-employment, substance use, and reduced likelihood of prosocial attachments (e.g., family, peers; Draine et al., 2002). Similarly, elevated rates of homelessness among people with mental illnesses and substance use disorders contribute to greater rates of victimization, as well as higher rates of arrest, particularly for disorderly conduct and property theft (La Vigne et al., 2002; Maniglio, 2009; Osher, 2013). The relationship is reciprocal: experiencing homelessness increases the risk of incarceration, and incarceration increases the risk of future homelessness (Moschion & Johnson, 2019). A prison sentence often jeopardizes any housing arrangements a person may have had prior to incarceration and may also isolate an individual from their community and other social ties that support housing stability (Zorzi et al., 2006).

Mental health–related stigma also mediates criminal justice system involvement and outcomes. As introduced in Chapter 6, health-related stigma is a social process in which groups are devalued, rejected, and excluded, which can occur on the basis of a socially discredited health condition (Goffman, 1963; Weiss et al., 2006). Police officers often express fear of people with mental illnesses because of the perceived unpredictability of their behaviour and the presumption of dangerousness (Kesic et al., 2010). Research further suggests that it is possible that correctional officers monitor people with mental illnesses more closely due to stigma-based fear, making them more likely to be caught for a technical parole violation (Skeem & Peterson, 2012). Indeed, among parolees, people with and without mental illnesses are equally likely to be rearrested, but people with mental illnesses are more likely to be returned to prison (Skeem et al., 2014). Recent studies have shown that enhanced mental health training is associated with more positive perceptions of people with mental illnesses (Lavoie et al., 2006), as well as reduced incidents involving use of force (Parker, 2009). While health literacy among the public has improved, stigma towards people with mental illnesses remains a pervasive problem (*The Lancet*, 2016).

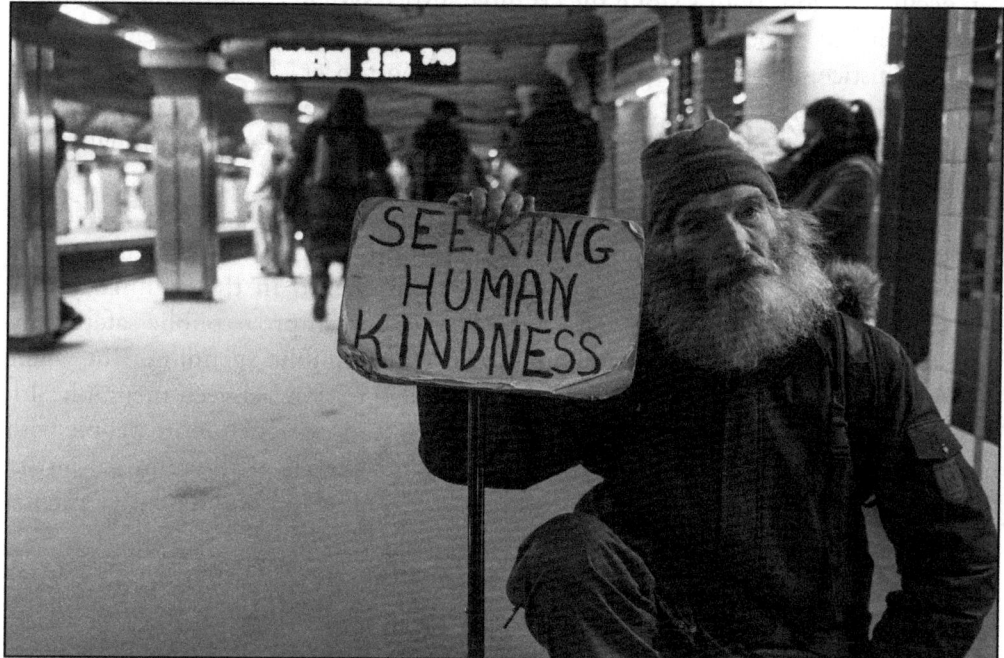

Figure 12.2: People with mental illnesses who have been incarcerated experience considerable stigma within the criminal justice system and in society. This stigma can prevent individuals from securing housing after release from prison, resulting in homelessness and increased risk for reincarceration.

Source: Unsplash/Matt Collamer

Entrenched social, structural, and economic disadvantage impact the likelihood and context under which persons with mental illnesses encounter the justice system (Hiday, 2006; MacPhail & Verdun-Jones, 2013). Effectively addressing the social determinants of health and ensuring access to appropriate treatment for people with mental illnesses, including substance use disorders, may help to reduce and prevent criminal offending.

Criminal Justice Diversion

Diversion refers to the redirection of people away from the criminal justice system and towards services believed to address the needs leading to offending (e.g., substance use, mental illnesses, poverty). The intention of diversion programs is to prevent low-risk offenders and individuals who are inappropriately overrepresented in custody (e.g., people with mental illnesses, Indigenous peoples) from becoming further entrenched in the criminal justice system. Diversion programs are also intended to improve the efficiency and effectiveness of the criminal justice system. Diversion can occur at various points along the criminal justice system "continuum" and often is accomplished through coordinated and integrated efforts between mental health, criminal justice, and social service systems (Livingston et al., 2008). An effective diversion model starts with a well-funded and comprehensive mental health and substance use services system so that people do not need to enter the criminal justice system before they are able to access mental health care.

Munetz and Griffin (2006) proposed the Sequential Intercepts Model as a framework for understanding the points of **interception** or opportunities to prevent an individual from entering or becoming further entrenched in the criminal justice system. Early intervention efforts have the potential to improve public safety, support positive health and social outcomes, and reduce public spending. But where community services are poorly developed and collaboration between mental health services and the criminal justice system is weak (or non-existent), more people with mental illnesses can be expected to move through all levels of the criminal justice system. The best intercept is described as an accessible and comprehensive mental health system (Munetz & Griffin, 2006).

> The system should have an effective base of services that include competent, supportive clinicians; community support services; medications; vocational and other role supports; safe and affordable housing; and crisis services. (Munetz & Griffin, 2006)

This model helps us understand the "big picture" of interactions between the criminal justice and mental health systems by breaking down the various steps involved in an individual's hypothetical path from first contact, to custody, and back to community. The complicated legislative framework governing the criminal justice

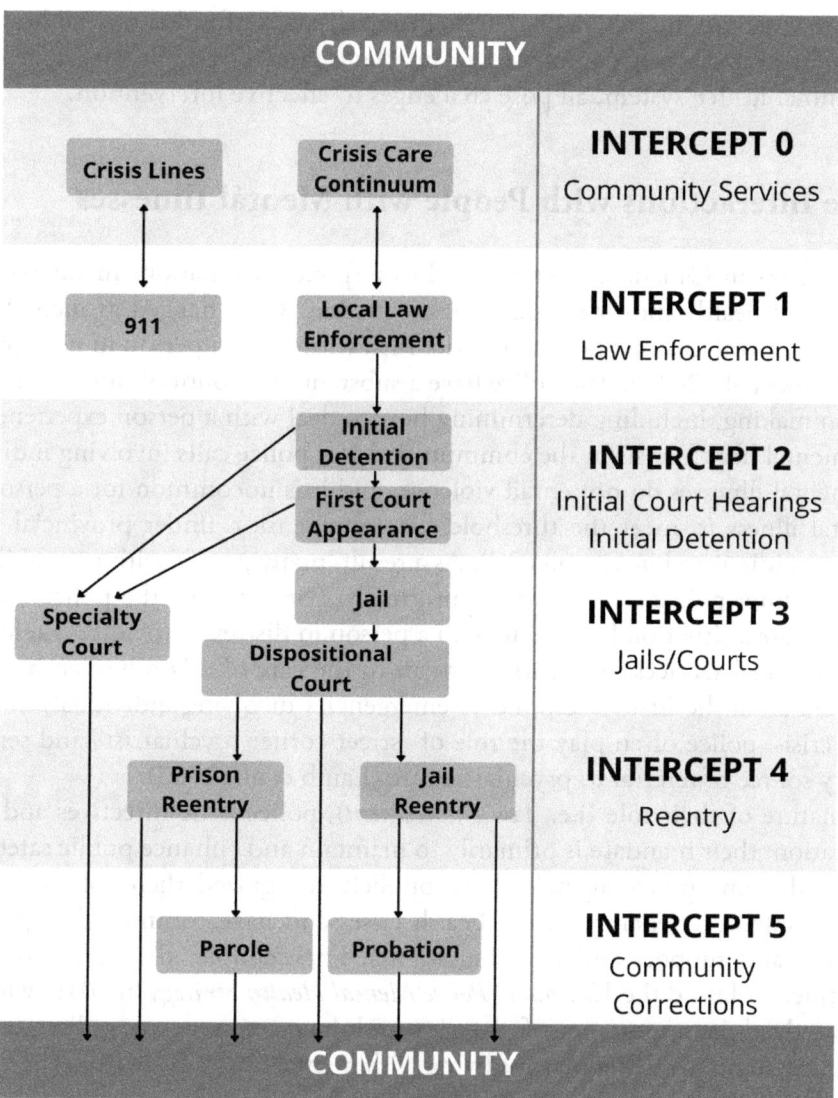

Figure 12.3: The Sequential Intercept Model illustrates different points at which people with mental illnesses and substance use disorders come into contact with the criminal justice system. The arrows show how people move through the criminal justice system and return to the community.

Source: Adapted from Substance Abuse and Mental Health Services Administration (SAMHSA). (2021). *The sequential intercept model (SIM)*. https://www.samhsa.gov/criminal-juvenile-justice/sim-overview

system in Canada, the fragmented and chronically underfunded mental health system, and the intersecting complex social problems faced by people who interact with the criminal justice system, all pose challenges to effective intervention.

Police Interactions with People with Mental Illnesses

Police officers in Canada are often called to respond to situations involving people with mental health and/or substance use concerns. Calls flagged as mental health related may involve someone who is a victim, a witness, or a person in need of assistance (Brink et al., 2011). The police have a substantial amount of discretion in their decision making, including determining how to deal with a person experiencing an acute mental health crisis in the community. Most police calls involving individuals with mental illnesses do not entail violence, and it is uncommon for a person with a mental illness to meet the threshold for apprehension under provincial mental health acts (discussed in Chapter 13). As a result, many people with mental illnesses who encounter police are dealt with informally. For example, the police may help to de-escalate a situation by talking with a person in distress, providing a referral for health or social services, or returning them to the care of a family member. Given police are often the first to respond to emergencies involving individuals in mental health crisis, police often play the role of "street corner psychiatrist" and serve as a primary source of referral to psychiatric care (Lamb et al., 2002).

By nature of their role (i.e., law *enforcement*), police issue directives and expect cooperation; their mandate is primarily to maintain and enhance public safety. That being said, some police agencies have publicly recognized their role in responding to people experiencing mental health crises and have committed to providing education and support and reducing stigma. For example, the Vancouver Police Department released the *Vancouver Police Mental Health Strategy* in 2016, wherein it acknowledged the importance of diversion and the prominent role police play: "The VPD is intent on diverting persons living with mental illness away from the criminal justice system when the circumstances of the criminal activity are minor in nature, have little immediate impact on the community at large, and are grounded in the individual's mental illness" (Wiebe, 2016).

The actions exhibited by someone in a mental health crisis can sometimes be misconstrued as aggressive or defiant (Parent, 2011), and/or people with mental illnesses may struggle to respond to police commands. This can lead to escalation and a coercive police response, especially when police officers have limited training and education about mental illnesses and their behavioural manifestations. Training in recognizing symptoms of mental illnesses and using de-escalation techniques can reduce the level of force and other negative outcomes of police intervention. Information on fatalities resulting from police officers' actions in Canada is not systematically collected, but at least 461 incidents occurred between 2000 and 2017 (Marcoux & Nicholson, 2018). It is estimated that more than 70 percent of the victims had mental health and/or substance use challenges (Marcoux & Nicholson, 2018).

In May 2020, George Floyd, a Black American man, was murdered by a white Minneapolis police officer, Derek Chauvin. Video footage of the murder, recorded by a witness, circulated widely, prompting demonstrations across the US and around the world (Buchanan et al., 2020). Advocacy groups are now putting new pressure on legislators and policymakers to "defund the police," a movement which has included calls ranging from cuts to police budgets, and the reallocation of those funds to community services, through to total abolition of police forces (Lum et al., 2021). Mr. Floyd's death reignited global discussions about police brutality, race-based violence, and the socioeconomic and political systems that are at the root of social and structural inequities (Weine et al., 2020).

Box 12.1: Police Use of Force: The Case of Robert Dziekański

Robert Dziekański died on October 14, 2007, following a police encounter at Vancouver International Airport in British Columbia (BC). Mr. Dziekański was in the process of immigrating to Canada from Poland to live with his mother and did not speak any English. After a lengthy customs process, he became distraught, agitated, and anxious, causing damage to property (Braidwood, 2010). Police were called and four RCMP officers arrived on scene. A conducted energy weapon (commonly referred to as a Taser) was deployed against Mr. Dziekański multiple times, and he died within minutes of being physically restrained (Braidwood, 2009). A video recording of the incident taken by a witness was initially retained by police, but later returned to the individual who then released it to the media, causing a public outcry (Braidwood, 2010).

The Province of BC appointed Justice Thomas R. Braidwood to conduct two Commissions of Inquiry. The first examined the use of conducted energy weapons in BC and concluded that the RCMP was not justified in using such a weapon against Mr. Dziekánski, and that officers had intentionally misrepresented the situation to justify their actions. The second focused on the circumstances relating to Mr. Dziekański's death and concluded that the deployment of a conducted energy weapon contributed to his death (Braidwood, 2010). An investigation by the BC Coroners Service (2013) ruled Mr. Dziekański's death a homicide, citing the cause of death as cardiac arrhythmia resulting from a physical altercation and multiple deployments of a conducted energy weapon by RCMP. All four RCMP officers involved in the incident were charged with perjury and, in 2010, the RCMP issued a formal apology to Mr. Dziekański's mother.

This case highlights issues in police training on responding to incidents involving people experiencing mental health crises; police use of force and conducted energy weapon technology; police oversight and accountability, including the conflict of interest that may arise when a police service investigates its own members; and loss of public confidence in the police. Braidwood's recommendations have had a significant impact on policy, training, and practice, especially with respect to the use of conducted energy weapons in BC and across Canada (BC Coroners Service, 2013).

A study looking at Canadian police organizations found that entry-level training on mental illnesses is widely available, but highly variable (Coleman & Cotton, 2010). At the time of the study in 2008, few police agencies were providing reasonably comprehensive training and education in responding to people with mental illnesses and, in many cases, a relatively small proportion of personnel received it (Coleman & Cotton, 2010). With the intention of providing a starting point for police organizations, the Canadian Association of Chiefs of Police released a set of guidelines for police working with people with mental illnesses. The guidelines begin with the following central tenet:

> Each police organization should foster a culture in which mental illness is viewed as a medical disability not a moral failure, and in which [people with mental illnesses] are treated with the same degree of respect as other members of society. (Cotton & Coleman, 2008)

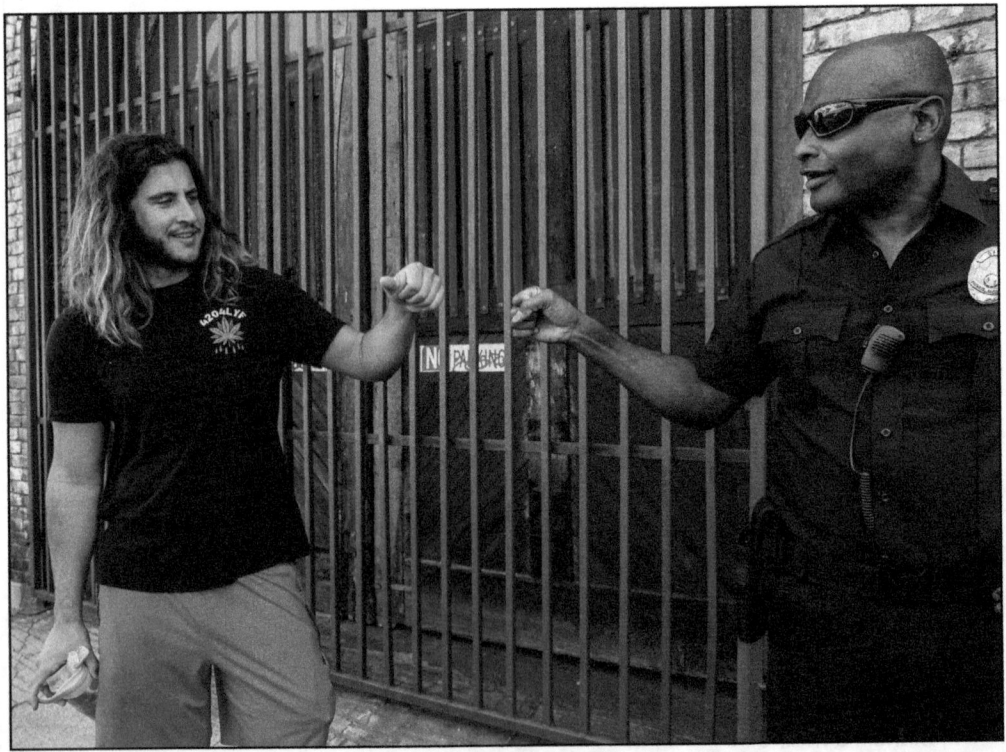

Figure 12.4: Police officers are often called to respond to people experiencing acute mental health crises in the community. Recent incidents involving police use of force with people experiencing mental health challenges illustrate the need for police to develop meaningful relationships with community mental health services and have a high level of knowledge and skill in verbal de-escalation.

Source: Pexels/Kindel Media

The principles indicate that police organizations should develop relationships with a primary contact person in the local mental health system, emergency services, and hospitals; have clearly defined policies and procedures for access to mental health expertise (e.g., a subset of specially trained officers); ensure all police and dispatching officers have sufficient knowledge and understanding of mental illnesses (e.g., ability to recognize symptoms and de-escalate situations involving mental health crisis); and systematically collect data on the nature, quantity, and outcomes of interactions with people with mental illnesses.

Common Pre-Arrest Diversion Models

In addition to police training, many police departments in Canada have developed formal strategies to improve interactions with people with mental illnesses and divert them away from the criminal justice system. Some of the most common pre-arrest diversion models are summarized in Table 12.1.

Crisis Intervention Training (CIT) was originally developed in the US following an incident in which a police officer shot and killed an individual with a history of a mental illness. Within a CIT approach, trained officers are dispatched to assist general patrol when the call has been flagged as mental health related, with the goals of safety, increased connection to mental health services, strategic use of law enforcement, and reduction of trauma (Usher et al., 2019). Studies in the US have found

Table 12.1: Pre-arrest diversion models/police–mental health collaboration

Model	Description
Crisis Intervention Teams (CIT)	Teams of officers receive specialized training to respond to mental health calls.
Co-Responder Teams	Specially trained officers and a mental health worker respond together. Most commonly, they ride in the same vehicle.
Mobile Crisis Teams	Teams of mental health professionals, skilled at stabilizing people during law enforcement encounters, are available to respond to calls for service at the request of police agencies.
Integrated Case Management Teams	Multidisciplinary teams that may include mental health workers, peers, social workers, nurses, psychiatrists, and police. The teams provide outreach, follow up, and ongoing case management to select priority people, such as repeat callers of emergency services. Officers do not treat or diagnose the individuals but work with mental health professionals to develop solutions to reduce repeat interactions.
Crisis Drop-Off Centres	Centralized sites available 24 hours per day to which police can bring a person in psychiatric crisis in need of formal assessment. Key features include no-refusal policies (police referrals always accepted) and streamlined intake (expedited drop-offs for police through separate entrance and/or specialized crisis response units).

that officers perceive CIT to be effective and beneficial in improving the response to people with mental illnesses (Bonfine et al., 2014; Canada et al., 2010), but there is not enough research to declare the model evidence-based practice (Jellicoe & Anderson, 2019). CIT has been adopted by police services across Canada, starting with the RCMP in 2016, and is now used in several jurisdictions including Toronto, Hamilton, Halifax, and Vancouver (Jellicoe & Anderson, 2019). To date, there are no studies on CIT effectiveness in the Canadian context.

The dominant mobile response in Canada is co-response triage (Cotton & Coleman, 2017). In a co-response model, a mental health professional assists the police during incidents either in person or remotely. The overall objectives are to de-escalate crises, prevent injuries, connect people quickly and effectively with mental health care, and reduce pressure on the mental health system (Shapiro et al., 2015). The rationale is that police and mental health workers together have the expertise required to appropriately handle mental health crises; police are equipped to respond to potential violence or injury, and the mental health professionals provide consultation and assessment. In Edmonton, the provincial health authority partnered with the Edmonton Police Service in 2004 to create the Police and Crisis Team (PACT), allowing the agencies to share information within the confines of privacy legislation. PACT has several teams comprised of a police officer and a trained mental health professional (e.g., psychologist, clinical social worker, registered psychiatric nurse; Jellicoe & Anderson, 2019). The teams work together to assess the individual, evaluate risk, and decide how best to respond. A similar partnership between the Vancouver Police Department and Mental Health Emergency Services, called "Car 87," pairs a mental health nurse with a plain-clothes police officer to respond to calls in an unmarked vehicle. The program provides follow-up, referral for services, and crisis intervention. There is a lack of controlled studies examining the effectiveness of co-response triage (Puntis et al., 2018), but preliminary evidence is promising. A Canadian study showed that such models may decrease injuries, increase escorts to hospitals and treatments, decrease involuntary commitments, and reduce the time officers spend at the hospital when compared with officers responding alone (Lamanna et al., 2018).

Forensic Mental Health Systems

After a person has been arrested and charged with a crime, their case goes to court and they and/or their lawyer attend a court hearing. Every person who comes before the court is presumed to be innocent, fit to stand trial, and mentally well. If, however, the accused's mental health is called into question, the court will seek guidance in determining whether it may have an impact on the administration of justice. The accused's mental health is considered in two manners: (1) the accused may be found unfit to stand trial because of a mental disorder; or (2) if the case proceeds to trial and during the proceedings the judge or jury determines the person did commit the act underlying the offence, the accused or Crown may raise the NCRMD defence. Alternatively, at the time of the verdict the judge may order a psychiatric assessment. Regardless of who raises the issue, the accused is typically remanded to a psychiatric hospital and an evaluation is conducted to determine if the person was acutely mentally ill at the time of the offence. The details of each of these procedures deserves further consideration and are described below.

Fitness to Stand Trial

An accused person is presumed to be fit to stand trial unless the court is satisfied that the person is unfit. If they are **unfit to stand trial (UST)**, Canadian law recognizes that it would be unfair to prosecute them. Section 2 of the *Criminal Code* stipulates that a person is UST if they are unable on account of mental disorder to: (a) understand the nature or object of the proceedings; (b) understand the possible consequences of the proceedings; or (c) communicate with counsel. The issue of fitness can be raised at any point, before or during court appearances, prior to a verdict being rendered, where there are reasonable grounds to believe that the accused is unfit. However, it generally occurs early in the proceedings, often at the person's first court appearance. The issue of mental fitness can be raised pursuant to the court's own motion or the accused's lawyer, or Crown counsel can recommend a psychiatric assessment. If the judge agrees a psychiatric evaluation is necessary, the court will order a fitness assessment to be conducted by a psychiatrist.

If a person is found UST, the court may make an initial disposition, but even then, the Review Board will review the disposition within 90 days. If the court is not satisfied that it can make a disposition, the disposition hearing is referred to the provincial/territorial Review Board, which must make an order within 45 days of the verdict of UST. There are only two disposition options for an individual found UST: conditional discharge or a detention order. If the person is still UST after the initial 90 days, the Review Board reviews the case on an annual basis. The trial remains on hold while the person receives treatment. If the treatment is likely to render the person fit to ultimately stand trial, the court may order treatment for 60 days or less following a finding of UST, regardless of whether the person consents. If the person is found fit to stand trial, the trial continues. An accused person may be found UST again at any point before the verdict is reached.

Criminal Responsibility

It is a fundamental principle of the criminal justice system in Canada and many other countries that an accused person must have the capacity to understand that their behaviour was wrong in order to be found guilty of a crime (Latimer & Lawrence, 2006). The *Criminal Code of Canada* stipulates that: "No person is criminally responsible for an act committed or an omission made while suffering from a mental disorder that rendered the person incapable of appreciating the nature and quality of the act or omission or of knowing that it was wrong" (Section 16). The court's ability to order an assessment of criminal responsibility is limited at the outset of the trial. Criminal responsibility can only be raised if the accused has put their mental condition in issue by raising the NCRMD defence or it is determined that the accused has committed the offence in question. This means that the Crown may only raise the issue of criminal responsibility after the judge has determined that the accused would otherwise be guilty of the offence. It is important to understand that a finding of NCRMD (or "NCR") is neither an acquittal nor a finding of guilt, but rather, it acknowledges that the person cannot be held criminally responsible for their actions (*Winko v. British Columbia*, 1999). In this case, a sentence is replaced by the least onerous and least restrictive option to protect both the accused individual and the public.

If an individual is found NCRMD, it is rare for the court to make an initial disposition; nonetheless, they may direct the accused to be detained in custody. NCR accused generally come under the purview of the Review Board system. Review Boards are specialized tribunals chaired by a judge, or an individual qualified for a judicial appointment, and comprised of at least five other members, one of whom must be entitled to practice psychiatry (672.38(1)). Under section 672.54 of the *Criminal Code*, there are three dispositions available to the court or Review Board following a finding of NCRMD: (1) absolute discharge; (2) conditional discharge; and (3) detention in custody. The conditions a person is subject to upon discharge may include supervision, treatment, counselling, prohibition on the possession of firearms/weapons, or prohibition on use of alcohol/drugs, among others. When making its decision, the Review Board must order the disposition that is "necessary and appropriate under the circumstances," and it is required to prioritize the safety of the public as well as considering the mental condition of the accused, the reintegration of the accused into society, and the other needs of the accused. If the Review Board orders detention, the accused will generally be placed in custody within a forensic hospital. In some cases (e.g., limited bed availability, minor offences) a person found NCRMD may be detained in a general tertiary psychiatric hospital (Crocker & Côté, 2009).

There are many misconceptions regarding people found NCR, and public fear is often fuelled by media coverage of rare, high-profile, often violent, cases. Common myths include that the designation is used frequently and conveniently, and that after a brief period of hospitalization those who are found NCR will be released into the community and promptly reoffend (Canadian Mental Health Association Ontario, 2015). In reality, NCR verdicts are rare: for example, they comprise only 1.34 per 1,000 judicial decisions in British Columbia and 0.95 in Ontario (Crocker et al., 2015). Further, individuals found NCR will on average spend more time in custody or under supervision than if they had been incarcerated, especially for minor offences (Silver, 1995). A comprehensive review of 1,800 patient files in Quebec, Ontario, and British Columbia revealed a much lower reconviction rate for NCR individuals (17 percent over 3 years of follow-up) compared to people who have been incarcerated in jails and prisons and treated for mental illness (70 percent over the same time period; Charette et al., 2015).

> **Box 12.2: Not Criminally Responsible: The Case of Matthew de Grood**
>
> On April 15, 2014, in Calgary, Alberta, five university students lost their lives at a year-end house party: Lawrence Hong (aged 27), Joshua Hunter (aged 23), Kaitlin Perras (aged 23), Zachariah Rathwell (aged 21), and Jordan Segura (aged 22). Each had been stabbed to death by 22-year-old Matthew de Grood, a student at the University of Calgary and the son of a Calgary police officer (*Canadian Press*, 2014). Mr. de Grood was charged with five counts of first-degree murder. On May 22, 2015, he was subjected to a psychiatric assessment and was found fit to stand trial. Mr. de Grood pled not guilty on all charges, though he did not deny stabbing the victims (Canadian Resource Centre for Victims of Crime, 2016).
>
> Prior to the incident, he had reportedly posted online about killing vampires, and he was found to be experiencing a psychotic episode at the time of the offence (Canadian Resource Centre for Victims of Crime, 2016). On May 25, 2016, Mr. de Grood was found Not Criminally Responsible on account of Mental Disorder (NCRMD). In 2018, the Alberta Review Board determined that his mental illness was in full remission, and he was granted a number of privileges. The victims' families called on the Alberta Review Board to keep Mr. de Grood in custody indefinitely, arguing that he should be rehabilitated but not reintegrated into the community ("Family Statement," 2018). A study examining Twitter activity related to Mr. de Grood's case demonstrated the perception that an NCR defence is a legal loophole (particularly relevant in a case involving the son of a local police officer), and that the defence is a miscarriage of justice (Goossens et al., 2021). A noteworthy finding was that, although the minority, some tweets expressed support and hope that the case would ignite public discussion about the need for mental health services, noting that stigma may have been at the root of Mr. de Grood not seeking support in the first place. Others expressed dismay at the nature of the opinions expressed, as one user remarked, "People are calling for the execution of individuals with mental illness. Stay classy internet" (user 56; Goossens et al., 2021).
>
> This case and the resulting research highlights issues concerning untreated mental illnesses, limited public awareness of the signs and symptoms of mental illnesses, and incomplete understanding of the mental health provisions in the *Criminal Code of Canada* and the rights and roles of victims (and their families) in the forensic mental health system. Misperceptions about the NCR defence and chronic, mental illness–related stigma demonstrate the need for public education and continued advocacy for, and with, people with mental illnesses.

In sum, the forensic system is designed to ensure that procedures are in place to protect both accused individuals who suffer from serious mental illnesses and the public. Unfortunately, it can be very difficult for victims, families, and the general public to understand the NCR verdict and the apparent lack of "responsibility" due to their illness. When there is no criminal conviction, a victim may feel a sense of injustice. Research on the needs and perceptions of victims is limited, but we know that inclusion in the process, timely information about Review Board dates, and presenting impact statements can increase victim satisfaction and a sense of justice. Restorative justice processes may also be beneficial, as they require "the joint engagement of victim and perpetrator so that they hear each other; understand feelings, concerns, and remorse; and aid in the recovery of both" (Quinn & Simpson, 2013).

Despite the availability of UST and NCRMD findings, a person with a mental illness who commits a crime is not necessarily exempt from criminal responsibility. This determination is based upon a strict legal test that requires the person to be acutely ill *at the time of the offence*. This means that many people with mental health issues who are charged with crimes will be tried and convicted within the criminal justice system, and often serve time in correctional facilities. However, diversion can take place at the court level via judicial discretion and specialty mental health court practices (Livingston et al., 2008).

Specialty Courts

A mental health court is one type of specialty court that is designed to better respond to accused persons who are experiencing mental health challenges. These courts are typically supported by psychiatrists, mental health workers, and other social services staff, and are intended to prevent the incarceration of people with mental illnesses. While mental health courts differ across jurisdictions, they share some common features: for example, they involve multidisciplinary teams that provide a treatment-oriented approach to address the needs of the individual, and they are based on holistic and therapeutic approaches, rather than punishment (MacDonald et al., 2014). Criminal justice and court staff work with mental health professionals to provide mental health services, such as medication and psychotherapy, as well as housing and job training. These services are often coordinated by case managers. Mental health courts accept referrals from lawyers, doctors, and others, with agreement from the person with a mental illness, who usually pleads guilty in order to access these services.

Mental health court staff and participants have provided strong anecdotal evidence that specialty courts are efficacious in connecting people to mental health resources and reducing substance use, costs, and **recidivism** (or reoffending; Schneider, 2013; Steadman et al., 2011). However, despite their potential, critics argue that they are paternalistic and that it is coercive to require a guilty plea from someone who has a mental illness. This is especially so for misdemeanor offences, where someone without mental illness may successfully have such charges dismissed (Seltzer, 2005). Furthermore, access to alternative courts may inadvertently "encourage" police to arrest people with mental illnesses with the intention of ensuring priority access to adequate mental health treatment. These two issues may ultimately result in the accused having a (longer) criminal record and being more likely to be incarcerated at some point. Importantly, mental health courts typically do not accept people charged with serious or violent offences. This means that if someone has committed a violent offence and does not meet the criteria for a NCRMD designation, they will likely be processed through the regular court system. Like pre-arrest diversion, the effectiveness of court support and diversion programs can be compromised by limited availability of community mental health services and a lack of dedicated funding (Centre for Addiction and Mental Health, 2013). Research on the value of mental health courts is limited in Canada; overall claims about effectiveness are challenging because there is significant variability in what jurisdictions define as a mental health court (Canada et al., 2019).

A few municipalities have developed other problem-solving courts (i.e., specialized dockets that seek to address the underlying problem(s) contributing to certain criminal offences). These courts deal with a spectrum of health and social issues that may include mental illnesses, including substance use, as well as homelessness and poverty. For example, Vancouver's Downtown Community Court (DCC), which opened in 2008, pioneered an approach that brings justice, health, and social services together, to help respond to individuals with complex needs. The court takes a problem-solving approach to address each person's unique needs and circumstances. An evaluation of the DCC compared DCC clients who were triaged to a case management team to a matched sample of those who received traditional provincial court outcomes (Somers et al., 2014). Those assigned to a case management team had significantly greater reductions in overall offending compared to the comparison group (Somers et al., 2014). However, concerns have been expressed about the fact that these services often stop when the individual's court obligations conclude, despite the fact that many of the people accessing these courts would benefit from ongoing support (Jackson et al., 2012). To the extent that mental health courts do reduce recidivism, the result may stem from the courts' ability to address needs that are unrelated to mental illness (e.g., challenges of everyday living; Butler et al., 2021; Han, 2019; Skeem et al., 2014).

Corrections

If an individual has not been diverted from the criminal justice system at the court stage, and has been convicted and sentenced, the next stage of the criminal justice process is corrections. **Correctional agencies** are responsible for supervising people who have been convicted and sentenced for committing a crime; this includes supervising people who are serving some or all of their sentence in the community (known as "community corrections"), as well as operating correctional facilities where people are detained in custody (i.e., jails, prisons). There are two branches to Canada's correctional system. Each province/territory has its own correctional system; as such, resource allocation, policies, and programs related to mental health vary considerably across the country. There is some consistency in federal custody because federal correctional facilities are managed by the Correctional Service of Canada (CSC). However, the Office of the Correctional Investigator (OCI) of Canada has repeatedly asserted that the provisions to support people with mental illnesses in prisons are inadequate and fragmented. The *Corrections and Conditional Release Act* outlines CSC's responsibility to provide health services to people in federal custody; however, it is unclear whether mental health services are considered *essential* health care, unless they significantly impact a person's functioning in the correctional setting or their reintegration into the community. It is important to note that health services, including mental health care for federal offenders, are not covered under the *Canada Health Act*. This leaves responsibility for the mental health care of federally sentenced offenders in custody and in the community to CSC. A great deal of research has been conducted regarding evidence-based practice in correctional psychology and psychiatry and in particular aspects of providing care in institutional settings (e.g., suicide and self-harm prevention, managing individuals at risk of violence; Ternes et al., 2018; Trestman et al., 2015). However, standards for mental health services in corrections have not kept pace with the research, and there are few judicial decisions clarifying the right to mental health treatment in custody in Canada.

The OCI found that between 1998 and 2007, the proportion of offenders in federal correctional facilities with significant, identified mental health needs more than doubled (Sapers, 2011). Incarcerated women are more likely than incarcerated men to experience a mental disorder in Canada: in 2014, 45.7 percent of women and 26 percent of men in federal prisons had an active psychotropic medication prescription (Farrell MacDonald et al., 2015). In 2004, CSC launched a Mental Health Strategy to better match mental health services with the needs of the population. The Strategy is based on five key components: (1) intake, (2) primary care, (3) intermediate care, (4) psychiatric hospital care, and (5) transitional care. Despite implementing key elements of the strategy, CSC has still not produced a comprehensive and official strategic planning document. A review of the strategy noted that the lack of an overarching plan compromises funding, implementation, accountability, and evaluation:

> There are obviously many important needs within CSC and society, however, mental health is among the most urgently in need of immediate and continued action as a result of longstanding neglect. (Service, 2010)

In 2015, CSC published a *Review of Mental Health Commitments*, describing progress made against the priorities in the Mental Health Strategy. Some of the commitments that were met included implementing computerized mental health screening at intake, filling community mental health job vacancies, providing mental health awareness training to frontline CSC staff, and securing funding for a complex needs units (CSC, 2015).

The Impacts of Imprisonment on Psychological Well-being

The psychological effects of incarceration vary across individuals, but many people who are incarcerated suffer long-term social and psychological consequences (Schnittker, 2013), including post-traumatic stress responses upon release (Hagan et al., 2018; Haney, 2017). Due to the criminalization of poverty, people who enter prison are more likely to have been living in entrenched disadvantage and have unmet mental health needs prior to admission to prison. As such, experiences of violence and victimization leading to trauma *prior* to incarceration are very common; the estimated lifetime prevalence of post-traumatic stress disorder (PTSD) is 18 percent for men and 40 percent for women in prison, compared to 5 percent for men and 10 percent for women in the general population (Barayani et al., 2018). Mental health concerns, including PTSD, may be exacerbated or caused by conditions of confinement, including lack of purposeful activity, overcrowding, exposure to violence, and separation from family (De Viggiani, 2007). While prison is arguably challenging for anyone, prisoners with mental illnesses may have diminished ability to cope with the stress of incarceration (Metzner & Fellner, 2010). Symptoms of some severe mental disorders include hallucinations, delusions, chaotic thought processes, and disruptions in memory and consciousness. As such, people with mental illnesses may exhibit behaviours that could be perceived by others as bizarre or annoying and act in ways that the prison systems consider punishable misconduct (Abramsky & Fellner, 2003). As a result, they typically have higher rates of disciplinary infractions than prisoners without mental illnesses (Metzner & Fellner, 2010).

The use of solitary confinement is a practice that has unfortunately been employed to control "difficult" prisoners, many of whom have mental illnesses. In solitary confinement, prisoners may spend 23–24 hours per day in small cells locked by solid steel doors. The units are often bare, under constant surveillance and security controls, and the prisoners engage in very little (if any) social interaction, recreation, vocational, or other purposeful activities (Metzner & Fellner, 2010). According to a US federal judge, placing a person with serious mental illness in solitary confinement "is the mental equivalent of putting an asthmatic person in a place with little air to breathe" (Metzner & Fellner, 2010). Prisoners in solitary confinement display signs and symptoms of helplessness, hostility and aggression, depression, paranoia, cognitive disturbances, self-harm, and suicide (Arrigo & Bullock, 2007; Haney, 2003; Shalev, 2014). The living conditions, such as limited exercise and extreme loneliness, are also known risk factors for adverse physical health outcomes such as cardiovascular disease (Williams et al., 2019).

Canada has come under intense scrutiny by both the Office of the Correctional Investigator and the United Nations for its segregation practices. The United Nations Committee Against Torture recommended that Canada "increase the capacity of treatment centres for prisoners with intermediate and acute mental health issues" and "abolish the use of solitary confinement for persons with serious or acute mental illness" (United Nations Committee against Torture, 2012). In 2019, CSC

Box 12.3: Death in Segregation: The Case of Ashley Smith

Ashley Smith died on October 19, 2007, at age 19, of "ligature strangulation and positional asphyxia" (Chief Coroner of Ontario, 2013). At the time of her death, she was on 24-hour suicide watch while in segregation at Grand Valley Institution for Women, a federal prison for women in Kingston, Ontario. Ms. Smith first came into contact with the youth criminal justice system at age 13 (Sapers, 2008) and was incarcerated at age 15 for breaching her probation (LeBlanc et al., 2015). She received 50 more criminal charges while in custody and was transferred from youth to adult custody less than one year before her death (Sapers, 2008). Ms. Smith was then transferred between institutions 17 times in the 11.5 months she was in federal custody and was held in administrative segregation for most of that time (Bingham & Sutton, 2012). Correctional staff documented 150 incidents of self-injurious behaviour while Ms. Smith was in federal custody (Bingham & Sutton, 2012; LeBlanc et al., 2015). She submitted seven formal grievances about her treatment to the CSC, all of which were denied (LeBlanc et al., 2015).

CSC failed to conduct a comprehensive mental health assessment or develop a comprehensive treatment plan despite Ms. Smith's history of mental health concerns (Sapers, 2008). Hours before her death, she had communicated to correctional staff that she wanted to end her life; she then tied a ligature around her neck (Sapers, 2008). A video recording of the incident showed that "correctional staff failed to respond immediately to this medical emergency" (Sapers, 2008). By the time they intervened, it was too late (LeBlanc et al., 2015). Several correctional workers were charged with criminal negligence causing death, and Ms. Smith's family later filed a wrongful death lawsuit against the federal government, which was settled out of court (Bromwich & Kilty, 2017). After a mistrial in the first inquest, a second inquest was ordered and, in 2013, the Chief Coroner of Ontario ruled Ms. Smith's death a homicide.

Investigations into the circumstances surrounding Ms. Smith's death exposed numerous individual and systemic failures, and resulted in dozens of recommendations to government related to the provision of mental health services in corrections, mental health training for correctional staff, the use and long-term impacts of segregation, responses to self-injurious behaviour, alternatives to custody, and organizational accountability (see Chief Coroner of Ontario, 2013; Richard, 2008; Sapers, 2008). These recommendations, and subsequent legal challenges regarding the use of segregation for prisoners experiencing mental illnesses, led to the introduction of Bill C-83, which became law in 2019 and includes "the elimination of the use of administrative segregation and its replacement by structured intervention units" (Casavant & Charron-Tousignant, 2019). The implementation and operation of these units have been heavily criticized.

abolished segregation and implemented Structured Intervention Units (SIUs) with the goal of promoting positive, intervention-based approaches to address individual needs and prison safety. According to CSC policy, SIUs are similar to a regular cell, and include a minimum of four hours per day outside of the cell and two hours per day of meaningful human interaction (e.g., cultural practices, family contact through video visitation), and a health assessment within 24 hours (CSC, 2021). However, reports conducted voluntarily by two prominent Canadian criminologists found that the SIUs were not operating in a manner consistent with the relevant law; prisoners were not getting their promised time out of cells or meaningful human contact, the SIUs lacked external oversight, and they noted regional differences in SIU implementation (Sprott & Doob, 2021). With respect to the use of solitary confinement, the authors concluded that: "the lack of accountability that appears to exist [from within CSC] does not look to us to be very different from what experts on this topic have been describing for at least 50 years ... it appears nothing much has changed."

Health Promotion in Prison

While the conditions of the prison environment may cause or exacerbate mental health issues, overall health improves (at least temporarily) for some people while in custody. Particularly for people living in entrenched disadvantage, incarceration may provide a period of stabilization, reduced access to and supported withdrawal from alcohol and drugs, and access to mental health care (Nicholls et al., 2018; Rich et al., 2014). This is of course contingent on correctional services having both the mandate and resources to support health and well-being. Many people will receive mental health services for the first time while in jails because they have not been able to access services in the community.

Contact with the criminal justice system represents an important opportunity to detect mental illnesses, assess treatment needs, and then link people with community-based resources. Most people cycle through custody for very short periods of time (often days to weeks), particularly in jails and remand centres (Butler et al., 2021; Kouyoumdjian et al., 2016). As such, efficient and effective intake, assessment and treatment within the institution, and discharge planning that includes linking people with community resources, are vital (for a model see, Nicholls et al., 2018; Nicholls et al., 2005). While health professionals have not traditionally viewed the criminal justice system as part of the care continuum, experts assert that jails and prisons hold enormous potential to play an active and beneficial role in the health care system (Rich et al., 2014). The World Health Organization (WHO) has championed the concept of "health-promoting prisons," whereby a whole-prison setting promotes health through: (1) prison policies; (2) an environment that is supportive of health; and (3) disease prevention, health education, and other health promotion initiatives (Baybutt et al., 2014). This paradigm shift from penal to health promoting policies has not been wholly adopted in Canadian corrections. That said, positive steps have been taken, including the adoption of therapeutic and person-centred practices in some jurisdictions. One example is BC Corrections' "Right Living Units," where staff and inmates work together to create an environment based on trust, communication, and accountability. While the units are not specifically focused on people with mental illnesses, they can support positive mental health by promoting healing rather than punishment. Right Living Units involve a therapeutic approach, a shared commitment to changing unhealthy lifestyles, setting shared rules, and working together to build a community (Office of the Auditor General of BC, 2019).

Community Corrections and Re-Entry

The community corrections system has a crucial role to play in the diversion of people with mental illnesses away from the criminal justice system. This system generally includes those serving their sentences in the community (i.e., conditional sentence, probation), and those who have been granted early release from federal custody by a parole board. Ideally, people on probation and parole are screened for mental illnesses and substance use concerns, and routinely evaluated (Lurigio & Swartz, 2006). In BC, for example, community corrections clients may be referred to Forensic Regional Community Clinics (six clinics and satellite services exist throughout the province). The clinics provide assessment, treatment, and ongoing monitoring for clients referred by the courts or forensic hospital.

Case management, discharge planning, and diversion efforts upon release from custody can prevent people from returning to custody. For example, **Assertive Community Treatment (ACT)** has shown promise as a model for providing services after discharge from jail for people with complex needs. The model calls for a "total team approach," and the core features include assertive outreach, multidisciplinary staffing models, direct provision of health and social services, high staff–participant ratios, long-term time-unlimited services, and client contact primarily at home or in the community (McGrew & Bond, 1995). Client eligibility is clearly defined, services are available 24 hours a day, each consumer's response to interventions is carefully monitored, and there is a focus on everyday problems in living in addition to clinical needs. ACT programs have demonstrated merit, in terms of reducing re-arrest and re-hospitalization (Lurigio et al., 2000). An adaptation of the ACT model for justice-involved clients is Forensic Assertive Community Treatment (FACT; Jennings, 2009). FACT builds on the ACT model by making adaptations based on criminal justice issues—namely, an added focus on addressing criminogenic needs and risks. FACT teams may involve criminal justice partners and peer specialists with lived criminal justice experience. In 2012, the Vancouver Police Department became part of the Vancouver ACT Team, an innovative approach, as most ACT teams in Canada do not include police (Public Safety Canada, 2015). Similar to specialty courts, the key features of case management approaches include successfully addressing social determinants of health in addition to providing treatment for mental illnesses and addressing criminogenic needs and risk. ACT teams are discussed further in Chapter 15.

Conclusion

The primary risk factors for involvement in the criminal justice system are largely shared by those with and without mental illness; and, as would be expected, people with mental illnesses tend to have more of these characteristics. Social and environmental contexts (e.g., poverty, homelessness, unemployment, drug use, stigma, racism, trauma) contribute to the relationship between mental illnesses and crime. Efforts to divert people with mental illnesses away from the criminal justice system exist at each interception point: pre-arrest, pre-trial, post-sentence, and post-incarceration. The best intercept is early intervention because becoming entrenched in the criminal justice system increases an individual's risk of adverse health, social, and justice outcomes. Given the overlap between social determinants of health and social determinants of criminal behaviour, the evidence is in favour of a public health approach to improving public safety. In other words, individuals' health and criminal behaviour should be of joint concern for health promotion and crime prevention interventions. Importantly, despite making progress in developing promising models, there continue to be opportunities for improvements on the whole to better meet the needs of people with mental illnesses and justice involvement in Canada. People with mental illnesses who are further marginalized by multiple, overlapping forms of structural inequity (e.g., systemic racism, poverty) suffer disproportionately, and there is a need for ongoing attention to the underlying conditions and circumstances that lead them to justice involvement.

Glossary

assertive community treatment (ACT): A model for providing services after discharge from jail for people with complex needs. ACT calls for a "total team approach" and the core features include assertive outreach, multidisciplinary staffing models, direct provision of health and social services, high staff-participant ratios, long-term time-unlimited services, and client contact primarily at home or in the community.

bail: The procedure to determine if a person charged with a criminal offence will be released or detained while awaiting trial.

correctional agencies: Responsible for supervising people who have been convicted and sentenced for committing a crime. This includes supervising people who are serving some or all of their sentence in the community (known as "community corrections") as well as operating correctional facilities where people are detained in custody (i.e., jails, prisons).

deinstitutionalization: Refers to a process of shifting mental health care from institutional to community-based outpatient settings.

disposition: The outcome of a criminal charge.

diversion: The redirection of people away from the criminal justice system and towards services believed to address the needs leading to offending.

interception: Opportunities to prevent an individual from entering or becoming further entrenched in the criminal justice system.

not criminally responsible on account of mental disorder (NCRMD): A disposition for crimes committed while an individual was suffering from a mental illness, or whose mental illness makes them unfit to stand trial on criminal charges.

probation: Allows a person to serve their sentence in the community with conditions prescribed in a probation order.

recidivism: A criminal justice term for reoffending.

Review Board: An administrative tribunal established to make decisions and orders concerning the liberty of individuals whom courts have found to be NCRMD.

transinstitutionalization: Refers to deinstitutionalization policy reforms resulting in the movement of people with mental illnesses to institutions that are not designed for or equipped to provide quality mental health care.

unfit to stand trial (UST): A disposition for individuals unable on account of mental disorder to: (a) understand the nature or object of the proceedings; (b) understand the possible consequences of the proceedings; or (c) communicate with counsel.

Critical Thinking Questions

1. How do the social determinants of health overlap with the social determinants of crime? What does a "public health approach to crime prevention" mean to you?
2. What are the various interception points of criminal justice system interaction? What are examples of diversion that can be used at each intercept (e.g., police, court, corrections)?
3. What is the role of the mental health system in the success of justice diversion?
4. Under what circumstances might someone be placed in the care of the forensic psychiatric system rather than prison? Why is the forensic psychiatric system an important component of the justice system?
5. The Correctional Service of Canada claims to have abolished solitary confinement, but critics argue that this is not necessarily true in practice. After reading Ashley Smith's story, what do you think about solitary confinement practices and reforms in Canada? How are people with mental illnesses uniquely impacted by these practices?

Recommended Readings

Bloom, H., & Schneider, R. D. (2017). *Mental disorder and the law: A primer for legal and mental health professionals.* Irwin Law.

Davies, M., Szigeti, Z., McMahon, M., & Presser, J. R. (2020). *A guide to mental disorder law in Canadian criminal justice.* LexisNexis Canada.

Dupuis, T., MacKay, R., & Nicol, J. (2013). *Current issues in mental health in Canada: Mental health and the criminal justice system.* Library of Parliament. https://publications.gc.ca/collections/collection_2014/bdp-lop/bp/2013-88-eng.pdf

Mental Health Commission of Canada. (2020). *Mental health and the criminal justice system: "What we heard."* https://www.mentalhealthcommission.ca/wp-content/uploads/drupal/2020-08/mental_health_and_the_law_evidence_summary_report_eng.pdf

Recommended Websites

Health Justice. www.healthjustice.ca

Homeless Hub—Assertive Community Treatment (ACT) Teams. www.homelesshub.ca/solutions/supports/assertive-community-treatment-act-teams

John Howard Society—Broken Record: The Continued Criminalization of Mental Health Issues. https://johnhoward.on.ca/brokenrecord

References

Abramsky, S., & Fellner, J. (2003). *Ill-equipped: U.S. prisons and offenders with mental illness.* Human Rights Watch.

Arrigo, B. A., & Bullock, J. L. (2007). The psychological effects of solitary confinement on prisoners in supermax units: Reviewing what we know and recommending what should change. *International Journal of Offender Therapy and Comparative Criminology, 52*(6), 622–640. https://doi.org/10.1177/0306624X07309720

Baranyi, G., Cassidy, M., Fazel, S., Priebe, S., & Mundt, A. P. (2018). Prevalence of posttraumatic stress disorder in prisoners. *Epidemiologic Reviews, 40*(1), 134–145. https://doi.org/10.1093/epirev/mxy007

Baybutt, M., Acin, E., Hayton, P., & Dooris, M. (2014). *Promoting health in prisons: A setting approach.* World Health Organization. http://www.euro.who.int/__data/assets/pdf_file/0018/249210/Prisons-and-Health,-21-Promoting-health-in-prisons-a-settings-approach.pdf

BC Coroners Service. (2013). *Coroner's Report into the death of Mr. Robert Dziekański.* https://www2.gov.bc.ca/assets/gov/birth-adoption-death-marriage-and-divorce/deaths/coroners-service/reports/investigative/robert-dziekanski.pdf

Bingham, E., & Sutton, R. (2012). *Cruel, inhuman and degrading? Canada's treatment of federally-sentenced women with mental health issues.* International Human Rights Program, University of Toronto. https://ihrp.law.utoronto.ca/sites/ihrp.law.utoronto.ca/files/documents/WorkingGroup_Clinic/Cruel%20and%20Inhuman_FINAL_Print.pdf

Bonfine, N., Ritter, C., & Munetz, M. R. (2014). Police officer perceptions of the impact of Crisis Intervention Team (CIT) programs. *International Journal of Law and Psychiatry, 37*(4), 341–350. https://doi.org/10.1016/j.ijlp.2014.02.004

Bonta, J., Blais, J., & Wilson, H. A. (2014). A theoretically informed meta-analysis of the risk for general and violent recidivism for mentally disordered offenders. *Aggression and Violent Behavior, 19*(3), 278–287. https://doi.org/10.1016/j.avb.2014.04.014

Braidwood, T. R. (2009). *Restoring public confidence: Restricting the use of conducted energy weapons in British Columbia.* Braidwood Commission on Conducted Energy Weapon Use. https://www2.gov.bc.ca/assets/gov/law-crime-and-justice/about-bc-justice-system/inquiries/braidwoodphase1report.pdf

Braidwood, T. R. (2010). *Why? The Robert Dziekanski Tragedy.* Braidwood Commission on the Death of Robert Dziekanski. https://www2.gov.bc.ca/assets/gov/law-crime-and-justice/about-bc-justice-system/inquiries/braidwoodphase2report.pdf

Brink, J., Livingston, J., & Desmarais, S. (2011). *A study of how people with mental illness perceive and interact with the police.* Mental Health Commission of Canada. https://www.mentalhealthcommission.ca/wp-content/uploads/drupal/Law_How_People_with_Mental_Illness_Perceive_Interact_Police_Study_ENG_1_0_1.pdf

Bromwich, R., & Kilty, J. M. (2017). Introduction: Law, vulnerability, and segregation: What have we learned from Ashley Smith's carceral death? *Canadian Journal of Law and Society, 32*(2), 157–164.

Buchanan, L., Bui, Q., & Patel, J. K. (2020, July 3). Black Lives Matter may be the largest movement in U.S. history. *New York Times.* https://www.nytimes.com/interactive/2020/07/03/us/george-floyd-protests-crowd-size.html

Butler, A., Nicholls, T. N., Samji, H., Fabian, S., & Lavergne, R. (2021). Prevalence of mental health needs, substance use, and co-occurring disorders among people admitted to prison in British Columbia. *Psychiatric Services.* https://doi.org/10.1176/appi.ps.202000927

Canada, K. E., Angell, B., & Watson, A. C. (2010). Crisis intervention teams in Chicago: Successes on the ground. *Journal of Police Crisis Negotiations, 10*(1–2), 86–100. https://doi.org/10.1080/15332581003792070

Canada, K. E., Barrenger, S., & Ray, B. (2019). Bridging mental health and criminal justice systems: A systematic review of the impact of mental health courts on individuals and communities. *Psychology, Public Policy, and Law, 25*(2), 73–91. https://doi.org/10.1037/law0000194

Canadian Mental Health Association Ontario. (2015). *Landmark study dispels "not criminally responsible" myths.* https://ontario.cmha.ca/news/landmark-study-dispels-not-criminally-responsible-myths/

Canadian Press. (2014, April 17). Father of murder suspect said he'd do anything to bring victims back. *Maclean's*. https://www.macleans.ca/news/father-of-mass-murder-suspect-says-hed-do-anything-to-bring-victims-back/

Canadian Resource Centre for Victims of Crime. (2016). Calgary man found not criminally responsible in killing of five young people at party. *National Justice Network Update, 23*(5), 3–4.

Casavant, L., & Charron-Tousignant, M. (2019). *Bill C-38: An act to amend the Corrections and Conditional Release Act and another Act* (Publication No. 42-1-C38-E). Library of Parliament. https://lop.parl.ca/staticfiles/PublicWebsite/Home/ResearchPublications/LegislativeSummaries/PDF/42-1/c83-e.pdf

Centre for Addiction and Mental Health. (2013). *Mental health and criminal justice policy framework*. https://www.camh.ca/-/media/files/pdfs---public-policy-submissions/mh_criminal_justice_policy_framework-pdf.pdf

Charette, Y., Crocker, A. G., & Billette, I. (2011). The judicious judicial dispositions juggle: Characteristics of police interventions involving people with a mental illness. *The Canadian Journal of Psychiatry, 56*(11), 677–685. https://doi.org/10.1177/070674371105601106

Charette, Y., Crocker, A. G., & Billette, I. (2014). Police encounters involving citizens with mental illness: Use of resources and outcomes. *Psychiatric Services, 65*(4), 511–516. https://doi-org.proxy.lib.sfu.ca/10.1176/appi.ps.201300053

Charette, Y., Crocker, A. G., Seto, M. C., Salem, L., Nicholls, T. L., & Caulet, M. (2015). The national trajectory project of individuals found not criminally responsible on account of mental disorder in Canada. Part 4: Criminal recidivism. *The Canadian Journal of Psychiatry, 60*(3), 127–134. https://doi.org/10.1177/070674371506000307

Chief Coroner of Ontario. (2013). *Inquest touching the death of Ashley Smith: Jury verdict and recommendations*. http://www.caefs.ca/wp-content/uploads/2014/01/A.S.-Inquest-Jury-Verdict-and-Recommendations1.pdf

Coleman, T. G., & Cotton, D. (2010). *Police interactions with persons with a mental illness: Police learning in the environment of contemporary policing*. The Mental Health and the Law Advisory Committee, Mental Health Commission of Canada. https://www.mentalhealthcommission.ca/sites/default/files/Law_Police_Interactions_Mental_Illness_Report_ENG_0_1.pdf

Conor, P., Carrière, S., Amey, S., Marcellus, S., & Sauvé, J. (2020). *Police resources in Canada, 2019*. Canadian Centre for Justice Statistics, Statistics Canada. https://www150.statcan.gc.ca/n1/en/pub/85-002-x/2020001/article/00015-eng.pdf?st=ZsYAqtHy

Correctional Service Canada [CSC]. (2015). *Review of mental health commitments. Internal audit sector*. https://www.csc-scc.gc.ca/005/007/092/005007-2535-eng.pdf

Correctional Service Canada [CSC]. (2021). *Structured intervention units*. https://www.csc-scc.gc.ca/acts-and-regulations/005006-3000-en.shtml

Cotton, D. & Coleman, T. G. (2008). Contemporary policing guidelines for working with the mental health system. Canadian Association of Chiefs of Police. Retrieved from: https://cacp.ca/human-resources-and-learning-committee.html?asst_id=131

Cotton, D., & Coleman, T. G. (2017). The evolution of police interactions with people with mental health problems: The third generation (strategic) approach. In C. L. Mitchell & E. H. Dorian (Eds.), *Police psychology and its growing impact on modern law enforcement* (p. 252–273). IGI Global.

Council of State Governments Justice Centre. (2012). *Improving outcomes for people with mental illnesses involved with New York City's criminal court and correction systems*. Council of State Governments. https://csgjusticecenter.org/wp-content/uploads/2013/05/CTBNYC-Court-Jail_7-cc.pdf

Criminal Code, R.S.C., C-46. (1985).

Crocker, A. G., & Côté, G. (2009). Evolving systems of care: Individuals found not criminally responsible on account of mental disorder in custody of civil and forensic psychiatric services. *European Psychiatry, 24*(6), 356–364. https://doi.org/10.1016/j.eurpsy.2009.07.008

Crocker, A. G., Nicholls, T. L., Seto, M. C., Côté, G., Charette, Y., & Caulet, M. (2015). The national trajectory project of individuals found not criminally responsible on account of mental disorder in Canada. Part 1: Context and methods. *The Canadian Journal of Psychiatry, 60*(3), 98–105. https://doi.org/10.1177/070674371506000304

De Viggiani, N. (2007). Unhealthy prisons: Exploring structural determinants of prison health. *Sociology of Health & Illness, 29*(1), 115–135. https://doi.org/10.1111/j.1467-9566.2007.00474.x

Douglas, K. S., Guy, L. S., & Hart, S. D. (2009). Psychosis as a risk factor for violence to others: A meta-analysis. *Psychological Bulletin, 135*(5), 679–706. https://doi.org/ 10.1037/a0016311

Draine, J., Salzer, M. S., Culhane, D. P., & Hadley, T. R. (2002). Role of social disadvantage in crime, joblessness, and homelessness among persons with serious mental illness. *Psychiatric Services, 53*(5), 565–573. https://doi.org/10.1176/appi.ps.53.5.565

Family Statement—Alberta Review Board hearing—De Grood. (2018, September 8). The City of Calgary Newsroom. https://newsroom.calgary.ca/family-statement—alberta-review-board-hearing—de-grood/

Farrell MacDonald, S., Keown, L.-A., Boudreau, H., Gobeil, R., & Wardrop, K. (2015). *Prevalence of psychotropic medication prescription among federal offenders. (Research Report R-373)*. Correctional Service of Canada. https://www.csc-scc.gc.ca/research/005008-r373-eng.shtml

Fazel, S., & Danesh, J. (2002). Serious mental disorder in 23 000 prisoners: A systematic review of 62 surveys. *The Lancet, 359*(9306), 545–550. https://doi.org/10.1016/S0140-6736(02)07740-1

Fazel, S., & Seewald, K. (2012). Severe mental illness in 33 588 prisoners worldwide: Systematic review and meta-regression analysis. *British Journal of Psychiatry, 200*(5), 364–373. https://doi.org/10.1192/bjp.bp.111.096370

Forchuk, C., Russell, G., Kingston-Macclure, S., Turner, K., & Dill, S. (2006). From psychiatric ward to the streets and shelters. *Journal of Psychiatric and Mental Health Nursing, 13*(3), 301–308. https://doi.org/10.1111/j.1365-2850.2006.00954.x

Goffman, E. (1963). *Stigma: Notes on the management of spoiled identity*. Prentice Hall.

Goossens, I., Jordan, M., & Nicholls, T. L. (2021). #AbolishNCR: A qualitative analysis of social media narratives around the insanity defense. *Canadian Journal of Criminology and Criminal Justice, 63*(2), 46–67. https://doi.org/10.3138/cjccj.2020-0019

Hagan, B. O., Wang, E. A., Aminawung, J. A., Albizu-Garcia, C. E., Zaller, N., Nyamu, S., Shavit, S., Deluca, J., Fox, A. D., & Transitions Clinic Network. (2018). History of solitary confinement is associated with post-traumatic stress disorder symptoms among individuals recently released from prison. *Journal of Urban Health, 95*, 141–148. https://doi.org/10.1007/s11524-017-0138-1

Han, W. (2019). Life changes matter more than satisfaction or sanctions/incentives: An examination of mental health court experience factors associated with arrest. *International Journal of Forensic Mental Health, 18*(4), 376–388. https://doi.org/10.1080/14999013.2019.1588434

Haney, C. (2003). Mental health issues in long-term solitary and "supermax" confinement. *Crime & Delinquency, 49*(1), 124–156. https://doi.org/10.1177/0011128702239239

Haney, C. (2017). "Madness" and penal confinement: Some observations on mental illness and prison pain. *Punishment & Society, 19*(3), 310–326. https://doi.org/10.1177/1462474517705389

Hiday, V. A. (2006). Putting community risk in perspective: A look at correlations, causes and controls. *International Journal of Law and Psychiatry, 29*(4), 316–331. https://doi.org/10.1016/j.ijlp.2004.08.010

Jackson, M., Glackman, W., Giles, C., & Buchwitz, R. (2012). *Compilation of research on the Vancouver Downtown Community Court 2008 to 2012*. Simon Fraser Universtiy. https://www2.gov.bc.ca/assets/gov/law-crime-and-justice/courthouse-services/community-court/dcc-research-compilation.pdf

Jellicoe, D., & Anderson, T. (2019). Mental health services and special intervention teams. In U. Williams, D. J. Jones, & J. R. Reddon (Eds.), *Police response to mental health in Canada* (pp. 245–256). Canadian Scholars.

Jennings, J. L. (2009). Does assertive community treatment work with forensic populations? Review and recommendations. *The Open Psychiatry Journal, 3*, 13–19. https://doi.org/10.2174/1874354400903010013

John Howard Society of Ontario. (2015). *Unlocking change: Decriminalizing mental health issues in Ontario*. http://www.johnhoward.on.ca/wp-content/uploads/2015/07/Unlocking-Change-Final-August-2015.pdf

Kesic, D., Thomas, S. D., & Ogloff, J. R. (2010). Mental illness among police fatalities in Victoria 1982–2007: Case linkage study. *Australia & New Zealand Journal of Psychiatry, 44*(5), 463–468. https://doi.org/10.3109/00048670903493355

Kim, D.-Y. (2014). Psychiatric deinstitutionalization and prison population growth: A critical literature review and its implications. *Criminal Justice Policy Review, 27*(1), 3–21. https://doi.org/10.1177/0887403414547043

Kouyoumdjian, F., Schuler, A., Matheson, F. I., & Hwang, S. W. (2016). Health status of prisoners in Canada: Narrative review. *Canadian Family Physician, 62*(3), 215–222.

Kouyoumdjian, F. G., Wang, R., Mejia-Lancheros, C., Owusu-Bempah, A., Nisenbaum, R., O'Campo, P., Stergiopoulos, V., & Hwang, S. W. (2019). Interactions between police and persons who experience homelessness and mental illness in Toronto, Canada: Findings from a prospective study. *The Canadian Journal of Psychiatry, 64*(10), 718–725. https://doi.org/10.1177%2F0706743719861386

La Vigne, N., Davies, E., Palmer, T., & Halberstadt, R. (2002). *Release planning for successful reentry*. Urban Institute Justice Policy Centre. https://www.urban.org/sites/default/files/publication/32056/411767-Release-Planning-for-Successful-Reentry.PDF

Lamanna, D., Shapiro, G. K., Kirst, M., Matheson, F. I., Nakhost, A., & Stergiopoulos, V. (2018). Co-responding police-mental health programmes: Service user experiences and outcomes in a large urban centre. *International Journal of Mental Health Nursing, 27*(2), 891–900. https://doi.org/10.1111/inm.12384

Lamb, H. R., Weinberger, L. E., & DeCuir, W. J. (2002). The police and mental health. *Psychiatric Services, 53*(10), 1266–1271. https://doi.org/10.1176/appi.ps.53.10.1266

The Lancet. (2016). The health crisis of mental health stigma [Editorial]. *The Lancet, 387*(10023), 1027. https://doi.org/10.1016/S0140-6736(16)00687-5

Langeveld, J., Bjørkly, S., Auestad, B., Barder, H., Evensen, J., ten Velden Hegelstad, W., Joa, I., Johannessen, J. O., Larsen, T. K., Melle, I., Opjordsmoen, S., Røssberg, I., Rund, B. R., Simonsen, E., Vaglum, P., McGlashan, T., & Friis, S. (2014). Treatment and violent behavior in persons with first episode psychosis during a 10-year prospective follow-up study. *Schizophrenia Research, 156*(2–3), 272–276. https://doi.org/10.1016/j.schres.2014.04.010

Large, M. M., & Nielssen, O. (2011). Violence in first-episode psychosis: A systematic review and meta-analysis. *Schizophrenia Research, 125*(2–3), 209–220. https://doi.org/10.1016/j.schres.2010.11.026

Latimer, J., & Lawrence, A. (2006). *The review board systems in Canada: An overview of results from the mentally disordered accused data collection study*. Department of Justice Canada. https://www.justice.gc.ca/eng/rp-pr/csj-sjc/jsp-sjp/rr06_1/p1.html

Lavoie, J. A., Connolly, D. A., & Roesch, R. (2006). Correctional officers' perceptions of inmates with mental illness: The role of training and burnout syndrome. *International Journal of Forensic Mental Health, 5*(2), 151–166. https://doi.org/10.1080/14999013.2006.10471239

LeBlanc, N., Kilty, J. M., & Frigon, S. (2015). Examining the preventable but predictable death of Ashley Smith. *International Journal of Prisoner Health, 11*(3), 126–140. https://doi.org/10.1108/IJPH-11-2014-0048

Livingston, J., Nicholls, T., & Brink, J. (2011). The impact of realigning a tertiary psychiatric hospital in British Columbia on other institutional sectors. *Psychiatric Services, 62*(2), 200–205. https://doi.org/10.1176/ps.62.2.pss6202_0200

Livingston, J., Weaver, C., Hall, N., & Verdun-Jones, S. (2008). *Criminal justice diversion for persons with mental disorders: A review of best practices.* Canadian Mental Health Association, BC Division. https://cmha.bc.ca/wp-content/uploads/2016/07/DiversionBestPractices.pdf

Lum, C., Koper, C. S., & Wu, X. (2021). Can we really defund the police? A nine-agency study of police response to calls for service. *Police Quarterly.* https://doi.org/10.1177%2F10986111211035002

Lurigio, A. J., Fallon, J. R., & Dincin, J. (2000). Helping the mentally ill in jails adjust to community life: A description of a postrelease act program and its clients. *International Journal of Offender Therapy and Comparative Criminology, 44*(5), 532–548. https://doi.org/10.1177/0306624X00445002

Lurigio, A. J., & Swartz, J. A. (2006). Mental illness in correctional populations: The use of standardized screening tools for further evaluation or treatment. *Federal Probation, 70*(2), 29–35.

MacDonald, S.-A., Bellot, C., Sylvestre, M.-E., Michaud, A.-A. D., & Pelletier, A. (2014). *Mental health courts: Processes, outcomes and impact on homelessness.* Government of Canada's Homelessness Partnering Strategy. https://www.homelesshub.ca/resource/mental-health-courts-processes-outcomes-and-impact-homelessness

MacPhail, A., & Verdun-Jones, S. (2013). *Mental illness and the criminal justice system.* Paper presented at the Re-Inventing Criminal Justice: The Fifth National Symposium Montreal, QC, Canada.

Maniglio, R. (2009). Severe mental illness and criminal victimization: A systematic review. *Acta Psychiatrica Scandinavica, 119*(3), 180–191. https://doi.org/10.1111/j.1600-0447.2008.01300.x

Marcoux, J., & Nicholson, K. (2018). Deadly force: Fatal encounters with police in Canada, 2000–2017. *CBC Radio-Canada.* https://newsinteractives.cbc.ca/longform-custom/deadly-force

McGrew, J., & Bond, G. (1995). Critical ingredients of assertive community treatment: Judgments of the experts. *The Journal of Mental Health Administration, 22*(2), 113–125. https://doi.org/10.1007/BF02518752

Messina, N., Burdon, W., Hagopian, G., & Prendergast, M. (2004). One year return to custody rates among co-disordered offenders. *Behavioral Sciences & the Law, 22*(4), 503–518. https://doi.org/10.1002/bsl.600

Metzner, J. L., & Fellner, J. (2010). Solitary confinement and mental illness in U.S. Prisons: A challenge for medical ethics. *Journal of the American Academy of Psychiatry and the Law Online, 38*(1), 104–108.

Moschion, J., & Johnson, G. (2019). Homelessness and incarceration: A reciprocal relationship? *Journal of Quantitative Criminology, 35*(4), 855–887. https://doi.org/10.1007/s10940-019-09407-y

Munetz, M. R., & Griffin, P. A. (2006). Use of the sequential intercept model as an approach to decriminalization of people with serious mental illness. *Psychiatric Services, 57*(4), 544–549. https://doi.org/10.1176/ps.2006.57.4.544

Nicholls, T. L., Butler, A., Kendrick-Koch, L., Brink, J., Jones, R., & Simpson, S. (2018). Assessing and treating offenders with mental illness. In M. Ternes, P.

Magaletta, & M. Patry (Eds.), *The Practice of Correctional Psychology* (pp. 9–37). Springer.

Nicholls, T. L., Roesch, R., Olley, M., Ogloff, J. R. P., & Hemphill, J. (2005). *Jail Screening Assessment Tool (JSAT): A guide for conducting mental health screening in jails and pretrial centres.* Simon Fraser University.

Office of the Auditor General of BC. (2019). *Progress audit: Correctional facilities and programs.* https://www.bcauditor.com/pubs/2019/progress-audit-correctional-facilities-and-programs

Osher, F. C. (2013). *Integrating mental health and substance abuse services for justice-involved persons with co-occurring disorders.* SAMHSA's GAINS Centre for Behavioural Health and Justice Transformation. http://www.antoniocasella.eu/archipsy/Osher_2013.pdf

Parent, R. (2011). The police use of deadly force in British Columbia: Mental illness and crisis intervention. *Journal of Police Crisis Negotiations, 11*(1), 57–71. https://doi.org/10.1080/15332586.2011.548144

Parker, G. F. (2009). Impact of a mental health training course for correctional officers on a special housing unit. *Psychiatric Services, 60*(5), 640–645. https://doi.org/10.1176/ps.2009.60.5.640

Public Safety Canada. (2015). *Mental illness in correctional populations: The use of standardized screening tools for further evaluation or treatment.* https://www.publicsafety.gc.ca/cnt/cntrng-crm/plcng/cnmcs-plcng/ndx/snpss-en.aspx?n=483

Puntis, S., Perfect, D., Kirubarajan, A., Bolton, S., Davies, F., Hayes, A., Harriss, E., & Molodynski, A. (2018). A systematic review of co-responder models of police mental health "street" triage. *BMC Psychiatry, 18*, Article 256. https://doi.org/10.1186/s12888-018-1836-2

Quinn, J., & Simpson, A. I. F. (2013). How can forensic systems improve justice for victims of offenders found not criminally responsible? *The Journal of the American Academy of Psychiatry and the Law, 41*(4), 568–574.

Rich, J. D., Chandler, R., Williams, B. A., Dumont, D., Wang, E. A., Taxman, F. S., Allen, S. A., Clarke, J. G., Greifinger, R. B., Wildeman, C., Osher, F. C., Rosenberg, S., Haney, C., Mauer, M., & Western, B. (2014). How health care reform can transform the health of criminal justice-involved individuals. *Health Affairs, 33*(3), 462–467. https://doi.org/10.1377/hlthaff.2013.1133

Richard, B. (2008). *A report of the New Brunswick ombudsman and child and youth advocate on services provided to a youth involved in the youth criminal justice system.* Office of the Ombudsman and Child and Youth Advocate. https://www.cyanb.ca/images/AshleySmith-e.pdf

Sapers, H. (2008). *A preventable death.* Office of the Correctional Investigator. https://www.oci-bec.gc.ca/cnt/rpt/pdf/oth-aut/oth-aut20080620-eng.pdf

Sapers, H. (2011). *Mental health and corrections.* Paper presented at the Department of Psychology Colloquium Series, Saint Francis Xavier University, Antigonish, Nova Scotia.

Schneider, R. D. (2013). Mental health courts. In A. Jamieson & A. Moenssens (Eds.), *Wiley Encyclopedia of Forensic Sciences*. John Wiley & Sons.

Schnittker, J. (2013). The psychological dimensions and the social consequences of incarceration. *The ANNALS of the American Academy of Political and Social Science, 651*(1), 122–138. https://doi.org/10.1177/0002716213502922

Seltzer, T. (2005). Mental health courts: A misguided attempt to address the criminal justice system's unfair treatment of people with mental illnesses. *Psychology, Public Policy, and Law, 11*(4), 570–586. https://doi.org/10.1037/1076-8971.11.4.570

Service, J. (2010). *Under warrant: A review of the implementation of the Correctional Service of Canada's "Mental Health Strategy."* Office of the Correctional Investigator of Canada. https://www.oci-bec.gc.ca/cnt/rpt/pdf/oth-aut/oth-aut20100923-eng.pdf

Shalev, S. (2014). Solitary confinement as a prison health issue. In S. Enggist, L. Moller, G. Galea, & C. Udesen (Eds.), *Prisons and health* (pp. 27–35). World Health Organization. https://www.euro.who.int/__data/assets/pdf_file/0005/249188/Prisons-and-Health.pdf

Shapiro, G., Cusi, A., Kirst, M., O'Campo, P., Nakhost, A., & Stergiopoulos, V. (2015). Co-responding police-mental health programs: A review. *Administration and Policy in Mental Health, 42*(5), 606–620. https://doi.org/10.1007/s10488-014-0594-9

Silver, E. (1995). Punishment or treatment? *Law and Human Behavior, 19*(4), 375–388. https://doi.org/10.1007/BF01499138

Skeem, J. L., & Peterson, J. K. (2012). Identifying, treating, and reducing risk for offenders with mental illness. In J. Petersilia & K. R. Reitz (Eds.), *The Oxford handbook of sentencing and corrections* (pp. 521–543). Oxford University Press.

Skeem, J. L., Winter, E., Kennealy, P. J., Louden, J. E., & Tatar, J. R. (2014). Offenders with mental illness have criminogenic needs, too: Toward recidivism reduction. *Law and Human Behavior, 38*(3), 212–224. https://doi.org/10.1037/lhb0000054

Somers, J. M., Moniruzzaman, A., Rezansoff, S. N., Patterson, M., & Franken, I. H. A. (2014). Examining the impact of case management in Vancouver's Downtown Community Court: A quasi-experimental design. *PLoS One, 9*(3). https://doi.org/10.1371/journal.pone.0090708

Sprott, J. B., & Doob, A. N. (2021). *Solitary confinement, torture, and Canada's Structured Intervention Units.* https://www.crimsl.utoronto.ca/sites/www.crimsl.utoronto.ca/files/Torture%20Solitary%20SIUs%20%28Sprott%20Doob%2023%20Feb%202021%29.pdf

Steadman, H. J., Redlich, A., Callahan, L., Robbins, P., & Vesselinov, R. (2011). Effect of mental health courts on arrests and jail days: A multisite study. *Archives of General Psychiatry, 68*(2), 167–172. https://doi.org/10.1001/archgenpsychiatry.2010.134

Substance Abuse and Mental Health Services Administration (SAMHSA). (2021). *The Sequential Intercept Model (SIM).* https://www.samhsa.gov/criminal-juvenile-justice/sim-overview

Ternes, M., Magaletta, P., & Patry, M. (Eds.). (2018). *The practice of correctional psychology*. Springer Nature Switzerland.

Trestman, R., Applebaum, K., & Metzner, J. (Eds.). (2015). *Oxford textbook of correctional psychiatry*. Oxford University Press.

United Nations Committee against Torture. (2012). *Convention against torture and other cruel, inhuman or degrading treatment or punishment. Consideration of reports submitted by States parties under article 19 of the Convention*. https://www.ohchr.org/en/professionalinterest/pages/cat.aspx

Usher, L., Watson, A. C., Bruno, R., Andriukaitis, S., Kamin, D., Speed, C., & Taylor, S. (2019). *Crisis Intervention Team (CIT) programs: A best practice guide for transforming community responses to mental health crises*. CIT International. https://www.citinternational.org/resources/Best%20Practice%20Guide/CIT%20guide%20desktop%20printing%202019_08_16%20(1).pdf

Weine, S., Kohrt, B., Collins, P., Cooper, J., Lewis-Fernandez, R., Okpaku, S., & Wainberg, M. (2020). Justice for George Floyd and a reckoning for global mental health. *Global Mental Health, 7*, E22. https://doi.org/10.1017/gmh.2020.17

Weiss, M. G., Ramakrishna, J., & Somma, D. (2006). Health-related stigma: Rethinking concepts and interventions. *Psychology, Health & Medicine, 11*(3), 277–287. https://doi.org/10.1080/13548500600595053

White, H. R., Conway, F. N., & Ward, J. H. (2019). Comorbidity of substance use and violence. In M. Krohn, N. Hendrix, G. Penly Hall, & A. Lizotte (Eds.), *Handbook on crime and deviance* (Vol. 2; pp. 513–532). Springer.

Wiebe, D. (2016). *Vancouver Police Mental Health Strategy: A comprehensive approach for a proportional police response to persons living with mental illness*. Vancouver Police Department. https://vpd.ca/wp-content/uploads/2021/06/mental-health-strategy.pdf

Williams, B. A., Li, A., Ahalt, C., Coxson, P., Kahn, J. G., & Bibbins-Domingo, K. (2019). The cardiovascular health burdens of solitary confinement. *Journal of General Internal Medicine, 34*(10), 1977–1980. https://doi.org/10.1007/s11606-019-05103-6

Wilson, A., Draine, J., Barrenger, S., Hadley, T., & Evans, A. (2014). Examining the impact of mental illness and substance use on time till re-incarceration in a county jail. *Administration and Policy in Mental Health, 41*(3), 293–301. https://doi.org/10.1007/s10488-013-0467-7

Winko v. British Columbia (Forensic Psychiatric Institute), [1999] 2 S.C.R. 625.

Zorzi, R., Scott, S., Doherty, D., Engman, A., Lauzon, C., McGuire, M., & Ward, J. (2006). *Housing options upon discharge from correctional facilities*. Canada Mortgage and Housing Corporation. https://publications.gc.ca/collections/collection_2011/schl-cmhc/nh18-1/NH18-1-332-2006-eng.pdf

Chapter 13

Mental Health Legislation and Patients' Rights

Iva W. Cheung

Introduction

Laws meant to protect public health, like seatbelt laws or mandatory vaccination laws, sometimes infringe on personal choices and liberties. In more extreme cases, such as quarantines of people with highly transmissible infections, for example, people might even be deprived of their freedom of movement. And in the realm of mental health care, each province and territory in Canada has legislation that allows hospitals to, under certain conditions, detain people with mental illnesses. In some cases, this legislation also allows the hospitals to administer psychiatric treatment without the patient's consent.

In this chapter, you will be introduced to some of the legal and ethical issues relating to this type of involuntary hospitalization, which is also referred to as civil commitment. In Canada, it is often called "certification," because patients are detained on the authority of a legal document called a *certificate*. Involuntary hospitalization is separate from the forensic psychiatric system discussed in Chapter 12, where people are detained in a psychiatric facility after having been found to be not criminally responsible or unfit to stand trial for a criminal offence. While individuals who receive involuntary care are referred to as *patients* in this chapter, some people may prefer terms such as *clients* or *consumers*. As we explore the history of mental health laws, please be aware that some of the historical legislation uses language to describe people with mental illnesses that we would now consider offensive.

This chapter first introduces the different approaches to involuntary hospitalization. We then examine the history of involuntary hospitalization in Britain and the United States and illustrate how it has shaped involuntary mental health care in Canada. Next, current approaches to mental health legislation across Canada will be discussed, including how criteria for involuntary hospitalization, treatment decisions, and involuntary outpatient treatment vary by jurisdiction. Patients' experiences with involuntary hospitalization will also be presented, illustrating the diversity of perspectives. Next, the protections built into mental health legislation, including Review Board panels and patient rights information, will be introduced, as well as violations of patients' rights. The chapter concludes with an exploration of procedural justice as it relates to patients' experiences of involuntary hospitalization and treatment.

Approaches to Involuntary Hospitalization

There is fierce debate about when it is justifiable to hospitalize people involuntarily for mental illnesses. This debate is largely driven by two competing ideological perspectives: (1) the civil libertarian approach and (2) the human needs approach. The **civil libertarian approach** is based on the view that individual freedoms are of the utmost importance. Proponents of this perspective argue that a person's freedom should be limited only if they are a physical danger to themselves or to others. Under detention in hospital, the threat to safety is removed, so the patient has the right to refuse treatment if they wish. Thus, according to this approach, the decision to detain is separate from the decision to treat. In many jurisdictions that use a civil libertarian model, the decision to detain a person is made by a judge, with a medical professional, such as a psychiatrist, assessing the risk that the person poses to themselves or to others. For this reason, the civil libertarian approach has been described as having a *judicial* view of involuntary hospitalization.

Some influential advocates and scholars hold a purist, literal interpretation of the civil libertarian approach and don't believe that involuntary hospitalization should exist at all. For example, Tina Minkowitz, a human rights lawyer who experienced forced psychiatric treatment, has argued for the complete abolition of involuntary hospitalization and treatment. Minkowitz (2006) wrote that "forced psychiatric interventions" violate articles 12, 25, 17, and 15 of the United Nations's *Convention on the Rights of Persons with Disabilities* (UN General Assembly, 2006), interfering with the right to "free and informed consent of persons with disabilities, and equal right to respect for physical and mental integrity, as well as the freedom from torture and cruel, inhuman or degrading treatment or punishment" (Minkowitz, 2006). Minkowitz considers any form of coercion in the psychiatric system a form of violence. Similarly, Thomas Szasz (1961), one of the most outspoken critics of state intervention, held the view that mental illnesses—such as schizophrenia—are social constructs that lack a biological basis. Szasz believed that involuntary hospitalization and psychiatric medication were used as tools for social control and for persecuting behavioural differences based on factors like a person's socioeconomic status. Other scholars, like H. Archibald Kaiser (2009), have acknowledged that mental illnesses have a medical cause but argue that treating them should involve "minimally coercive legislation" that supports people in achieving their recovery goals as they define them, instead of imposing treatment.

In contrast, the **human needs approach** focuses on a person's need for psychiatric treatment. Proponents of this perspective argue that mental illnesses have a clear biological basis and that a chief symptom of some mental illnesses—such as psychosis—is anosognosia, or a "lack of insight." In other words, the illness itself makes the person incapable of recognizing that they are ill, leading them to reject voluntary treatment that could help them regain function and autonomy. As a result, involuntary treatment is seen as the only way to alleviate psychological suffering. What's more, treatment should begin as soon as possible, because early treatment is associated with a better prognosis (Perkins et al., 2005). Unlike the civil libertarian approach, where detention and treatment are considered separately, the human needs approach asserts that the purpose of detaining someone is to treat them, so involuntary patients are given psychiatric treatment whether they want it or not. This approach takes a *medical* view (as opposed to a judicial view) of involuntary hospitalization, where the decision to detain is made by a medical professional (instead of a judge) who acts not as a risk assessor but as a clinician serving the patient's best interests. Someone given involuntary treatment may object at first, but the belief underpinning this approach is that the patient will recover to the point where they recognize their illness and seek out voluntary care in the future.

Outspoken advocates of the human needs model include John Gray, who wrote that tying treatment to detention allows people to receive care and recovery quickly, whereas giving patients a right to refuse treatment leads to a situation where they might be detained indefinitely or "warehoused" because they never recover (Gray et al., 2008). He cites the case of *Sevels v. Cameron* in Ontario as an example, where Edwin Sevels, hospitalized for symptoms of schizophrenia and violence, refused treatment and was kept in seclusion for 404 days. Sevels was finally treated after he attacked and seriously injured a staff member. Following this treatment, his mental health slowly improved to the point where he could be released to receive care in the community. Gray argues that Sevels would have been able to begin his recovery much earlier if he had not had the option of refusing treatment.

Gray also argues that using physical dangerousness as a criterion for detention, as the civil libertarian approach does, increases stigma against people with mental illnesses because it implies that people hospitalized for a mental illness are a threat. American psychiatrists Appelbaum and Gutheil (1979) made a similar argument, writing that the "majority of legal arguments in support of the right to refuse medication" do not "fit the clinical reality" and that allowing patients to refuse treatment will mean that many will be detained and suffer from symptoms perhaps indefinitely, essentially "rotting with their rights on." Psychiatrist Richard O'Reilly (1998) has written extensively about mental health law and says that the focus on legal rights interferes with patients' right to get well, sometimes resulting in long delays in treatment or agonizing waits until one deteriorates to the point where emergency intervention is needed. "Mental health legislation must protect a patient's right to appropriate treatment in addition to the patient's right to autonomy," wrote O'Reilly, and "It behoves all psychiatrists to continue to insist that the law serve our patients' best interests."

Table 13.1: Key differences between the civil libertarian and human needs approaches

Civil Libertarian Approach	Human Needs Approach
Detention based on dangerousness	Detention based on need for treatment
Detention separate from treatment	Treatment is the reason for detention
Decision to detain is made by the court (judicial view)	Decision to detain is made by a medical professional (medical view)

History of Involuntary Hospitalization

In practice, different jurisdictions' approaches to involuntary hospitalization fall somewhere along a spectrum between a civil libertarian and human needs approach. To better understand the orientation to involuntary hospitalization in Canada, it is helpful to explore the history of this practice in both the United Kingdom (UK), which leans towards a human needs approach, and the United States (US), which adopts a more civil libertarian stance.

Involuntary Hospitalization in Britain

In mid-18th century Britain, people deemed "insane" were either kept in the family home or were detained in *madhouses*—private residences where the owners would collect fees in exchange for housing the person (Unsworth, 1993). This system led to severe abuses: not only were people with mental illnesses subject to horrendous conditions with no medical oversight, but many detainees did not actually have a mental illness and were falsely imprisoned. Reports of these cases prompted the British government to enact its first piece of legislation related to mental health, the *Madhouses Act* of 1774, which required that all madhouses be licensed and inspected. In 1808, the *County Asylums Act* established the first public asylums to house "pauper lunatics," who otherwise lived on the streets or in prisons or workhouses. At this point in history, effective treatments for mental illnesses were not yet available, and the function of these asylums was to manage and detain people with mental illnesses. The act was replaced in 1845 with a revised *County Asylums Act* and a new *Lunacy Act*, which for the first time explicitly addressed treatment: All asylums would have to have a resident physician and written regulations to uphold living and treatment standards.

Unfortunately, without clear criteria for detention, people were sometimes held for seemingly arbitrary reasons. The 1853 *Lunatic Asylums Act* tried to correct this problem. It outlined a clear legal procedure, allowing police to take people suspected of a mental illness to appear before a judge, who could then order an examination by a "Physician, Surgeon, or Apothecary." The person could then be detained in an asylum if the medical professional signed a certificate stating that they were a "Lunatic, or an Idiot, or a Person of unsound Mind." The legislation gave patients no room to

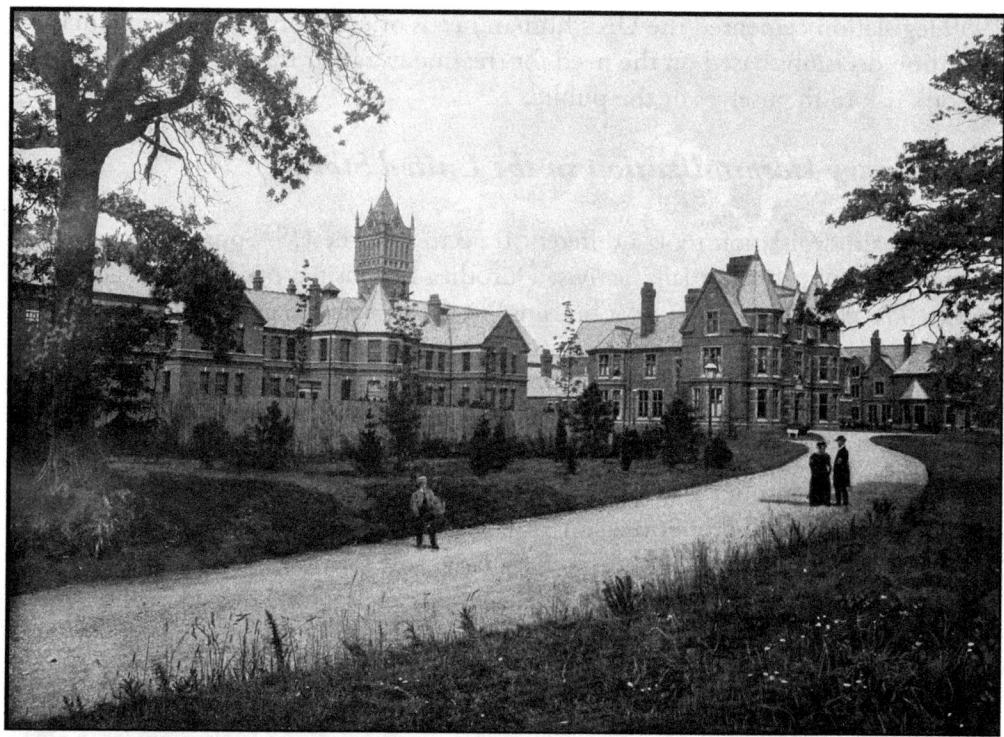

Figure 13.1: Claybury Asylum was opened in 1893 in Woodford Bridge, UK. In keeping with the function of asylums to manage and detain people with mental illnesses, the site was described as "perfectly secluded" from nearby communities.

Source: iStockphoto/ilbusca

challenge their detention, which could be extended indefinitely. The 1890 *Lunacy Act* limited the length of the first detention to one year.

Around the turn of the 20th century, mental illnesses became the focus of more scientific study, with researchers beginning to classify different categories of illness and modern psychiatry gaining a foothold. As a result, more emphasis was put on treating—rather than simply detaining—people with mental illnesses. In 1930, the *Mental Treatment Act* marked the first time that mental health legislation included provisions for people seeking voluntary or outpatient treatment. It also modernized much of the terminology: *asylum* was changed to *hospital*, and *lunacy* was changed to *mental illness*.

With the UK's first *Mental Health Act*, enacted in 1959, physicians, rather than judges, made the decision to detain. A person could be involuntarily hospitalized based on the recommendation of two doctors, one of whom had to have psychiatric experience. The law also established a Medical Review Tribunal that allowed patients to challenge their hospitalization if they believed they were wrongly detained. Although the UK's mental health legislation has been updated since, the

1959 legislation cemented the UK's human needs orientation, with doctors making detention decisions based on the need for treatment, rather than on perceptions of a person's risk to themselves or the public.

Involuntary Hospitalization in the United States

Mental health legislation took a different trajectory in the US. Spurred by reports of mistreatment of people in jails, activist Dorothea Dix visited prisons, jails, and almshouses (i.e., charitable or low-cost housing) in the eastern US and argued that people with mental illnesses should have safe and peaceful refuges where they can recover. Her work inspired states to build psychiatric hospitals as alternatives to the horrendous conditions of the jails and almshouses. Unfortunately, psychiatric hospitals eventually developed their own reputations for their poor treatment of patients. By the early 20th century, institutions across North America were experimenting with questionable treatments such as lobotomy (i.e., surgical severing of connections in the prefrontal cortex of the brain) and malarial fever therapy, and in some settings, patients were experimented on or sterilized against their will. Adverse effects of treatment, hospital

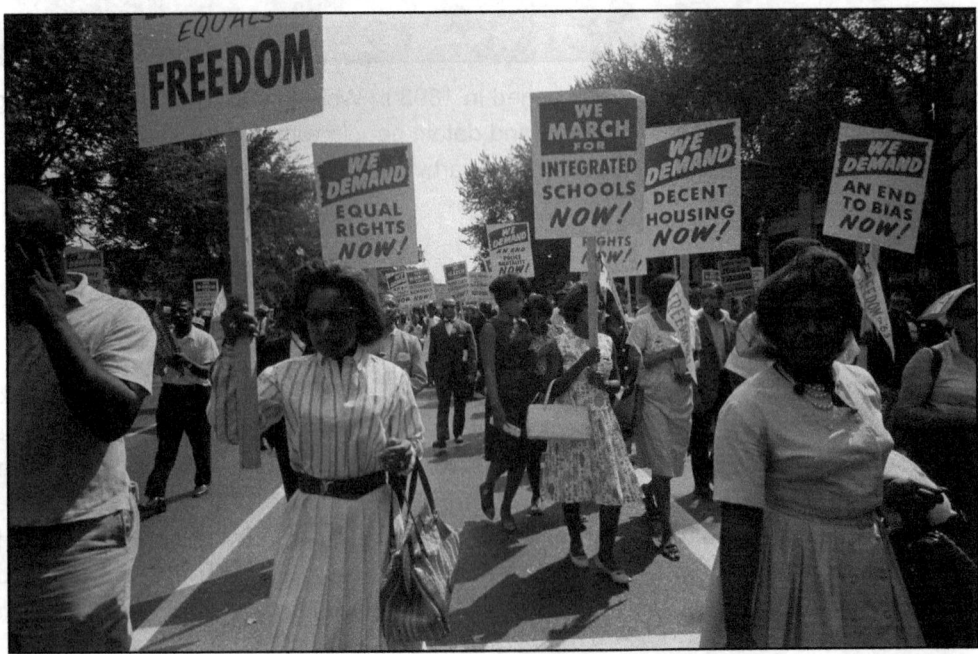

Figure 13.2: In the US, the civil rights movement in the 1960s emphasized individual liberties and civil rights, as seen in these signs carried during the Civil Rights March on Washington, DC. The civil rights movement further supported a civil libertarian approach to mental health policies, which continues to dominate in the US.

Source: Library of Congress

overcrowding, and documented abuses sowed the seeds for a movement to change how the state treated people with mental illnesses (Gelman, 2003).

The post–Second World War period saw conditions ripen for this movement, which coincided with the civil rights movement in the US and emphasized individual rights and civil liberties. Advocates argued in favour of self-determination, and accounts of people being wrongly institutionalized for dissenting religious or political beliefs (Curtis, 2001) underscored the need for strong safeguards against abuses of power by state intervention. At the same time, the first antipsychotic medications became available and made deinstitutionalization a possibility, as discussed in previous chapters (Gordon, 1993). The civil libertarian perspective was codified into law in the District of Columbia in 1964, at which time, lawmakers passed a bill stipulating that involuntary hospitalization could only be mandated for people who were a physical threat to themselves or others. This "physical dangerousness" criterion became the basis of civil commitment in the rest of the US by 1979 (Isaac & Brakel, 1992). Because a detained person was no longer considered a threat, the state could not justify mandating treatment. As a result, refusing psychiatric treatment became a right in the US. Although many states have since broadened their involuntary hospitalization criteria to include a need for treatment, the civil libertarian approach still dominates US mental health policies.

Involuntary Hospitalization in Canada

Due to Canada's history as a British colony and its proximity to the US, it has been heavily influenced by both countries' approaches to involuntary hospitalization. Early Canadian mental health legislation was based on the UK's 1853 *Lunatic Asylums Act*, and detentions were made on a person's apparent need for treatment, assessed by a doctor and ordered by a judge. An involuntary patient's consent was not needed before they were treated. As the civil rights and deinstitutionalization movements grew in the US, their tenets of individual rights and autonomy influenced policies in Canada to varying degrees. Each province and territory has since developed its own mental health legislation, which falls at varying points across the civil libertarian–human needs spectrum.

Criteria for Involuntary Hospitalization across Jurisdictions

Each province or territory's Mental Health Act sets out criteria that a person has to meet before they can be involuntarily hospitalized. In all jurisdictions, a person must be "unsuitable" for voluntary admission. This criterion usually applies to people who refuse voluntary psychiatric treatment. In practice, people seeking voluntary care at a hospital may find themselves involuntarily hospitalized, sometimes because their treatment team is concerned that they might change their mind and leave when they need intervention, and sometimes because the facility does not have the resources to justify treating voluntary patients. Patients seeking voluntary treatment might be told that the only way they can access care is to become an involuntary patient.

The different provincial and territorial jurisdictions in Canada also vary in what they consider a "mental disorder." Ontario, for example, defines "mental disorder" as "any disease or disability of the mind," which is quite broad. In contrast, Prince Edward Island more narrowly defines "mental disorder" as "a substantial disorder of thought, mood, perception, orientation or memory that seriously impairs judgment, behaviour, capacity to recognize reality or ability to meet the ordinary demands of life." In other words, a person's function must be seriously impaired for them to meet the criterion of having a "mental disorder." Ontario, Quebec, and Yukon have admission criteria based on the likelihood that a person with a mental disorder would cause *bodily* harm. All other provinces and territories specify "harm" only, which in some jurisdictions has been broadly interpreted to include not only physical or bodily harm but also financial, social, and vocational harm. For example, if someone with bipolar disorder had a manic episode and was spending their life savings, a British Columbia court has ruled that this behaviour would constitute financial harm and that the person would meet this criterion for involuntary hospitalization.

In many provinces and territories, people may also be involuntarily hospitalized if they are at risk of "substantial mental or physical deterioration." Examples of deterioration risk include a person who believes their food is poisoned and stops eating or a person who exhibits extreme social withdrawal and neglects their basic hygiene to the point where they endanger their well-being. New Brunswick, Prince Edward Island, Quebec, and Yukon do not have a deterioration criterion.

Quebec is the only jurisdiction where involuntary hospitalization decisions are made by a court rather than by a health care professional.

Treatment Decisions

In British Columbia, Manitoba, Nova Scotia, Newfoundland, Nunavut, and Saskatchewan, people can be detained only if their mental disorder is amenable to treatment, and the purpose of hospitalization is to treat rather than detain. A person with a mental disorder that has no known effective treatment would not meet this "need for treatment" criterion. In most cases, patients deemed "incompetent" can receive involuntary treatment, but Canadian jurisdictions assess competency at different points in the hospitalization process. For example, Newfoundland and Labrador, Nova Scotia, and Saskatchewan will not detain people deemed competent, meaning that all patients who are involuntarily hospitalized have already been assessed to be incompetent to make treatment decisions and can be treated involuntarily. Alberta, New Brunswick, Northwest Territories, Quebec, and Yukon allow patients to refuse treatment but have ways of overriding that refusal, such as through an independent review panel. Nunavut, Manitoba, Ontario, and Prince Edward Island have no override, meaning competent patients can refuse treatment and that refusal must be respected, even if it means the person is detained indefinitely. Finally, British Columbia is the only jurisdiction in Canada with no test for competence: anyone involuntarily hospitalized under its Mental Health Act may be treated against their wishes. For this reason, BC's legislation is considered by many to be the country's most paternalistic (Davis, 2013; Fraser, 2015; Johnston, 2017).

In five provinces—British Columbia, New Brunswick, Newfoundland and Labrador, Quebec, and Saskatchewan—the government authorizes treatment of involuntary patients, either through a tribunal (New Brunswick) or court (Quebec) or through a medical professional or hospital administrator. In all other jurisdictions, a *substitute decision maker*—often a family member or caregiver—consents to or refuses treatment on the patient's behalf. In Nunavut, Ontario, and Yukon, the substitute decision maker must respect the patient's previously expressed wishes about treatment, if the patient stated those wishes when they were competent. In all other provinces and territories, the substitute decision maker may authorize treatment based on what they believe are the patient's best interests. If we consider the involuntary hospitalization criteria and approaches to treatment, the jurisdiction closest to the civil libertarian end of the spectrum is Quebec, and the one closest to the human needs end of the spectrum is British Columbia, with all other provinces lying somewhere in between.

Involuntary Outpatient Treatment

All Canadian jurisdictions except for New Brunswick have provisions in their mental health legislation for providing people with involuntary treatment in the community, which can take the form of **conditional leave** or community treatment orders. Under this kind of involuntary outpatient treatment, patients are allowed to live at their homes in the community rather than stay in the hospital, but they must follow a list of conditions, which might include regularly visiting a health care professional for follow-up and receiving treatment they do not want. If a patient does not meet the conditions of their leave or treatment order, they could be detained and taken to hospital to be treated as an inpatient. Conditional leave is initiated when the patient is in the hospital, whereas community treatment orders can sometimes be initiated in the community and may require that the patient have had previous hospitalizations. Alberta is the only jurisdiction where a person may be placed on a community treatment order without ever having been hospitalized.

Involuntary outpatient treatment is meant to support patients who respond well to treatment in the hospital but who might lack the insight or skills to maintain treatment once discharged. Such patients are at high risk of relapse and re-hospitalization, and the aim of involuntary outpatient treatment is to prevent this cycle and offer patients the treatment they need in a less restrictive setting. Proponents of involuntary outpatient treatment say that it is a necessary and acceptable consequence of de-institutionalization and that merely offering—rather than forcing—treatment is not enough for people who lack insight into their mental illness. Opponents of involuntary outpatient treatment argue that it extends coercion beyond hospital settings in ways that can drive patients away from the mental health system or be used for social control to compel certain behaviours (O'Reilly, 2004).

Patients' Experiences with Involuntary Hospitalization

So far, what has been presented reflects a theoretical discussion about legal and ethical considerations and ideological approaches to involuntary hospitalization. But how do patients who have been involuntarily hospitalized feel about their experience? Their opinions, as one might expect, are diverse. Some patients recall being terrified of forced injections and restraints when they were hospitalized yet believe in retrospect that the treatment was necessary and helped them get well. Erin Hawkes Emiru, who detailed her own experiences of involuntary hospitalization in *When Quietness Came: A Neuroscientist's Personal Journey with Schizophrenia*, has written about how involuntary treatment was necessary for her. Giving people whose illness interferes with their judgment the right to refuse treatment, she says, is like allowing children to play with knives:

> But we must have the right to harm ourselves, have we not? Such reasoning parades as a constitutional right, the right to choose what happens to our bodies and brains. Move beyond that and find that the right to refuse psychiatric treatment is a growing movement. This group insists that any treatment for a mental illness is exceedingly harmful to the person—if indeed there is such a thing as mental illness. "Mental illness," they say, is a "personal journey," something special that must not be crushed by involuntary medication or hospitalization ... Unmedicated "journeys" for me are a hell of hallucinations, paranoia, and delusion. Please, I do want the drugs, even though I tantrum against the injections. Please, someone, make choices for me when I cannot: choose to give me the treatment that, for me, has worked in the past. Medicate me. Don't leave me to myself; I will play with those knives and may not learn until I bleed to death what harm I have the "right" to do.

Bryn Ditmars, who lives with schizophrenia and has been hospitalized several times in British Columbia, told the *Globe and Mail*: "A few times I was in agreement, but most of the time I was given no choice." He recalled being held in seclusion and in restraints and injected with antipsychotic medications against his will. He states, "That being said, I strongly believe that, were it not for these interventions, I would not be alive today. I was a danger to myself and others." Ditmars said that involuntary hospitalization was "the best thing that could have happened ... Doctors and nurses and police officers, they never hear this side of the story. They never hear the voice of people saying, 'Thank you for arresting me, thank you for taking me to hospital, thank you for committing me under the Mental Health Act.'"

A 2012 evaluation of Ontario's community treatment order program included focus groups and interviews with the program's stakeholders. Some people who were placed on a community treatment order credited the treatment and services they received with improving their quality of life, with one person saying, "I was paranoid for four years. It's an awful feeling. My meds changed all that." Another said, "If I didn't have it, I wouldn't be where I am today. I'd still be in the hospital."

But not all patients are grateful for involuntary hospitalization and treatment. Many have found the experience dehumanizing, even traumatic. Ethan, Deborah, and Jasmine had all experienced involuntary hospitalization and participated in a study about the Mental Health Act in British Columbia. What Ethan found most frightening about his experience was that he was never told what the Mental Health Act was and what the legislation authorized the hospital to do:

> It's like, OK, I'm being committed under some legislation that I don't know, and I don't know what being committed entails, and I don't know what the legislation allows ... It kind of felt like they could have done anything and told me, "Oh yeah, we can do this under the Mental Health Act," and I wouldn't have known.

Deborah sought help as a voluntary patient but found herself involuntarily hospitalized without her knowledge, which eroded her trust in the mental health system:

> I've been hospitalized three times. I walked in on my own accord on all three and didn't find out till I wanted to leave that they'd certified me. Didn't really know how that had happened when I'd walked in under my own steam. Not entirely sure me leaving at that point would have been a good idea or a bad idea. They might have been right, they might have been wrong, but, yeah, didn't like the feeling that I had no control or information over that at all ... The worst thing about going in as a voluntary and having such a horrible experience is, I don't trust that system ... Sure, you want to keep me out of the hospital—that's all our goals—but I shouldn't be scared of going there, right? That's not a good system if I'm scared of going there.

For both Ethan and Deborah, the lack of information and clear communication about their situation made them feel as though they did not have agency or control over their situation, which caused fear and resentment about their hospital experience. Jasmine was involuntarily hospitalized several times for symptoms of bipolar disorder and recalls her experiences in the hospital as humiliating:

> There are times that they've given me medications that have made me defecate myself, that have made me urinate myself, that have made me lethargic to the point where I cannot speak to my own mother, that I cannot recognize my own family ... Is that the way the Canadian systems want to recognize how to treat mental illness? There's got to be a better way ...

Jasmine did, however, say that staff who showed a genuine concern left a much more positive impression: "There's been some people in my life who really have helped me ... And they really do genuinely care."

These patients' experiences show that although involuntary hospitalization seems to be a necessary part of our mental health system, the way staff treat patients after they are certified can make a big impact on their experience as well as their future assessment of their illness and treatment needs. The loss of autonomy and an unfamiliar setting can be scary and confusing, and finding ways to mitigate those feelings and respect the rights that involuntary patients still have—including clearly communicating with them about their situation, as well as their legal and treatment options—can help patients stay engaged with the health care system and invested in their own recovery.

Involuntary Patients' Rights: *The Canadian Charter of Rights and Freedoms*

The *Canadian Charter of Rights and Freedoms,* enacted in 1982, is part of the Constitution, and all laws throughout the country must conform to it. But *Charter* rights are not absolute: a law may limit certain rights if the government can show that it protects other rights or balances the interests of individuals and society. For example, the right to free expression does not protect you from prosecution for distributing hate propaganda.

Moreover, any law that does not conform to the *Charter* risks being challenged in court. If the court determines that a law violates the *Charter* that law can be struck down for being unconstitutional. In the realm of mental health legislation, a few sections of the *Charter* are especially important:

- section 7: Everyone has the right to life, liberty, and security of person.
- section 9: Everyone has the right not to be arbitrarily detained.
- section 10: Everyone who is detained has the right to be told why they are being detained, to consult a lawyer, and to challenge the validity of their detention in court.
- section 12: Everyone has the right not to be subjected to any cruel and unusual treatment or punishment.
- section 15: Everyone has the right to equal protection of the law without discrimination, including against mental disability.

Mental health laws must balance individual autonomy, a person's right to safety (including from self-harm), and public safety. Because involuntary hospitalization involves curtailing a person's liberty and may include confinement in a seclusion room or restraint of their movement, which could be considered cruel and unusual treatment, legislation governing involuntary hospitalization must include procedural safeguards to protect patients' rights.

Protections and Safeguards in Mental Health Legislation

Section 10 of the *Charter* states that involuntary patients have the right to a lawyer and the right to challenge their detention in court. However, most jurisdictions have special mental health tribunals or review boards that patients can appeal to if they want to challenge their detention. These are usually less costly, easier to access, and more time efficient than taking a case to court. The review boards are responsible for organizing panels to conduct hearings to determine whether a patient meets the criteria for involuntary hospitalization. If the panel decides that the patient does not meet the criteria, it can order that the patient be discharged. In some jurisdictions, the review panel may also make judgments about other issues, such as the following:

- the patient's capacity to consent to treatment
- the patient's competence to manage their affairs or property
- the patient's treatment plan
- the validity of a patient's advance directive (where the patient can document their health care preferences in case they become incapable of making decisions about their health)
- the choice of a substitute decision maker for the patient
- the patient's access to health records and other communication

Treatment decisions may be handled by separate mechanisms in some provinces and territories. For example, in British Columbia, the review panel hearings do not address treatment plans, but a patient can apply for a second medical opinion to review their treatment.

Section 10 of the *Charter* also says that involuntary patients have the right to know why they have been hospitalized. However, how detailed that information must be has been a matter of debate. Some scholars have argued that patients only need to be told that they meet the jurisdiction's criteria for involuntary hospitalization (Gray et al., 2008). In contrast, advocates for patient rights believe that patients ought to have access to their medical records and to know *how* the criteria of the Mental Health Act apply to their specific situation (Johnston, 2017). Opponents to this open, accessible approach have expressed that it could cause harm—for example, if the record contains references to events or people that could endanger third parties or cause an escalation in a patient's agitation.

The mental health legislation in all provinces and territories requires the hospital to tell patients about their rights, but they differ in their specifics. For example, in all jurisdictions, patients must be told, usually by clinician staff, about their Section 10 rights, but in Alberta, New Brunswick, Newfoundland and Labrador, Nova Scotia, Nunavut, Ontario, and Saskatchewan, patients have an added layer of rights information from advisors who are independent of the treatment team. Independent rights advisors help eliminate the conflict of interest of a clinician giving patients' rights information. The concern is that a clinician who believes a patient should stay in the hospital might not be completely transparent or forthcoming, whether consciously or unconsciously, about ways the patient could challenge their detention or treatment.

Other differences in approach to rights information relate to whether the information must be repeated, posted, or offered in a language the patient understands. Sometimes when patients are first admitted, they refuse rights information or are not in a state of mind to absorb or understand new information. In British Columbia, Manitoba, Newfoundland and Labrador, the Northwest Territories, Nunavut, Prince Edward Island, and Yukon, rights information must be repeated if the patient appears not to understand it the first time. There is no such requirement in other jurisdictions, although in the provinces with automatic independent rights advice, patients are guaranteed to hear about their rights more than once.

Posting the rights in a high-traffic area of the hospital gives patients another opportunity to learn about their rights. The mental health legislation in British Columbia, Manitoba, Newfoundland and Labrador, the Northwest Territories, Nova Scotia, and Prince Edward Island requires that rights information be posted. Other jurisdictions do not have this requirement.

Finally, patients in Alberta, Manitoba, Newfoundland and Labrador, the Northwest Territories, Nunavut, Prince Edward Island, and Yukon have the right to receive rights information in a language they understand. In contrast, British Columbia, New Brunswick, Nova Scotia, Ontario, Quebec, and Saskatchewan make no such guarantee in their mental health legislation. Individual health authorities or institutions may have policies to accommodate patients with different language needs, but the legislation itself does not require it. This issue is important because patients who face language barriers and who do not have access to an interpreter face a "higher risk of misdiagnosis, misunderstanding, and mismanagement" (Dhand, 2016).

Violations of Patients' Rights

Despite what is written in the legislation to protect patients' rights, rights violations have occurred—some relatively recently. For example, a 2001 report shed light on physical and sexual abuses at Woodlands School, a facility for children with mental illnesses and developmental disabilities in British Columbia that closed in 1996 (McCallum, 2001). The province apologized to residents in 2003 and set aside more than $15 million in compensation in 2018 (Urquhart, 2018). In 2019, the BC Office of the Ombudsperson released a report detailing its investigation into how well the province's health authorities were following the legal requirements of the Mental Health Act. According to the legislation, every involuntary patient's file must contain five forms:

- the certificate, including a detailed description of how the person meets the certification criteria,

- a consent to treatment form,
- a form explaining the patient's Mental Health Act rights,
- a form for the patient to name a near relative to receive information about the patient's hospital stay, and
- a form to notify the near relative of the patient's hospitalization and rights.

The Office of the Ombudsperson was disappointed to find the required legal forms in only 28 percent of the patient files they reviewed. They rebuked the health authorities for not having "developed a culture within the mental health care system that places sufficient emphasis on the importance of an involuntary patient's legal rights" (BC Office of the Ombudsperson, 2019). Their report told the story of Florence and Albert:

> Florence had Alzheimer's disease and was admitted involuntarily under the Mental Health Act after she was brought to the hospital's emergency department. The hospital completed a Medical Certificate (Form 4) that authorized her initial admission and detention for up to 48 hours. However, there was no evidence that a second Form 4 was completed, meaning that the hospital did not have legal authority to keep her admitted once the 48 hours had expired. Florence ended up being involuntarily admitted for just over three weeks. During this time, the hospital did not notify Florence of her rights as an involuntary patient, nor did it provide her with an opportunity to nominate a near relative to receive notification of her detention and rights. Her file contained no written notification to a near relative and, in particular, there was no evidence that a Form 16 had been provided to Florence's husband, Albert, who was her caregiver. There was also no completed Consent for Treatment (Form 5) in Florence's file. At least three times during the three-week detention, the hospital refused to discharge Florence when she or Albert requested that she go home. On one occasion, staff called security. The hospital refused these discharge requests despite having no legal authority to continue to detain Florence … The lack of information on her rights caused considerable distress for both Florence and Albert and, given the facility's failure to observe other key procedures in relation to both of Florence's admissions, adversely affected Albert's ability to advocate for Florence's discharge.

In Alberta, Justice Kristine Eidsvik ruled in 2019 that parts of Alberta's *Mental Health Act* were unconstitutional, based on the case brought forth by JH, a man who was in the hospital recovering from physical injuries from a hit and run in 2014. When he asked to be released, he found himself involuntarily hospitalized and treated with psychiatric medications without his consent, even though he had no history of a mental illness. He was not released until May 2015, and only after an appeal in court. "According to Eidsvik's ruling," wrote Adam MacVicar for Global News, "there were multiple issues with JH's detention, including 'vague and incomplete' admission certificates, and the fact JH nor his family received written notice about why he was being held in hospital" (MacVicar, 2019).

A case from Newfoundland and Labrador shows how mental health legislation can be used as a tool for social control (*CBC News*, 2018). In 2018, a court ruled that the six-day detention of Andrew Abbass under the *Mental Health Care and Treatment Act* was unlawful. Abbass was taken into custody after publishing posts on social media expressing anger against the Royal Newfoundland Constabulary for the fatal shooting of Newfoundland resident Don Dunphy. Although he won his case, Abbass blames the hospitalization for a derailed business plan, several moves owing to threats of violence against his family, and the end of his relationship with his child's mother. Abbass's case shows that even though people who are wrongly certified do have legal recourse, it is often a long process (his hospitalization was in 2015), and the detention itself, even if it is relatively brief, can have a major influence on a person's life course.

Procedural Justice in Involuntary Hospitalization

People with mental illnesses have a long history of experiencing powerlessness within society related to stigma that excludes them from opportunities. When they become involuntary patients, they find themselves on the disadvantaged end of even more sources of power imbalance: (a) between health care professional and patient (Gluyas, 2015; Joseph-Williams et al., 2014; Koeck, 2014), and (b) between detainer (the hospital, in this case) and detainee (Bhui, 2017; Goodstein et al., 1984). This combined disempowerment can lead to a number of adverse consequences, including mistrust and avoidance of the health system (Kirby & Keon, 2006). Practices that empower patients have been found to have therapeutic effects, and a key way to promote empowerment and to reduce negative experiences with involuntary hospitalization and treatment is to increase patients' sense of **procedural justice**, which is their perception of fairness in the decision-making process to detain and treat them. As Donald Linhorst (2006) wrote:

> Procedural justice is enforced when people with mental illness are able to express their views; when their views are given serious consideration by those contemplating the coercive action; when they are treated with dignity and respect; when they are given accurate, relevant, and understandable information; and when people contemplating coercion express genuine concern for their well-being.

Perception of procedural justice "bears the strongest relationship to satisfaction with outcome" (Sydeman et al., 1997). A patient's belief that the admissions process was fair is important to their satisfaction with their hospitalization experience and may help them to accept the outcome of being involuntarily hospitalized.

Exercising a right can itself be therapeutic for patients, even if the outcome is not what they had hoped for. For example, suppose an involuntary patient applies for a hearing with a review panel. Even if the review panel decides that the patient must remain hospitalized, going through the process of the review panel hearing and feeling as though they had a voice can reduce the patient's perceptions of coercion and in some cases persuade them to accept treatment (Winick & Lerner-Wren, 2003). Roche et al. (2014) found that if a patient has a stronger sense of procedural justice, they will likely have a better therapeutic relationship with their treatment team, which in turn leads to better health outcomes, including adherence to treatment, satisfaction with mental health services, and quality of life. Reducing feelings of coercion and increasing trust can encourage patients to stay engaged with the health system and take an active role in working towards their own recovery (Dixon et al., 2016; Kreyenbuhl et al., 2009). More recent research, based on recovery principles (more on this in the next chapter!) and Trauma and Violence Informed Practice (TVIP), suggests that giving people a say in their treatment and care can provide a sense of connection that makes them more likely to accept treatment (Linhorst, 2006).

Historically, in the age of institutionalization, involuntary hospitalization and treatment could go on for years and, in some people's cases, for the rest of their lives. With more widely available effective psychiatric treatments and the growth of community-based care, involuntary stays are now much shorter—the average length of involuntary hospitalization in British Columbia, for example, is 14 days (BC Office of the Ombudsperson, 2019). But those 14 days can define the recovery trajectory of the patient in the long term. A positive experience built on a trusting therapeutic relationship between patient and staff may be the foundation for a period of stability and wellness in physical and mental health. A negative experience that traumatizes the patient and makes them want to avoid contact with the health system may set them up for repeated mental health crises, each of which furthers their experience of trauma and mistrust.

Conclusion

In this chapter, we explored involuntary hospitalization and treatment for mental illnesses in Canada, including historical and current approaches. Civil libertarian and human needs approaches to involuntary mental health care operate on different ends of a spectrum. Patient perspectives illustrate a diversity of opinion about the benefits and challenges of each of these approaches. Debates between these approaches should not ignore the therapeutic role that respecting and promoting patients' rights can play in long-term recovery. Developing strategies to promote procedural justice can be an important strategy in supporting people who are experiencing involuntary mental health care in hospital or in the community.

Glossary

civil libertarian approach: The view that individual freedoms are of the utmost importance. Proponents of this perspective argue that a person's freedom should be limited only if they are a physical danger to themselves or to others.

conditional leave: A form of involuntary outpatient treatment in which patients are allowed to live at their homes in the community rather than stay in the hospital, but they must follow a list of conditions, which might include regularly visiting a health care professional for follow-up and receiving treatment. Also known as community treatment orders.

human needs approach: Focuses on a person's need for psychiatric treatment.

procedural justice: A patient's perception of fairness in the decision-making process to detain and treat them.

Critical Thinking Questions

1. Compare and contrast civil libertarian and a human needs approaches to mental health legislation.
2. Describe some arguments that involuntary psychiatric hospitalization and treatment can be used as "social control."
3. How does involuntary psychiatric hospitalization affect stigma towards people with severe mental illnesses?
4. Describe the concept of procedural justice, including the ways in which the process can contribute therapeutic benefits.
5. Identify strategies that can make involuntary psychiatric hospitalization and treatment more trauma-informed and recovery-oriented.

Recommended Readings

BC's Representative for Children and Youth. (2021). *Detained: Rights of children and youth under the Mental Health Act*. https://rcybc.ca/reports-and-publications/detained

Chandler, J. A., & Flood, C. M. (Eds.). (2016). *Law and mind: Mental health law and policy in Canada*. LexisNexis.

Government of Nunavut. (2017). *Mental Health Act review—What we heard from Nunavummiut*. https://www.gov.nu.ca/sites/default/files/mental_health_act_review_-summary-report_-_en.pdf

Mehler Paperny, A. (2019). Opinion: In bad form? The rise of coercive care in Canada. *The Globe and Mail*. https://www.theglobeandmail.com/opinion/article-in-bad-form-the-rise-of-coercive-care-in-canada

Recommended Websites

BC Mental Health Rights. www.bcmentalhealthrights.ca
Éducaloi—Forced Hospitalization: Three Types. https://educaloi.qc.ca/en/capsules/forced-hospitalization-three-types
Health Justice. www.healthjustice.ca
Psychiatric Patient Advocate Office. www.ontario.ca/page/psychiatric-patient-advocate-office

References

Appelbaum, P. S., & Gutheil, T. G. (1979). "Rotting with their rights on": Constitutional theory and clinical reality in drug refusal by psychiatric patients. *Journal of the American Academy of Psychiatry and the Law Online, 7*(3), 306–315. http://jaapl.org/content/jaapl/7/3/306.full.pdf

BC Office of the Ombudsperson. (2019). *Committed to change: Protecting the rights of involuntary patients under the Mental Health Act.* https://bcombudsperson.ca/sites/default/files/OMB-Committed-to-Change-FINAL-web.pdf

Bhui, H. S. (2017). Inspecting immigration detention: Her Majesty's Inspectorate of Prisons. In M. J. Flynn & M. B. Flynn (Eds.), *Challenging immigration detention: Academics, activists and policy-makers* (pp. 82–96). Edward Elgar Publishing.

CBC News. (2018, May 3). Man unlawfully detained in psychiatric unit for tweets, Supreme Court rules. https://www.cbc.ca/news/canada/newfoundland-labrador/abbass-supreme-court-unlawful-detention-1.4646917

Curtis, A. (2001). Involuntary commitment. *Bad Subjects, 58.* http://psychrights.org/states/Maine/InvoluntaryCommitmentbyAliciaCurtis.htm

Davis, S. (2013). *Community mental health in Canada, revised and expanded edition: Theory, policy, and practice.* UBC Press.

Dhand, R. (2016). Race, culture and ethnicity in mental health law and policy. In J. A. Chandler & C. M. Flood (Eds.), *Law and mind: Mental health law and policy in Canada.* LexisNexis.

Dixon, L. B., Holoshitz, Y., & Nossel, I. (2016). Treatment engagement of individuals experiencing mental illness: Review and update. *World Psychiatry, 15*(1), 13–20. http://doi.org/10.1002/wps.20306

Fraser, G. (2015). *Governing madness: Coercion, resistance and agency in British Columbia's mental health law regime* (Doctoral dissertation).

Gelman, S. (2003). Looking backward: The twentieth century revolutions in psychiatry, law and public mental health. *Ohio Northern University Law Review, 29,* 531–586.

Gluyas, H. (2015). Patient-centred care: Improving healthcare outcomes. *Nursing Standard, 30*(4), 50. https://doi.org/10.7748/ns.30.4.50.e10186

Goodstein, L., MacKenzie, D. L., & Shotland, R. L. (1984). Personal control and inmate adjustment to prison. *Criminology, 22*(3), 343–369. https://doi.org/10.1111/j.1745-9125.1984.tb00304.x

Gordon, R. M. (1993). Out to pasture: A case for the retirement of Canadian mental health legislation. *Canadian Journal of Community Mental Health, 12*(1). https://doi.org/10.7870/cjcmh-1993-0003

Gray, J. E., Shone, M. A., & Liddle, P. F. (2008). *Canadian mental health law and policy* (2nd ed.). LexisNexis.

Isaac, R. J., & Brakel, S. J. (1992). Subverting good intentions: A brief history of mental health law reform. *Cornell Journal of Law and Public Policy, 2,* 89.

Johnston, L. (2017). *Operating in darkness: BC's Mental Health Act detention system.* Community Legal Assistance Society. https://d3n8a8pro7vhmx.cloudfront.net/clastest/pages/1794/attachments/original/1527278723/CLAS_Operating_in_Darkness_November_2017.pdf?1527278723

Joseph-Williams, N., Edwards, A., & Elwyn, G. (2014). Power imbalance prevents shared decision making. *BMJ, 348*(3), g3178. https://doi.org/10.1136/bmj.g3178

Kaiser, H. A. (2009). Canadian mental health law: The slow process of redirecting the ship of state. *Health Law Journal, 17,* 139–194.

Kirby, M. J. L., & Keon, W. J. (2006). *Out of the shadows at last: Transforming mental health, mental illness and addiction services in Canada.* Standing Senate Committee on Social Affairs, Science and Technology. http://www.parl.gc.ca/content/sen/committee/391/soci/rep/rep02may06-e.htm

Koeck, C. (2014). Imbalance of power between patients and doctors. *BMJ, 349,* g7485. https://doi.org/10.1136/bmj.g7485

Kreyenbuhl, J., Nossel, I. R., & Dixon, L. B. (2009). Disengagement from mental health treatment among individuals with schizophrenia and strategies for facilitating connections to care: A review of the literature. *Schizophrenia Bulletin, 35*(4), 696–703. http://doi.org/10.1093/schbul/sbp046

Linhorst, D. M. (2006). *Empowering people with severe mental illness: A practical guide.* Oxford University Press.

MacVicar, A. (2019, July 18). Sections of Alberta's Mental Health Act deemed unconstitutional, court rules. *Global News.* https://globalnews.ca/news/5654753/alberta-mental-health-act-unconstitutional/

McCallum, D. (2001). *The need to know: Administrative review of Woodlands School.* Government of British Columbia, Ministry of Children and Family Development.

Minkowitz, T. (2006). The United Nations Convention on the Rights of Persons with Disabilities and the right to be free from nonconsensual psychiatric interventions. *Syracuse Journal of International Law and Commerce, 34,* 405.

O'Reilly, R. (2004). Why are community treatment orders controversial? *The Canadian Journal of Psychiatry, 49*(9), 579–584. https://doi.org/10.1177/070674370404900902

O'Reilly, R. L. (1998). Mental health legislation and the right to appropriate treatment. *The Canadian Journal of Psychiatry, 43*(8), 811–815. https://doi.org/10.1177/070674379804300805

Perkins, D. O., Gu, H., Boteva, K., & Lieberman, J. A. (2005). Relationship between duration of untreated psychosis and outcome in first-episode schizophrenia: A critical review and meta-analysis. *American journal of psychiatry, 162*(10), 1785–1804. https://doi.org/10.1176/appi.ajp.162.10.1785

Roche, E., Madigan, K., Lyne, J. P., Feeney, L., & O'Donoghue, B. (2014). The therapeutic relationship after psychiatric admission. *Journal of Nervous and Mental Disease, 202*(3), 186–192. https://doi.org/10.1097/NMD.0000000000000102

Sydeman, S. J., Cascardi, M., Poythress, N. G., & Ritterband, L. M. (1997). Procedural justice in the context of civil commitment: A critique of Tyler's analysis. *Psychology, Public Policy, and Law, 3*(1), 207–221. https://doi.org/10.1037/1076-8971.3.1.207

Szasz, T. S. (1961). *The myth of mental illness*. Harper & Row.

United Nations General Assembly. (2006). Convention on the Rights of Persons with Disabilities. https://www.un.org/development/desa/disabilities/convention-on-the-rights-of-persons-with-disabilities/convention-on-the-rights-of-persons-with-disabilities-2.html

Unsworth, C. (1993). Law and lunacy in psychiatry's "golden age." *Oxford Journal of Legal Studies, 13*(4), 479–507.

Urquhart, C. (2018, October 8). Decades after its closure, survivors of abuse at Woodlands receive compensation. *Global News*. https://globalnews.ca/news/4527566/decades-after-its-closure-survivors-of-abuse-at-woodlands-receive-compensation/

Winick, B. J., & Lerner-Wren, G. (2003). Do juveniles facing civil commitment have a right to counsel?: A therapeutic jurisprudence brief. *University of Cincinnati Law Review, 71*, 115–126.

Chapter 14

Treatment Approaches for Mental Health and Substance Use Challenges

Courtney Devane, Allie Slemon, and Emily Jenkins, adapted from original chapter by Elliot M. Goldner, Emily Jenkins, and Dan Bilsker

> Respond intelligently even to unintelligent treatment.
> —Lao-tzu (Chinese philosopher, writing in the 6th century BC)

Introduction

In this chapter, we provide a brief overview of some of the treatments currently used to promote mental health and well-being and to treat mental and substance use disorders. These may be classified broadly as biological, psychological, social, or spiritual in nature. Some approaches to treatment reflect a combination of these orientations. Biological treatments include the use of medications and other approaches that target what is believed to be the physical origin of the illness, largely centring on altering brain chemistry (e.g., neurotransmitter levels). Psychological approaches include various forms and traditions of psychotherapy, which aim to enhance coping, identify and/or avoid problematic thought or behavioural patterns, and improve interpersonal relationships. Social approaches represent an effort to respond to the social etiology of mental and substance use disorders. This includes strategies to redress the social determinants or "root causes" of poor mental health, such as isolation and poverty. Spiritual approaches to finding meaning in the experience of mental illness include those provided by organized religions, distinct cultural traditions, meditative practices, or other unique spiritual routines and paths. Following discussion of these established treatment modalities, we introduce some emergent approaches to treating mental health and substance use challenges, particularly those that have not responded to other more widely utilized forms of treatment.

At the end of the chapter, we have listed recommendations for further reading so that you may obtain more complete information about the treatments listed here and others that are not included. We also provide a personal mental health toolkit aimed at helping you to cope with stress and enhance mental health and well-being;

this is written with *students* in mind (since readers of this book will often be students), but it is applicable to people in all walks of life.

Psychopharmacotherapy

The advent of psychopharmacotherapy, that is, the use of medications for the treatment of psychiatric symptoms, occurred during the 1950s when chlorpromazine was first marketed for the treatment of psychotic symptoms. Since that time, pharmacotherapy has become the predominant mode of treatment for mental illnesses. The main classes of psychiatric medications and their established uses are described below, but note that medications are sometimes prescribed "off label" (i.e., used in the treatment of illnesses for which the medication has not been approved by the official regulatory body, Health Canada).

Antipsychotic Medications

The discovery of chlorpromazine as an effective treatment for psychotic symptoms (i.e., delusions and hallucinations) changed the course of psychiatric therapy. It was a surgeon in France, Henri Laborit, who was studying the potential use of chlorpromazine in anaesthesia, and who wondered whether it might soothe agitated patients in psychiatric wards. The improvements that psychiatrists saw in patients who were administered the new medication were so profound that they considered chlorpromazine to be a miracle drug. This treatment "breakthrough" ushered in the rapid development and marketing of other "first generation" antipsychotic medications (Ban, 2007), which significantly improved the prognosis for individuals with psychotic illnesses. Indeed, it was partly responsible for the deinstitutionalization policies that soon swept across Canada (Dyck, 2011). These and many of the more recently developed antipsychotic medications appear to act by blocking dopamine receptors in various areas of the brain. Over the past few decades, first-generation antipsychotics have lost favour as treatments for psychosis, partly because of the side effects associated with these medications. A common set of side effects are **extrapyramidal symptoms**—movement disorders resulting from the inhibition of dopamine activity. These include dystonia, which is characterized by muscle spasms resulting in distorted or twisted body positions; akathisia, which results in restlessness and inability to sit still; and Parkinsonism, which involves slowed movements, stiff posture, and emotionless facial expression. In addition, some patients may experience tardive dyskinesia, a sometimes irreversible condition consisting of unusual involuntary movements (e.g., lip-smacking, and "pill-rolling" finger movements); and oculogyric crisis, which is a medical emergency that presents as a fixed upward stare of the eyes lasting for several minutes to an hour, sometimes treated with intramuscular injections of anticholinergic medications (which block the action of the neurotransmitter acetylcholine, helping to minimize involuntary muscle movements).

More recently, atypical or second- and third-generation antipsychotics have become the standard treatment for psychotic disorders. The first of these so-called atypical antipsychotic medications, clozapine, was patented in the 1960s. Unfortunately, a very serious side effect called agranulocytosis (i.e., dangerously low levels of white blood cells resulting in increased risk for acquiring life-threatening infections) was found to be associated with this medication. Clozapine use initially declined, but its effectiveness in treating psychotic symptoms in patients not responding to other treatments led to its reintroduction to clinical practice, although with extra monitoring. Atypical antipsychotics are now recommended as an initial treatment for psychosis because they are less likely to induce the serious side effects that result from the first-generation medications. However, an additional harmful side effect of these medications is metabolic syndrome, in which individuals experience substantial weight gain and are at a significantly increased risk of health comorbidities, including diabetes mellitus and hypertension.

Antidepressant Medications

Antidepressant medications are used in the treatment of mood disorders, such as depression and several anxiety disorders (e.g., panic disorder and generalized anxiety disorder). They may also be used in the treatment of bipolar disorder, though they are prescribed with caution as they can increase the risk of "rapid cycling" mood states between depression and mania (Cheniaux & Nardi, 2019). Antidepressants are believed to exert their effects by altering levels of various neurotransmitters in the brain as well as by increasing or decreasing the actions of surrounding neurons. Depending on the particular group or class of antidepressant medication, the neurotransmitters targeted include serotonin, norepinephrine, noradrenaline, and dopamine (Andrade & Rao, 2010).

The first group of antidepressant medications identified were the monoamine oxidase inhibitors (MAOIs) followed shortly thereafter by the tricyclic antidepressants (TCAs). While both are associated with good treatment response, these classes of medications fell out of popular use due to their respective side effect profiles. Specifically, the MAOIs bring the potential for dangerous interactions with certain foods (e.g., aged cheeses, cured meats) and other drugs, and the TCAs have a high level of lethality in overdose.

Currently, selective serotonin reuptake inhibitors (SSRIs) are the most frequently prescribed class of antidepressants, though serotonin and norepinephrine reuptake inhibitors (SNRIs) and atypical antidepressants (i.e., those that don't fall within the other antidepressant classes) are also commonly used. Antidepressant medication is generally considered to be effective for individuals with moderate to severe forms of depression. However, the effectiveness of antidepressant medications has, at times, been called into question. In a review of clinical trial data, researchers concluded that they may be no more effective than a placebo for many individuals (Fournier et al., 2010). Other research has found that compared to placebo, antidepressants reduce symptoms by an additional 25 to 30 percent among adults diagnosed with depression; however, they are associated with high levels of symptom relapse (Safer, 2019). The side effects associated with antidepressant medications can be quite bothersome and include sexual dysfunction, weight gain, agitation, and hypertension. Further, there is growing acknowledgment that cessation of these medications can result in pronounced and uncomfortable discontinuation symptoms for some, including sensory disturbances, insomnia, hyperarousal, and flu-like symptoms. Many people find that they need to try a number of different antidepressant medications before finding one that works for them.

Mood Stabilizers

Mood stabilizers are primarily prescribed for patients diagnosed with bipolar disorder, helping to control abnormally high mood states (i.e., mania). Their mechanism of action is not well understood, though it is hypothesized that they work by helping to stabilize and reduce activity in areas of the brain that have become overstimulated. Lithium carbonate was the first medication approved for this purpose and continues to be widely used. Other commonly used mood stabilizers include divalproex sodium, carbamazepine, and lamotrigine. The side effects associated with mood stabilizers vary widely by medication, but some require close monitoring of blood levels to avoid toxicity.

Sedatives

Sedative medications include several classes of drugs that cause drowsiness when given in higher dose. They can be used to induce sleep or to reduce agitation and anxiety. Sedatives operate by increasing the activity of the neurotransmitter gamma-aminobutyric acid (GABA) in the brain, which produces feelings of relaxation. Of the different types of sedative drugs available, the benzodiazepines (e.g., lorazepam, diazepam, or clonazepam) are the most commonly used. Although considered safe for short-term treatment, extended use of benzodiazepines can lead to dependence and withdrawal and so are prescribed with caution.

Substitution Therapy for Substance Use Dependence

Substitution therapy is a pharmacotherapy offered to people experiencing substance use disorders. This treatment involves replacing one drug (illicit or prescription) with another drug to reduce associated harms and prevent withdrawal symptoms. This approach has been used most commonly in the treatment of opioid dependence, in which people who are dependent on heroin, morphine, or other opiates are prescribed alternatives. These alternatives bind to the same opioid receptors in the brain as the previously used opioids would have, helping to reduce cravings and withdrawal; however, they do so more slowly, which tends to limit feelings of euphoria. Referred to collectively as opioid agonist therapies (OATs), these prescribed medications such as buprenorphine/naloxone and methadone, are typically taken orally, though there are programs that offer prescribed injectable opioids (e.g., diacetylmorphine or hydromorphone) for people with significant opioid dependence. The use of OATs has been associated with sharp reductions in rates of infection and overdose associated with injection and the use of drugs of unknown potency and composition (Bahji & Bajaj, 2018).

Managed Alcohol

Managed alcohol is a treatment approach used to decrease the harms related to severe alcohol dependence. Managed alcohol programs provide individuals at high risk of harm due to the risky nature of their alcohol use (e.g., consumption of non-beverage alcohol products such as mouthwash and hand sanitizer) with regular doses of alcohol at consistent intervals. The goals of a managed alcohol treatment approach are to maintain or reduce alcohol use, prevent withdrawal, minimize non-beverage alcohol consumption, and promote safer use of alcohol (BC Centre on Substance Use, 2020). Managed alcohol programs can operate in the community or within supportive residential settings. A managed alcohol approach may also be used within the hospital setting to support patients in avoiding withdrawal.

Issues in Psychopharmacotherapy

In recent years, medications have become the dominant form of treatment provided to people living with mental health challenges (Gask, 2018; Jenkins, 2014). This has occurred for a number of reasons, including the introduction of relatively effective medication therapies for certain mental illnesses, the development of new technologies that have enhanced understandings of relationships between neurochemistry and mental illnesses, and the effective use of marketing strategies by the pharmaceutical industry (Jenkins, 2014; Smith & Grant, 2016). Although psychopharmacotherapies benefit many individuals, enthusiasm must also be balanced by appropriate prudence in the use of medications outside the bounds of current knowledge. Medications can be combined in a "pharmacological cocktail" to address various symptoms and enhance response (Mojtabai & Olfson, 2010). However, such **polypharmacy** increases the risk of significant side effects, and the effectiveness of some frequently used medication combinations is questionable (Iversen et al., 2018). Side effects and other potential harms that may be caused by psychiatric medications must be prevented wherever possible. Another important concern is that psychopharmacotherapy has become such a predominant mode of treatment that other evidence-based approaches may be underutilized (Khouzam, 2017), with negative consequences for quality of life and experiences with mental health care.

> **Box 14.1: Thalidomide**
>
>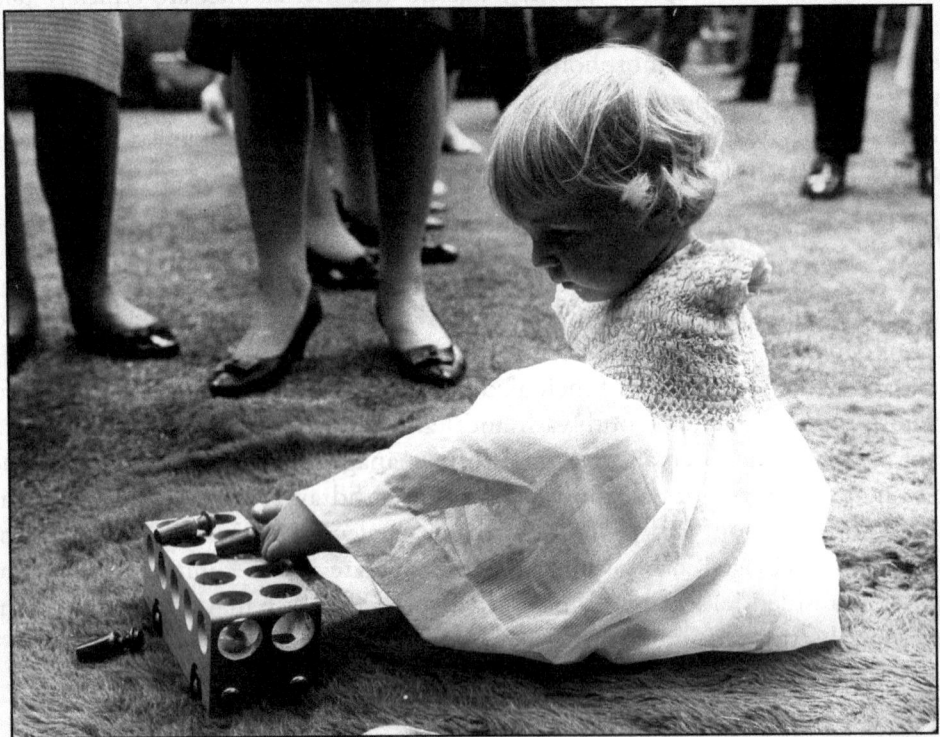
>
> **Figure 14.1:** Thalidomide caused birth defects resulting in short, unformed limbs.
>
> *Source*: GetStock
>
> There is often pressure to quickly introduce medications with the potential for improving mental health challenges (Hoffman, 2017). However, the need for caution is highlighted by the case of thalidomide, a medication prescribed to thousands of pregnant women during the late 1950s and early 1960s as a treatment for anxiety as well as morning sickness (Vargesson, 2015). It was learned too late that thalidomide use during pregnancy can cause birth defects. As many as 20,000 children were born with severe physical disabilities as a result of exposure to this medication in utero. The disabilities associated with thalidomide use are characterized by short, unformed limbs. In response to this tragedy, the process for developing, testing, and marketing new medications became stricter and more closely regulated in the hope of preventing such a disaster in the future.

Electroconvulsive Therapy and Magnetic Seizure Therapy

Electroconvulsive therapy (ECT), first developed in the 1930s, is perhaps the most controversial treatment to be used commonly in modern psychiatry. ECT involves passing an electric current through the brain to induce a seizure. In its early use, ECT was somewhat barbaric, as seizures were induced without anesthesia, often resulting in convulsions and causing substantial discomfort or injury. In current practice, a very brief-acting anesthetic agent is given in preparation for ECT to induce sedation and block muscular response (thereby reducing the physical impact of seizures).

ECT is used primarily in the treatment of severe depression, for which it is considered quite effective. Indeed, it has been proposed that ECT may be safer and more effective than antidepressants for older adults, a patient population with relatively poor treatment response to antidepressant medications (Zilles, 2018). Some patients respond well to a brief course of ECT treatment, while others receive regular treatments (i.e., maintenance ECT) to reduce the likelihood of symptom relapse. The mechanism of action is not understood, but it is hypothesized to involve an increase in the release of specific neurotransmitters. Side effects include short-term memory loss and confusion, and some ECT recipients report lasting impairment of their memory (Vann Jones & McCollum, 2019).

More recently, a newer form of convulsive therapy, magnetic seizure therapy, has been developed. Since evoking a seizure by using magnetic stimulation allows for more control of seizure activity, there appear to be fewer cognitive side effects than with ECT, including memory loss (Daskalakis et al., 2019; Peterchev et al., 2015). Studies indicate that this treatment is effective at reducing depressive symptoms and researchers are hopeful that this therapy could prove to be a good alternative to ECT.

Neurostimulation

There has been a surge of interest in the potential utility of various newer treatment approaches for mental illnesses that deliver more focal stimulation to discrete areas of the brain. These modalities include transcranial magnetic stimulation (TMS), vagus nerve stimulation (VNS), trigeminal nerve stimulation (TNS), and deep-brain stimulation (DBS). In TMS, a magnetic coil is placed over a specific area of the patient's scalp while the patient is awake. A magnetic field is induced that passes directly through the skull, resulting in a depolarizing of the brain cells directly below (at the junction of the grey and white matter of the cerebral cortex). For the most part, TMS is used as a second-line treatment for patients with depression who have not responded to first-line treatments (i.e., medication, psychotherapy). VNS involves placement of an electrode in the patient's neck that stimulates the vagus nerve repeatedly through use of a pacemaker. It is thought to transmit stimulation to subcortical brain areas. VNS has previously been used extensively to treat epilepsy but is now being examined as a potential treatment for depression and other mental

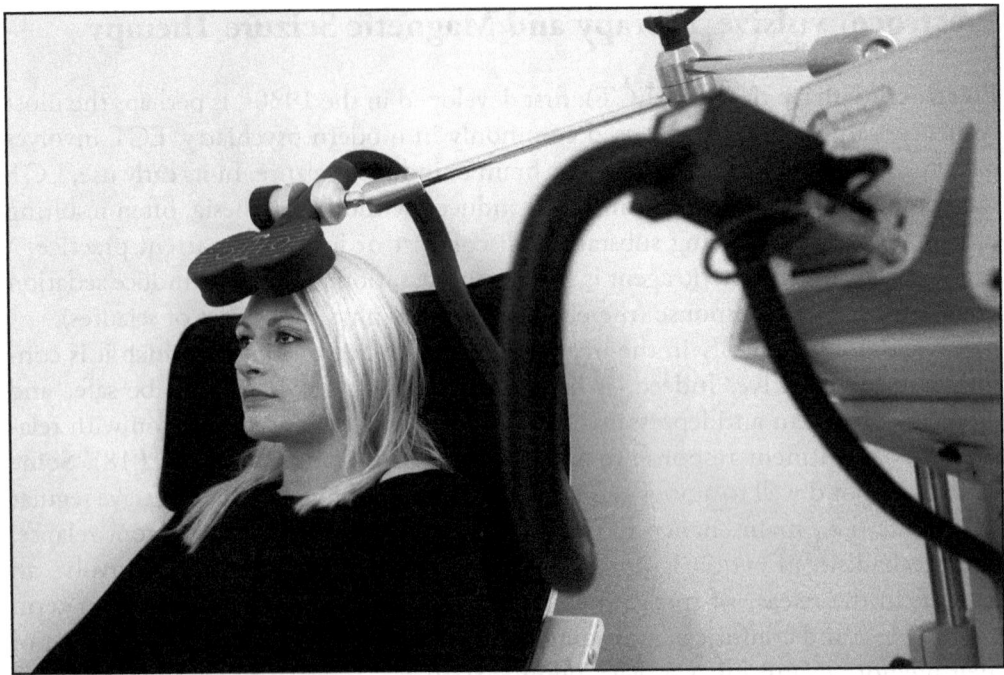

Figure 14.2: Transcranial magnetic stimulation (TMS).

Source: GetStock/AMELIE-BENOIST/BSIP

illnesses (Kong et al., 2018). TNS similarly transmits neurostimulation to the brain but does so through implantation of an electrode that activates the trigeminal nerve, which is located in the cranial area. In DBS, a surgical procedure is undertaken to place an electrode in a specific location in the brain. Through use of a pacemaker, the implanted electrode will deliver repetitive stimulation to deep brain structures. This experimental procedure has been studied in patients with severe mental illnesses and who have not responded to conventional treatment. To date, the relative benefits and risks of DBS remain unclear (Fitzgerald & Segrave, 2015).

Psychotherapy and Other Psychologically Oriented Treatments

Psychotherapy and other psychologically oriented treatments have been developed in line with a series of ideas and theories about mental function. Although there is good evidence that such approaches result in substantial improvements to mental health and reductions in the symptoms of mental illnesses, there remains debate about which approaches are most effective. There are hundreds of psychotherapy methods that have been developed and applied. In the following, we discuss a few commonly used approaches, beginning with a discussion of psychological self-management.

Self-Management

Prior to seeking any form of professional consultation or treatment for mental health challenges, many people explore "self-help" resources. There are books, toolkits, movies, groups, and websites, all devoted to helping people cope with stress and build skills for managing their mental health. It is estimated that two-thirds of internet users seek mental health information. A Google search for "self-help mental health" turns up thousands of sites devoted to providing mental health guidance and resources.

So, are mental health self-management resources effective? The simple answer is yes, reasonably so. Research has demonstrated moderate effectiveness of self-management programs when compared to no-treatment, wait-list, or placebo control groups (Lean et al., 2019). Many individuals report that self-help books have played a central role in their psychological improvement, and psychologists often recommend self-help materials or groups to their patients (Carty et al., 2016). Self-management resources are also inexpensive, compared to professional treatment. Moreover, many people fear stigma and discrimination when seeking professional help, while self-management resources offer privacy and anonymity. But we shouldn't be putting mental health professionals out to pasture just yet. Self-help does not work for everyone; there are many cases where a mental health challenge is severe enough that immediate professional help is necessary. Furthermore, self-help tools are most effective when accompanied by coaching and support (Corrigan & Mueser, 2012; Johnson et al., 2018), which brings us to **supported self-management** (SSM).

SSM involves a workbook or online program that teaches skills for coping more effectively with mental health challenges. The approach is usually based on cognitive behavioural therapy (CBT) principles (described in more detail below) and is to be accompanied by coaching and encouragement from a health care provider, family member, or peer counsellor. It is a "low-intensity" intervention suitable for a broad range of common mental health challenges, including depression, anxiety, and eating disorders. SSM focuses on such skills as setting goals to become more behaviourally active, systematic problem solving, thinking in a fairer and more realistic way, managing worry or physical tension, and identifying warning signs of symptom relapse. SSM builds upon people's own coping strengths and enhances their sense of personal competence. In this way, it helps to address feelings of disempowerment and builds self-efficacy and a sense of agency. SSM has performed well in controlled research, showing good effect in those experiencing mild to moderate depression, for example. However, it is important to note that SSM requires active participation in the therapeutic process, which may not be feasible for individuals experiencing more severe symptoms.

Cognitive Behavioural Therapy

Cognitive behavioural therapy (CBT) is the form of psychotherapy that has the strongest evidence for its effectiveness in the treatment of a wide variety of conditions. CBT represents a merger of "old-school" behavioural therapy (i.e., focused on the use of situational rewards to increase the frequency of adaptive behaviours and decrease maladaptive ones) and cognitive therapy (i.e., focused on helping individuals to identify unrealistic/unfair thinking patterns and replace them with more beneficial ones). It has been shown to be effective in the treatment of a wide variety of mental illnesses including depression, substance dependence, panic disorder, and bulimia nervosa (Carpenter et al., 2018; Linardon, 2018). Through individual or group CBT sessions, clients are taught to recognize maladaptive behaviours (such as withdrawal from social contact when feeling depressed) and distorted thought patterns (such as harsh or critical self-labelling) and to develop skills to change these habits of thought and behaviour. Homework is assigned between sessions, encouraging the individual to try out new ways of acting or thinking in different situations. In fact, most therapeutic progress is made via these "behavioural experiments" outside of the clinical sessions.

Crucial features of CBT are (1) a focus on the present, how someone is thinking and acting in the current situation; (2) an emphasis on the collaborative relationship between therapist and client; (3) treatment goals that are concrete, specific, and measurable (e.g., "rate mood as 20 percent improved"; "participate in fitness activity for 15 minutes, three times each week"); and (4) time-limited intervention, working within 6 to 12 sessions for most common mental health challenges.

A distinct form of CBT-derived therapy is **dialectical behaviour therapy (DBT)**, an intervention that first emerged as a treatment for individuals experiencing borderline personality disorder. In fact, it is considered one of the few interventions to be effective in reducing suicidal behaviour and self-harm in patients diagnosed with this condition (Lakeman & Emeleus, 2020). Its use has since spread to other patient populations, with good effect. It is described as follows:

> DBT evolved from standard cognitive-behavioral therapy ... The theoretical orientation to treatment is a blend of three theoretical positions: behavioral science, dialectical philosophy, and Zen practice. Behavioral science, the principles of behavior change, is countered by acceptance of the client (with techniques drawn both from Zen and from Western contemplative practice); these poles are balanced within the dialectical framework. (Barlow, 2008)

DBT differs from CBT's focus on changing problematic thought and behaviour patterns, instead focusing on helping individuals learn how to live more presently (i.e., avoid past- and future-oriented thinking), establish healthy ways of managing stress, regulate intense emotions, and enhance their interpersonal relationships. Outcomes associated with DBT include reductions in hospital and emergency department use as well as positive impacts for health care staff who deliver the intervention (De Cou et al., 2019).

In more recent years, other CBT-variants have also emerged as more focused or specialized modalities for particular mental health challenges. Some examples include Trauma-Focused CBT, which as the name suggests, is used in the treatment of trauma-related symptoms or disorders, and Exposure and Response Prevention, which has become the gold standard psychotherapeutic approach to reducing the symptoms of obsessive compulsive disorder.

Psychoanalytic Therapies

Psychoanalytic therapies refer to psychotherapeutic approaches that apply the theories of Sigmund Freud and the many other theorists who further developed and extended the original ideas of psychoanalysis. We have discussed psychoanalytic theory in Chapter 3; it aims to solve deep-seated conflicts that are purported to operate unconsciously (without our awareness). Once the most common approach to psychotherapy, psychoanalytic therapies have decreased in popularity as a result of their perceived impracticality as brief interventions and their inconclusive demonstrations of effectiveness in reducing symptoms (Paris, 2005). However, there continues to be considerable interest in more structured forms of psychoanalytic therapy, such as "brief dynamic therapy" and "short-term psychodynamic psychotherapy." Such approaches are of shorter duration than traditional psychoanalytic treatment and have shown reasonable effectiveness in the treatment of certain conditions (Steinert et al., 2017).

Play Therapy

Typically used with children between the ages of 3 and 12, play therapy allows children to express thoughts and feelings in a way that is natural and familiar to them—through play. The assumption behind play therapy is that children who are allowed to play freely will engage in play that reveals the issues with which they are struggling. Play therapy has been used effectively to treat a broad range of children's mental health challenges, including anxiety, aggressive behaviour, and trauma (Pester et al., 2019), and can be combined with other approaches, such as CBT. Parents and caregivers are typically the first to initiate contact with a play therapist, who conducts a number of one-on-one sessions using toys, art, games, and stories to communicate with the child. For example, the therapist and child might role-play a game of "house" to explore family relationships and the home environment, or a therapist might ask the child to use toy cars to show what happened in a car accident.

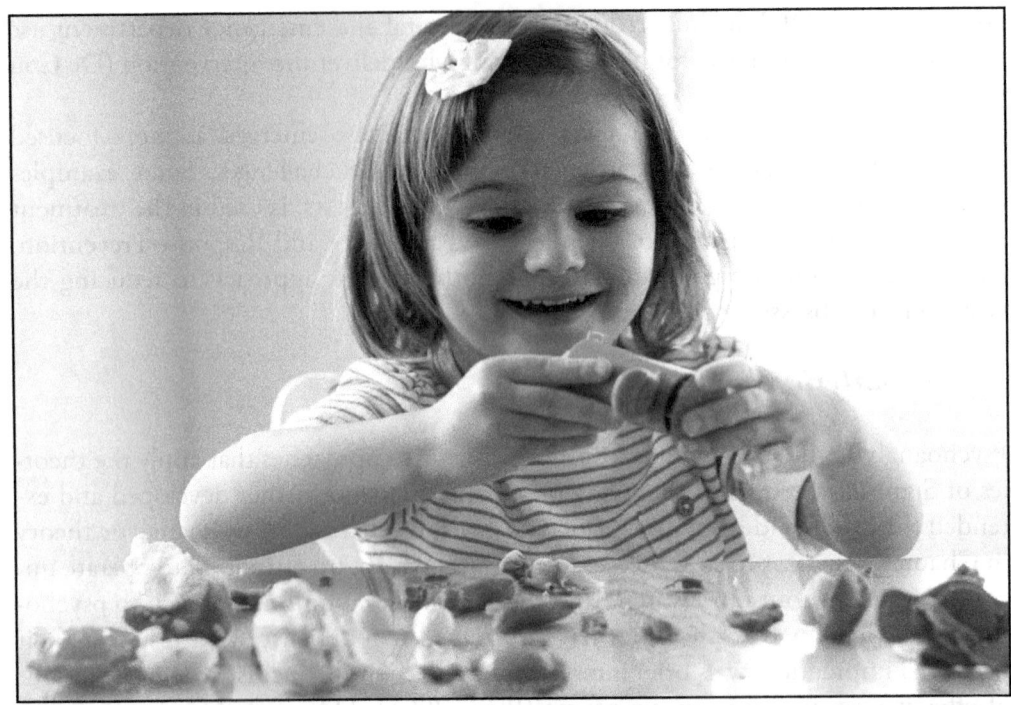

Figure 14.3: Play therapy has been shown to enhance children's self-concept, accelerate cognitive development, reduce anxiety, and improve social skills. Here, a young girl uses playdough to express her feelings during play therapy.

Source: iStockphoto/GeorgeBurba

Family Therapy

Although various family therapy approaches have been developed, they all consider the involvement of "families" as a critical element of treatment. In addition to relatives, families may include close friends and others in an individual's social network. The theoretical frameworks that inform family therapy have a rich history and many creative applications have been developed, including structural, systems, intergenerational, solution-focused, and narrative therapies. Family therapy may occur as a stand-alone intervention, or alongside other forms of mental health treatment (Gelin et al., 2018; Henderson et al., 2019).

Motivational Interviewing

Motivational Interviewing is a psychotherapeutic approach that was initially developed as a therapeutic response to substance use disorders and has since been applied more widely to address a variety of mental health challenges (Miller & Rose, 2009). A central feature is a focus on helping clients to consider their current situations and envisage the changes they would like to put in place. This is undertaken through a non-judgmental and non-adversarial approach. Motivational interviewing acknowledges that individuals are at various states of readiness for change and seeks to meet people "where they are."

Social Approaches to Mental Health

When thinking about treatment for mental illnesses or substance use disorders, it is likely that medications or psychological therapies will be the first to come to mind. Indeed, these are by far the most widely used approaches to addressing mental health challenges—the ones that most people are familiar with. However, social approaches are a critical component of a comprehensive mental health "treatment" strategy. Social approaches aim to address the social roots of mental or substance use challenges, attending to the social determinants of mental health such as inclusion and connection, access to housing, income, and employment.

Peer Support

In recent years, the prominence of peer support has increased exponentially in mental health and substance use treatment contexts. Peer support is based on the premise that individuals with lived experience of mental health or substance use challenges are uniquely positioned to provide social, emotional, and practical supports to others who are experiencing similar struggles. Through the development of a respectful, trusting, and amicable relationship between the peer supporter and the recipient of this support, there is a growth in feelings of empowerment and the capacity to make changes that will enhance quality of life alongside a reduction in hospital admissions (Repper & Carter, 2011). Interestingly, these benefits appear to be reciprocal, with peer supporters also reporting improved outcomes such as enhanced self-esteem and confidence, feelings of empowerment, and the ease that accompanies stable employment, such as feeling like a "valued and contributing citizen" (Hutchinson, et al., 2006).

Social Prescriptions

As discussed in Chapter 1, mental health is a product of complex interactions between an individual and their family, community, and society. Therefore, it is important to consider these broader social contexts—in addressing individual treatment needs, and also in responding to mental health and well-being at a population level. It is not uncommon for people who have mental health or substance use challenges to also experience difficulties with employment or income, housing, relationships, as well as encounters with discrimination and exclusion, for example. Yet how do we treat these larger issues? This is a question that often weighs heavy on the minds of health and social service professionals working with this client population. One approach is to provide social care to address social needs—a practice known as social prescribing. Brilliant! Social prescribing, while not a new concept, has yet to be widely taken up, though there is evidence to suggest it works (Teuton, 2015). Social prescribing involves the health care provider writing a "prescription" to link an individual to social resources or supports (Nowak & Mulligan, 2021). For example, a clinician may prescribe an exercise group to help someone with symptoms of depression to engage in activities and connect socially, or a prescription may be written to connect an individual to financial aid or supportive housing services if they are struggling with these issues. A prescription for volunteering may be helpful for someone who is experiencing loneliness and isolation that is contributing to suicidal thoughts or feelings that their life lacks purpose. It is important that these social prescriptions be tracked, much like a prescription for medication would be, to monitor uptake and document improvements.

Social Justice

While social prescriptions provide a mechanism to connect people with mental illnesses and substance use disorders to relevant social resources, this represents only one piece of a larger puzzle. This is because the social determinants of health are estimated to contribute to approximately 80 percent of our overall health and well-being. When these social determinants are not working in our favour, that is, the organization of our society is unfair and leads to disparities in access to the social determinants of good health—for example, income, education, health care services, and/or employment—then broader social justice actions are required. Such actions aim to address issues of human rights, access, representation, and equity. Taking action in the name of social justice isn't easy—it involves trying to change big systems and structures that scaffold our society. However, it is critical to addressing some of the root causes of poor mental health and mental health inequities. Examples of social justice efforts that can improve mental health include advocacy to address systemic racism in health care settings, efforts to change policies to provide universal coverage for psychological therapy, or the legal battles that have been fought to preserve the operation of supervised consumption sites in Canada. Though not an easy road, taking action in the name of social justice holds benefits for those fighting the cause as well as for society as a whole.

Religious, Spiritual, and Meditative Approaches

Many people consider mental health challenges in a religious or spiritual context and may seek support from religious or spiritual advisors. For some, this may include group prayer, meditation, or pastoral counselling. People who are Indigenous may practice traditional healing, including ceremonies, natural medicines (i.e., originating from plants, animals, or minerals), smudging, and other approaches to supporting mental health and wellness (First Nations Health Authority, 2014). Mental health professionals are sometimes criticized as being antagonistic towards spiritual practices that people adopt to cope with their mental health challenges; however, there is growing awareness of the importance of spirituality to mental health (Dilmaghani, 2018; Koenig, 2015).

Mindfulness

A relatively recent approach to supporting mental health and addressing symptoms of mental ill health is **mindfulness**. Mindfulness is a practice that combines Buddhist meditation with principles of CBT. It involves a set of skills designed to increase one's capacity to be clearly aware of their immediate situation, ongoing thoughts, and bodily sensations, without feeling the need to "fix" them. The aim of this approach is to be "present" in a non-judgmental way, observing the flow of thoughts and feelings without getting caught up in these experiences. It represents a form of awareness practice that promotes acceptance and openness, which in turn helps to relieve psychological symptoms and improve one's ability to manage psychological pain. A growing body of research supports the effectiveness of this therapeutic approach for mental health challenges, including anxiety and depression (Goldberg et al., 2018; Sundquist et al., 2015)

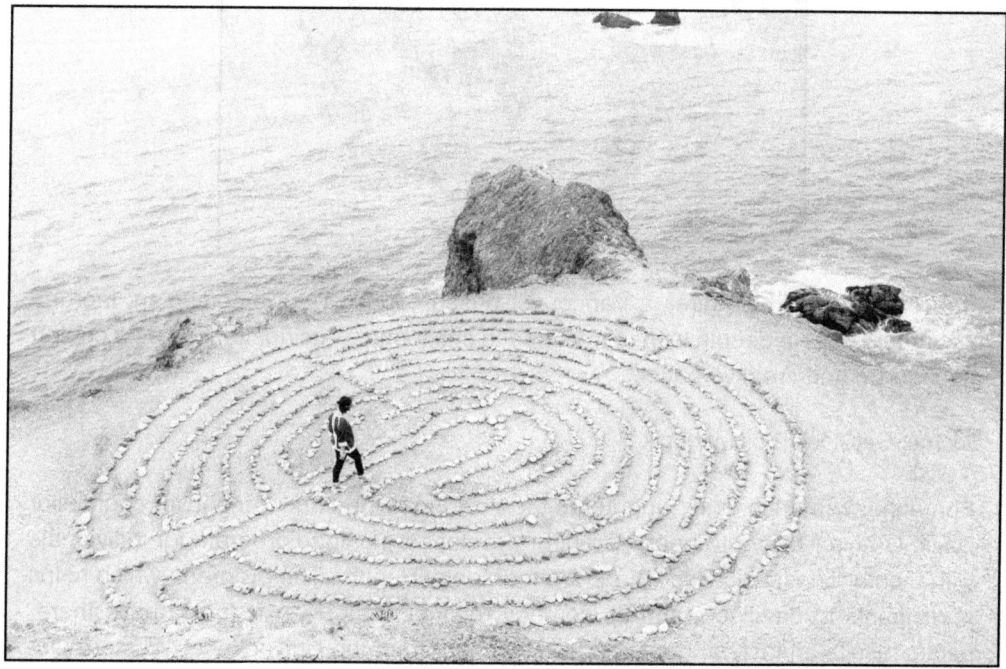

Figure 14.4: Labyrinth walking is an ancient meditative practice that continues to be used today. The labyrinth is not a maze and has no dead ends; continually winding through the path helps the walker quiet the mind, encourage self-reflection, and reduce stress.

Source: Unsplash/Ashley Batz

Combining Treatments

When it comes to the treatment of mental health or substance use challenges, there is no "one size fits all" approach. Selecting the most appropriate treatment depends on the pattern, duration, and severity of the problem; the availability of social or financial supports in the person's life; the presence of other physical or mental challenges; and other factors. Commonly, there is value in combining various treatment approaches, whether biological, psychological, social, or spiritual.

Box 14.2: Stand Up for Mental Health

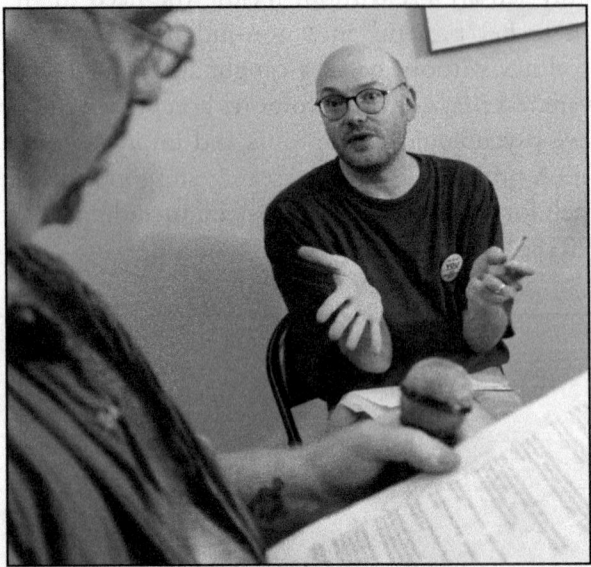

Figure 14.5: David Granirer, a Vancouver-based counsellor and comedian, merges his careers to help people with mental health challenges—using comedy as a coping mechanism and creative outlet.

Source: GetStock/Rick Madonik

Someone wise once said "laughter is the best medicine," and Vancouver counsellor David Granirer took it to heart. Granirer developed a unique program for individuals with mental illnesses called "Stand Up for Mental Health." The program, which helps participants to develop stand-up comedy routines, has been found to have therapeutic results. In fact, students and researchers from the University of Western Ontario have studied the benefits of participating in the program. The program has had such a positive response that Granirer is unable to accommodate everyone wanting to participate. If only all therapy could be so much fun! In an interview, Granirer joked, "People don't want to hear from a stand-up comic that's happy and well adjusted ... That would be really boring" (Carletti, 2010).

Emerging Practices

Many treatment approaches for mental health are well-established and widely practiced, with years—or even decades—of evidence supporting their effectiveness. Yet despite the many treatment approaches available, there are innovative practices continually being developed. This section describes some of these newer approaches to treatment, many of which focus on mental health challenges that have not responded to other forms of treatment.

Psychedelics

The use of psychedelics (also known as hallucinogens) has been around for thousands of years. Indigenous peoples used psychedelics to promote health and wellness. In the 1950s and 60s, psychedelics such as LSD were used experimentally to treat a variety of mental health and substance use challenges, including trauma symptoms and severe alcohol use. While health professionals noted considerable benefits of therapeutic psychedelic use, these substances were banned in Canada and globally in the 1960s. In 2020, however, Health Canada granted limited exemptions to this ban, allowing a small number of health organizations to proceed with psychedelics research and to administer psychedelic-assisted psychotherapy. Additionally, a small number of individuals have been granted permission to use psychedelic substances therapeutically, mostly to address mental health challenges related to terminal conditions. Since government bans on the testing of psychedelic substances have eased, we are seeing a growing body of peer-reviewed research and therapeutic clinical application of psychedelic substances including psilocybin, lysergic acid diethylamide (LSD), ketamine, ayahuasca, and 3,4-methylenedioxymethamphetamine (MDMA). MDMA has been used successfully to treat post-traumatic stress disorder and anxiety, and psilocybin (also known as "magic mushrooms") has been shown to be effective in the treatment of depression, anxiety, obsessive compulsive disorder, and some substance use challenges (Winkelman & Sessa, 2019). Numinus, a clinic based in British Columbia, is currently offering ketamine therapy for the treatment of depression, with the plan to expand the treatment to other conditions, including anxiety, substance use, and eating disorders. However, until regulatory bodies approve their medicinal use, access to psychedelics will remain restricted. Advocacy groups such as Decriminalize Nature Canada are petitioning the government to expand the availability of psychedelics, particularly as treatments for mental health and substance use challenges.

Cognitive Remediation Therapy

People living with psychotic disorders such as schizophrenia or bipolar disorder often develop profound and disabling cognitive deficits, which in some cases, can be even more challenging to live with than positive or negative symptoms of these illnesses. Cognitive losses associated with psychotic disorders can significantly impair daily functioning, contributing to chronic disability and unemployment. However, there is a growing evidence-base for cognitive remediation therapy. Described as being akin to physical exercise for your mind, cognitive remediation therapy aims to help people with mental illnesses improve their cognitive skills in order to achieve better functional outcomes. In recent years, there has been a proliferation of online exercises (games) that clinicians can assign to their patients as part of this therapeutic process.

Digital Phenotyping

A phenotype is a description of your physical, observable characteristics, such as height and hair colour, overall health and disease history, and behaviours. These features develop from interactions between a person's environment and their unique genetic composition. Digital phenotyping is emerging as a clinical approach to mental health and illness, drawing on data from smartphones and wearable technology to capture patterns of human behaviour—including those that might constitute early signs of mental ill health. Techniques to collect this information can be passive (e.g., a sensor on a smartwatch reading your heart rate) or active (e.g., calls, texts, emails, social media engagement). For example, a few years ago Facebook announced that they had developed an algorithm that scans posts to see if users' language patterns suggest that they are experiencing suicidal thoughts or behaviours. If the algorithm detects concerning language, it alerts a Facebook review team and responds to the user, including sending suicide helpline info or even working with local authorities to conduct a "wellness check" (Singer, 2018). While Facebook uses "active" information, machine-learning techniques are being used to determine if passive information collected from digital phenotyping can aid in early diagnosis and treatment of various mental illnesses.

The Recovery Model

Ultimately, the intention of any form of treatment is to help people who experience mental health challenges to achieve recovery. In the mental health context, recovery refers to "a way of living a satisfying, hopeful, and contributing life even with the limitations caused by illness" (Anthony, 1993), which is guided by the principles of the Recovery Model. At the centre of the Recovery Model are the concepts of *hope* and *empowerment*, which are believed to be essential to achieving health. Traditionally, the term "recovery" may have been viewed as synonymous with remission, that is, the absence of clinical symptoms. However, within this model, recovery refers to the "process of growth and transformation as the person moves beyond acute distress often associated with mental health problems or illness and develops new-found strengths and new ways of being" (Mental Health Commission of Canada, 2009). In fact, the Recovery Model has nothing to do with being "cured," but rather with achieving a full and productive life and optimal functioning.

The Recovery Model first emerged within the field of addictions within 12-step programming, and it was used primarily within this program until the late 1980s (Deegan, 1988). At that time, the process of deinstitutionalization was well underway, and mental health services that had previously operated within institutions were being established in the community. With this move into the community, many of the inadequacies of the mental health system became more evident and it was clear that there was a long way to go in terms of meaningful inclusion of people with mental illnesses. People living with mental illnesses responded to this adversity by demanding a shift in services and approach, advocating for the incorporation of the Recovery Model into mental health policy and service delivery (Deegan, 1988). Since this time, the Recovery Model has been gradually embraced by various sectors in a number of countries as a component of their efforts to reform mental health systems. In Canada, the *Out of the Shadows at Last* report advocated for recovery to be "placed at the centre of mental health reform" (Kirby & Keon, 2006), a call that has since been embraced by the Mental Health Commission of Canada in its strategy framework (Mental Health Commission of Canada, 2009; see Chapter 15).

One of the appealing aspects of the Recovery Model is that they place emphasis on the importance of valuing every person's individuality and unique life experience. Health care services are oriented towards supporting clients in achieving health, and health professionals learn that they can promote recovery "by helping a person to understand their experience, while strengthening their sense of meaning and purpose" (Mental Health Commission of Canada, 2009). The Mental Health Commission of Canada has summarized the key principles of recovery as the following:

- Finding, maintaining, and repairing hope: believing in oneself; having a sense of being able to accomplish things; being optimistic about the future.
- Re-establishing a positive identity: finding a new identity which incorporates illness but retains a core, positive sense of self.
- Building a meaningful life: making sense of illness; finding a meaning in life, despite illness; being engaged in life and involved in the community.
- Taking responsibility and control: feeling in control of illness and in control of life.

Figure 14.6 displays 10 fundamental components that have been included in the Recovery Model. Although various health professionals have embraced this paradigm of care, additional effort will be required to achieve a more complete adoption of these principles and practices throughout mental health and substance use services in Canada.

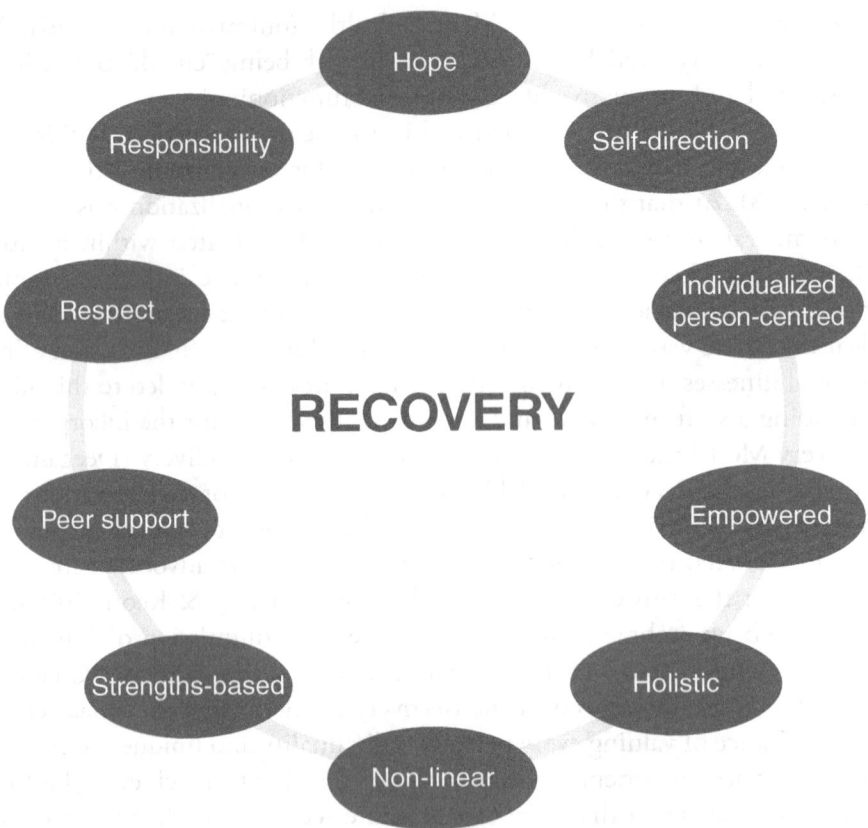

Figure 14.6: Components of recovery.

Source: Substance Abuse and Mental Health Services Administration. (n.d.). *National consensus statement on mental health recovery*. http://store.samhsa.gov/shin/content/SMA05-4129/SMA05-4129.pdf

Personal Mental Health Toolkit

At various times in our lives, we all deal with high levels of stress, whether at school, work, home, or in our interpersonal relationships. When stress becomes difficult to manage, we are liable to experience some psychological difficulty, which can manifest in various ways including worry, poor sleep, low mood, excessive drinking, harmful substance use, or irritability. Sometimes you have a trusted friend, family member, or counsellor who you can talk to, but often you work to manage these experiences on your own. Here are some strategies to help you deal with the stress of life. But remember, if you think you might be having serious difficulties with your mental health, reach out for professional help. This personal mental health toolkit is not a replacement for getting professional treatment when you need it.

Learning to Set Action Goals

Dealing with stress in a healthy manner involves setting goals, trying out new ways of coping, and then practising and sustaining these new coping behaviours over time. To be successful in your efforts, you will need to learn how to set goals in the most effective way. Often people set goals that are not likely to be carried forward and achieved. Let's say a friend of yours sets an ambitious goal to begin a fitness program, determined to go from no exercise to working out for an hour every day at the local fitness centre. This is not very effective goal setting because it is just too ambitious. Your friend will probably attend fitness classes for a couple of days, then miss one or two, then feel guilty and find reasons not to go. In the end, they not only fail to improve their fitness but are also left feeling discouraged.

An effective goal has three characteristics: it is *specific* (i.e., states exactly what you are going to do), *realistic* (i.e., within your capability and likely to be carried out), and *scheduled* (i.e., you write down when and how often you are planning to do it). Table 14.1 offers an example of an effective goal. You can create a similar table to help you in articulating your goals.

Finding a Means to Ground and Balance Yourself

It is helpful to find an approach to grounding, balancing, or centring yourself—something that you can do regularly as a source of pleasure and mental health promotion. It may be an activity like yoga; a sport such as swimming, martial arts, or running; or an artistic hobby such as making music or painting. At least one of the grounding approaches that you select should likely be physical, and you should find one that you truly enjoy and want to do at least once every week, even if it is only for a brief period of time. Ensure that the activity you choose really is one that is calming, grounding, and promotes feelings of happiness. It is important to find a way to consistently engage in these activities.

Relaxation

Knowing how to relax yourself mentally and physically is one of the most useful things you can learn. One way to do so is through a systematic relaxation method and, to make this easier, we've posted a free online audio file (see Positive Coping with Health Conditions in the Recommended Websites section at the end of this

Table 14.1: Example of an effective goal

What I'm Going To Do	When
30-minute workout at the fitness centre	*Mondays and Wednesdays, after my last class*

chapter) to guide you. It explains how to let go of tension and calm anxious thoughts. Find a quiet spot and listen to the audio file. The relaxation procedure is about 17 minutes long. Each time you listen to the relaxation audio, you'll learn more about how to achieve a relaxed state. Perhaps start by setting a goal of listening twice per week for the next several weeks. After a few weeks, it will be time to find a portable relaxation method, a short version of the relaxation procedure that you can do in any setting. An example of this could be to use the part of the relaxation audio where you slowly say "deeply relaxing" to yourself while breathing out. You can then continue this with each exhalation. We call this procedure the "slow breathing method." You might also figure out your own portable relaxation method, using the relaxation audio file, mobile apps, or podcasts with guided mindfulness or meditation sessions, or other mental strategies that help you achieve feelings of calm. Perhaps there is a particular image that has always been comforting for you, such as a sunny beach or a cool pond. Go with whatever works for you, as long as it helps you to relax and can be used easily in different situations.

Worry Management

You might have a worry "issue" if you worry so much that it interferes with other activities, you frequently experience a high level of anxiety, or you have difficulty falling or staying asleep because of worry. If this sounds familiar to you, start by writing down a problem that you have been worrying about. Next to the problem, jot down all the "worry thoughts" that are making you anxious. For example, perhaps you've been worrying about an impending exam for a course called "Mental Health in Canada," and you're having the "worry thought": "I'll never be able to learn this stuff. I'll fail the course and the program, and I'll never get a job." Then use the reality questions in the left-hand column of Table 14.2 to rethink the situation and come up with more realistic thoughts about the exam, the course, and your employment prospects.

Once you've used these questions to come up with thoughts that more accurately reflect the situation, you'll need to deliberately practise bringing them to mind. Whenever you notice yourself starting to worry too much about a problem, deliberately practise calm and realistic thinking. Tell yourself how to look at the situation, and advise yourself, just as you might a friend. Talk back to the worry thinking. Every time you talk back, you make the worry thinking weaker and the realistic thinking stronger.

A big problem with worry is that it often occurs while you're trying to do something else—watch a movie, talk with a friend, or concentrate on a book. Two things happen: first, it's hard to enjoy these activities or do them properly; and second, you can't focus on the problems you're worrying about because you're so distracted! Trying to force yourself to "stop thinking it" doesn't usually work. But what you can do is schedule a particular time during the week when you will concentrate on

Table 14.2: Questions to help manage worry

Question	Rationale
Can I get more evidence, maybe by asking someone about the situation?	It's often helpful to get another person's opinion about the situation.
Would most people agree with this thought? If not, what would most people think?	Just by imagining how most people would react to a "worry thought," you might be able to come up with a fair and realistic way of thinking.
What would I say to a friend if my friend were in a similar situation?	If a friend of yours were worrying too much, what would you say to them? It's likely that you would be able to help them think about the situation more fairly by looking at it in a more balanced way.
What will happen if I continue to think this way?	It's important to understand what results are likely if you continue to worry excessively. Consider the effect of worry on your enjoyment of time with other people, willingness to try activities, ability to get restful sleep, physical symptoms, etc. What might be the results for you and others if you continue to worry excessively?
What is a more encouraging or useful way of thinking?	Can you come up with another thought that would have better results? Is there a way of thinking that would be more encouraging and helpful in improving the situation?

worrying about your problems. During this "worry time," you're not allowed to do anything that would distract you from worrying. Write it into your schedule and make sure you won't be interrupted.

The aim of this scheduled worry time is to allow you to worry towards a solution instead of in circles. In order to fully benefit from this time, set yourself up in a comfortable spot, maybe at a desk in a quiet area, and make sure you have paper and pen or a computer—whatever helps you to think about problems and capture solutions. A useful way to organize your worry time is by using structured problem solving, outlined below.

Structured Problem Solving

First, write down a particular problem you've been dealing with—don't start with a huge problem, but a relatively small one. Next, write down three actions you might take that would help you get closer to a solution, though not necessarily solve it. For each of the actions, write down its advantages and disadvantages. Choose one of these actions to try out, the best or least bad of the three. Table 14.3 offers an example of structured problem solving.

Now make a goal, in the way we've described above, to carry out the action you have selected.

Table 14.3: Examples of structured problem solving

Problem: I have a big exam coming up, and I've been worrying so much that I'm sleeping badly.		
Possible Actions	**Advantages**	**Disadvantages**
Have three or four drinks each night to calm me down so I can sleep.	• It seems to help me sleep. • It calms my worrying.	• I've been suffering from a hangover in the morning, so I haven't been concentrating very well. • If I keep relying on drinking to get to sleep, I'll become dependent on this strategy—now I've started worrying about my drinking. • I've been told that this kind of drinking only works for a short while, then it makes anxiety and sleep even worse. • I don't like to need to use alcohol to sleep.
Get some sleep medication from my family doctor.	• It would help me sleep and relax at night.	• Sleep medication is to be used only for a short while; just like with alcohol, I might become physically and mentally dependent. • Also like alcohol, I might still feel the effect in the morning and have trouble concentrating.
Use relaxation and worry management to deal with my anxiety.	• This would help my worry and sleep. • There is no risk of physical or mental dependence. • There's no hangover in the morning.	• I'll need to practice these new skills. • It might take a while to see the effect.

Identify a Social Support Network

It helps to have one or more people who you can trust to provide support when you are facing challenges in your life. This can be a friend, a partner, a relative, a teacher or professor, a coach, a counsellor or therapist, or members of a peer support group. Our problems often become more burdensome and difficult when we keep them to ourselves. Aim to sustain connections with people whom you find to be helpful, non-judgmental, and uplifting and don't be shy about reaching out to such people and sharing your personal concerns and struggles. They may also call on you when they are facing their own life stresses—we all experience such times. There may be periods when it is harder to identify good sources of social support, such as when you have been in a close relationship that has broken up or when you are travelling or have moved to a new environment. These are times when it can be helpful to find a support group or see a therapist or counsellor.

Check Out Our Free Online Self-Care Workbooks

You can learn more about mental health self-care by downloading one of our free workbooks in the Publications section of the Centre for Applied Research in Mental Health & Addiction (CARMHA) website (see the Recommended Websites section at the end of this chapter).

Conclusion

Treatments or other responses to mental health challenges may be informed by biological, psychological, social, or spiritual perspectives. In Western society, the biological approach has become dominant, typically involving the use of medications to reduce symptoms of mental illness and related suffering. Commonly used medications include antidepressants, mood stabilizers, sedatives, and antipsychotics. Other forms of biological treatment involve procedures that alter the neurochemistry of the brain, such as ECT, used mainly for severe depression. Biological treatments have also included lobotomy and the administration of thalidomide; these were dark chapters in the history of mental health treatment, alerting us to the importance of carefully evaluating our interventions before implementing them widely. Psychological treatments include self-help approaches, such as workbooks or online programs (most effective when supported by a health care provider or coach) and various kinds of psychotherapy. Social approaches aim to address the inequities in access to the social determinants of mental health and may be administered on an individual basis, such as through social prescriptions, or at a population level, through social justice efforts. Recently, there has been an increased openness by mental health professionals to the use of spiritual practices to support mental health. Combined treatments are often beneficial. As each of us experiences stressors, the use of evidence-based tools and coping strategies, such as effective goal setting or relaxation exercises, can be helpful in minimizing the consequences to our mental health.

Glossary

cognitive behavioural therapy (CBT): A widely practiced form of psychotherapy that merges behavioural therapy and cognitive therapy to provide a goal-oriented therapy.
dialectical behavioural therapy (DBT): A distinct form of therapy derived from CBT, focusing on helping individuals learn how to live more presently, establish healthy ways of managing stress, regulate intense emotions, and enhance their interpersonal relationships.

electroconvulsive therapy (ECT): An invasive treatment that involves electrically induced seizures to treat a variety of mental illnesses.

extrapyramidal symptoms: Movement disorders resulting from the inhibition of dopamine activity during the use of antipsychotic medications.

mindfulness: A set of skills designed to increase one's capacity to be clearly aware of one's immediate situation, ongoing thoughts, and bodily sensations without feeling the need to "fix" them.

polypharmacy: The use of multiple medications of various sorts to address varied symptoms and hopefully enhance response.

supported self-management: A low-intensity intervention that involves a program to teach individual skills for coping more effectively with mental health challenges, in addition to coaching and encouragement provided by a health care provider, family member, or peer counsellor.

Critical Thinking Questions

1. Describe a form of psychotherapy discussed in this chapter as well as the mental health challenges that it is commonly used to treat.
2. Compare and contrast typical and atypical antipsychotic medications. Be sure to provide an example for each.
3. What are some examples of social approaches to mental health "treatment"?
4. What is the recovery model and how does it guide mental health practices?
5. Why is self-care important? What are some specific strategies that might be effective in helping you deal with the stress of student life?

Recommended Readings

Gabbard, G. O. (2014). *Gabbard's treatments of psychiatric disorders: DSM-5 edition*. American Psychiatric Association.

Goldbloom, D. S. (2010). *Psychiatric clinical skills*. Centre for Addiction and Mental Health.

Stahl, S. M. (2013). *Stahl's essential psychopharmacology: Neuroscientific basis and practical applications* (4th ed.). Cambridge University Press.

Recommended Websites

Canadian Mental Health Association. www.cmha.ca
CARMHA—Publications. www.sfu.ca/carmha/publications.html
Mental Health Commission of Canada. www.mentalhealthcommission.ca
Psychosocial Rehabilitation and Recovery Canada. www.psrrpscanada.ca

Wellness Together Canada. www.wellnesstogether.ca
National Coalition for Mental Health Recovery. www.ncmhr.org

References

Andrade, C., & Rao, N. S. K. (2010). How antidepressant drugs act: A primer on neuroplasticity as the eventual mediator of antidepressant efficacy. *Indian Journal of Psychiatry, 52*(4), 378–386. https://doi.org/10.4103/0019-5545.74318

Anthony, W. A. (1993). Recovery from mental illness: The guiding vision of the mental health service system in the 1990s. *Psychosocial Rehabilitation Journal, 16*(4), 11–23. https://doi.org/10.1037/h0095655

Bahji, A., & Bajaj, N. (2018). Opioids on trial: A systematic review of interventions for the treatment and prevention of opioid overdose. *Canadian Journal of Addiction, 9*(1), 26–33. https://doi.org/10.1097/CXA.0000000000000013

Ban, T. A. (2007). Fifty years chlorpromazine: A historical perspective. *Neuropsychiatric Disease and Treatment, 3*(4), 495–500.

Barlow, D. (2008). *Clinical handbook of psychological disorders: A step-by-step treatment manual* (4th ed.). Guilford Press.

British Columbia Centre on Substance Use. (2020). *Operational guidance for implementation of managed alcohol for vulnerable populations.* https://www.bccsu.ca/wp-content/uploads/2020/10/Operational-Guidance-Managed-Alcohol.pdf

Carletti, F. (2010). A funny thing happened to me on the way to mental illness. *The Tyee.* https://thetyee.ca/News/2010/03/01/CarlettiLaugherMedicine/

Carpenter, J. K., Andrews, L. A., Witcraft, S. M., Powers, M. B., Smits, J. A., & Hofmann, S. G. (2018). Cognitive behavioral therapy for anxiety and related disorders: A meta-analysis of randomized placebo-controlled trials. *Depression and Anxiety, 35*(6), 502–514. https://doi.org/10.1002/da.22728

Carty, S., Thompson, L., Berger, S., Jahnke, K., & Llewellyn, R. (2016). Books on Prescription—community-based health initiative to increase access to mental health treatment: An evaluation. *Australian and New Zealand Journal of Public Health, 40*(3), 276–278. https://doi.org/10.1111/1753-6405.12507

Cheniaux, E., & Nardi, A. E. (2019). Evaluating the efficacy and safety of antidepressants in patients with bipolar disorder. *Expert Opinion on Drug Safety, 18*(10), 893–913. https://doi.org/10.1080/14740338.2019.1651291

Corrigan, P. W., & Mueser, K. T. (2012). *Principles and practice of psychiatric rehabilitation: An empirical approach.* Guildford Press.

Daskalakis, Z. J., Dimitrova, J., McClintock, S. M., Sun, Y., Voineskos, D., Rajji, T. K., Goldbloom, D. S., Wong, H. C., Knyahnytska, Y., Mulsant, B. H., Downar, J., Fitzgerald, P. B., & Blumberger, D. M. (2019). Magnetic seizure therapy (MST) for major depressive disorder. *Neuropsychopharmacology, 45*, 276–282. https://doi.org/10.1038/s41386-019-0515-4

De Cou, C. R., Comtois, K. A., & Landes, S. J. (2019). Dialectical behavioural therapy is effective for the treatment of suicidal behaviour: A meta-analysis. *Behavior Therapy, 50*, 60–72. https://doi.org/10.1016/j.beth.2018.03.009

Deegan, P. E. (1988). Recovery: The lived experience of rehabilitation. *Psychosocial Rehabilitation Journal, 11*(4), 11–19. https://doi.org/10.1037/h0099565

Dilmaghani, M. (2018). Importance of religion or spirituality and mental health in Canada. *Journal of Religion and Health, 57*(1), 120–135. https://doi.org/10.1007/s10943-017-0385-1

Dyck, E. (2011). Dismantling the asylum and charting new pathways into the community: Mental health care in twentieth century Canada. *Histoire Sociale/ Social History, 44*(88), 181–196. https://doi.org/10.1353/his.2011.0016

First Nations Health Authority. (2014). *Traditional wellness strategic framework*. https://www.fnha.ca/WellnessSite/WellnessDocuments/FNHA_Traditional-WellnessStrategicFramework.pdf

Fitzgerald, P. B., & Segrave, R. A. (2015). Deep brain stimulation in mental health: Review of evidence for clinical efficacy. *The Australian and New Zealand Journal of Psychiatry, 49*(11), 979–993. https://doi.org/10.1177/0004867415598011

Fournier, J. C., DeRubeis, R. J., & Hollon, S. D. (2010). Antidepressant drug effects and depression severity: A patient-level meta-analysis. *Journal of the American Medical Association, 303*(1), 47–53. https://doi.org/10.1001/jama.2009.1943

Gask, L. (2018). In defence of the biopsychosocial model. *The Lancet Psychiatry, 5*(7), 548–549. https://doi.org/10.1016/S2215-0366(18)30165-2

Gelin, Z., Cook-Darzens, S., & Hendrick, S. (2018). The evidence base for multiple family therapy in psychiatric disorders: A review (Part 1). *Journal of Family Therapy, 40*(3), 302–325.

Gitlin, M. J. (2019). Antidepressants in bipolar depression: An enduring controversy. *Focus, 17*(3), 278–283. https://doi.org/10.1111/1467-6427.12178

Goldberg, S. B., Tucker, R. P., Greene, P. A., Davidson, R. J., Wampold, B. E., Kearney, D. J., & Simpson, T. L. (2018). Mindfulness-based interventions for psychiatric disorders: A systematic review and meta-analysis. *Clinical Psychology Review, 59*, 52–60. https://doi.org/10.1016/j.cpr.2017.10.011

Henderson, C. E., Hogue, A., & Dauber, S. (2019). Family therapy techniques and one-year clinical outcomes among adolescents in usual care for behavior problems. *Journal of Consulting and Clinical Psychology, 87*(3), 308. https://psycnet.apa.org/doi/10.1037/ccp0000376

Hoffman, E. (2017). The competitive dynamics of the generic drug manufacturing industry. *Business Economics, 52*(1), 68–75. https://doi.org/10.1057/s11369-017-0026-4

Hutchinson, D. S., Anthony, W. A., Ashcraft, L., Johnson, E., Dunn, E. C., Lyass, A., & Rogers, E. S. (2006). The personal and vocational impact of training and employing people with psychiatric disabilities as providers. *Psychiatric Rehabilitation Journal, 29*(3), 205–213. https://doi.org/10.2975/29.2006.205.213

Iversen, T. S. J., Steen, N. E., Dieset, I., Hope, S., Mørch, R., Gardsjord, E. S., Jørgensen, K. N., Melle, I., Andreassen, O. A., Molden, E., & Jönsson, E. G. (2018). Side effect burden of antipsychotic drugs in real life—impact of gender and polypharmacy. *Progress in Neuro-Psychopharmacology and Biological Psychiatry, 82*, 263–271. https://doi.org/10.1016/j.pnpbp.2017.11.004

Jenkins, E. K. (2014). The politics of knowledge: Implications for understanding and addressing mental health and illness. *Nursing Inquiry, 21*(1), 3–10. https://doi.org/10.1111/nin.12026

Johnson, S., Lamb, D., Marston, L., Osborn, D., Mason, O., Henderson, C., Ambler, G., Milton, A., Davidson, M., Christoforou, M., Sullivan, S., Hunter, R., Hindle, D., Paterson, B., Leverton, M., Piotrowski, J., Forsyth, R., Mosse, Goater, N., ... Lloyd-Evans, B. (2018). Peer-supported self-management for people discharged from a mental health crisis team: A randomised controlled trial. *The Lancet, 392*(10145), 409–418. https://doi.org/10.1016/S0140-6736(18)31470-3

Khouzam, H. R. (2017). Psychiatrists as prescribers versus holistic providers of mental health treatment. *Theranostics of Brain, Spine & Neural Disorders, 1*(1), 1–5. https://doi.org/10.19080/TBSND.2017.01.555551

Kirby, M. J. L., & Keon, W. J. (2006). *Out of the Shadows at Last: Transforming mental health, mental illness and addiction services in Canada*. Retrieved from: https://mentalhealthcommission.ca/wp-content/uploads/2021/09/out_of_the_shadows_at_last_-_full_0_0.pdf

Koenig, H. G. (2015). Religion, spirituality, and health: A review and update. *Advances in Mind-Body Medicine, 29*(3), 19–26.

Kong, J., Fang, J., Park, J., Li, S., & Rong, P. (2018). Treating depression with transcutaneous auricular vagus nerve stimulation: State of the art and future perspectives. *Frontiers in Psychiatry, 9*, 20. https://doi.org/10.3389/fpsyt.2018.00020

Lakeman, R., & Emeleus, M. (2020). The process of recovery and change in a dialectical behaviour therapy programme for youth. *International Journal of Mental Health Nursing, 29*(6), 1092–1100. https://doi.org/10.1111/inm.12749

Lean, M., Fornells-Ambrojo, M., Milton, A., Lloyd-Evans, B., Harrison-Stewart, B., Yesufu-Udechuku, A., Kendall, T., & Johnson, S. (2019). Self-management interventions for people with severe mental illness: Systematic review and meta-analysis. *The British Journal of Psychiatry, 214*(5), 260–268. https://doi.org/10.1192/bjp.2019.54

Linardon, J. (2018). Meta-analysis of the effects of cognitive-behavioral therapy on the core eating disorder maintaining mechanisms: Implications for mechanisms of therapeutic change. *Cognitive Behaviour Therapy, 47*(2), 107–125. https://doi.org/10.1080/16506073.2018.1427785

Mental Health Commission of Canada (MHCC). (2009). *Toward recovery and well-being*. https://www.mentalhealthcommission.ca/wp-content/uploads/drupal/FNIM_Toward_Recovery_and_Well_Being_ENG_0_1.pdf

Miller, W. R., & Rose, G. S. (2009). Toward a theory of motivational interviewing. *American Psychologist, 64*(6), 527–537. https://doi.org/10.1037/a0016830

Mojtabai, R., & Olfson, M. (2010). National trends in psychotropic medication polypharmacy in office-based psychiatry. *Archives of General Psychiatry, 67*(1), 26–36. https://doi.org/10.1001/archgenpsychiatry.2009.175

Nowak, D. A. & Mulligan, K. (2021). Social prescribing: A call to action. *Canadian Family Physician, 67*(2), 88–91. https://doi.org/10.46747/cfp.670288

Paris, J. (2005). *The fall of an icon: Psychoanalysis and academic psychiatry*. University of Toronto Press.

Pester, D., Lenz, A. S., & Dell'Aquila, J. (2019). Meta-analysis of single-case evaluations of child-centered play therapy for treating mental health symptoms. *International Journal of Play Therapy, 28*(3), 144–156. https://psycnet.apa.org/doi/10.1037/pla0000098

Peterchev, A. V., Krystal, A. D., Rosa, M. A., & Lisanby, S. H. (2015). Individualized low-amplitude seizure therapy: Minimizing current for electroconvulsive therapy and magnetic seizure therapy. *Neuropsychopharmacology, 40*(9), 2076–2084. https://doi.org/10.1038/npp.2015.122

Repper, J., & Carter, T. (2011). A review of the literature on peer support in mental health services. *Journal of Mental Health, 20*(4), 392–411. https://doi.org/10.3109/09638237.2011.583947

Safer, D. J. (2019). Overprescribed medications for US adults: Four major examples. *Journal of Clinical Medicine Research, 11*(9), 617–622. https://doi.org/10.14740/jocmr3906

Singer, N. (2018, February 25). How companies scour our digital lives for clues to our health. *New York Times*. https://www.nytimes.com/2018/02/25/technology/smartphones-mental-health.html

Smith, S., & Grant, A. (2016). The corporate construction of psychosis and the rise of the psychosocial paradigm: Emerging implications for mental health nursing. *Nurse Education Today, 39*, 22–25. https://doi.org/10.1016/j.nedt.2016.01.007

Steinert, C., Munder, T., Rabung, S., Hoyer, J., & Leichsenring, F. (2017). Psychodynamic therapy: As efficacious as other empirically supported treatments? A meta-analysis testing equivalence of outcomes. *American Journal of Psychiatry, 174*(10), 943–953. https://doi.org/10.1176/appi.ajp.2017.17010057

Substance Abuse and Mental Health Services Administration. (n.d.). *National consensus statement on mental health recovery*. http://store.samhsa.gov/shin/content/SMA05-4129/SMA05-4129.pdf

Sundquist, J., Lilja, Å., Palmér, K., Memon, A. A., Wang, X., Johansson, L. M., & Sundquist, K. (2015). Mindfulness group therapy in primary care patients with depression, anxiety and stress and adjustment disorders: Randomised controlled trial. *The British Journal of Psychiatry, 206*(2), 128–135. https://doi.org/10.1192/bjp.bp.114.150243

Teuton, J. (2015). *Social prescribing for mental health: Background paper*. NHS Health Scotland. http://www.healthscotland.com/uploads/documents/26712-Social%20Prescribing%20for%20Mental%20Health%20Background%205614.pdf

Vann Jones, S., & McCollum, R. (2019). Subjective memory complaints after electroconvulsive therapy: Systematic review. *BJPsych Bulletin, 43*(2), 73–80. https://doi.org/10.1192/bjb.2018.45

Vargesson, N. (2015). Thalidomide-induced teratogenesis: History and mechanisms. *Embryo Today: Reviews, 105*(2), 140–156. https://doi.org/10.1002/bdrc.21096

Winkelman, M., & Sessa, B. (Eds.). (2019). *Advances in psychedelic medicine: State-of-the-art therapeutic applications*. Praeger.

Zilles, D. (2018). Beneficial effects of electroconvulsive therapy in elderly people. *The Lancet Psychiatry, 5*(9), 697–698. https://doi.org/10.1016/S2215-0366(18)30264-5

Chapter 15

Mental Health Services in Canada

Erin Michalak and Rebecca Zappelli, adapted from original chapter by Elliot M. Goldner, Emily Jenkins, and Dan Bilsker

> I came to believe that health services ought not to have a price tag on them, and that people should be able to get whatever health services they required irrespective of their individual capacity to pay.
> —Tommy Douglas (Canadian politician)

Introduction

In this chapter, we examine the services provided to address mental health and illness within the Canadian health care system. However, when it comes to mental health, it has been noted that the available services are actually not much of a "system" at all. Instead, we see a patchwork of different programs and services that are not completely integrated or interconnected (and, in some circumstances, may be badly disintegrated or fragmented; Kirby & Keon, 2006). To understand mental health services in Canada, we first discuss the overall organization of health care delivery in the country and then describe how mental health services fit into this larger framework. An important focus of this chapter will be a description of efforts that have been put in place to strengthen and improve mental health services in Canada, including the pivotal work of the Mental Health Commission of Canada with its mission to "raise awareness of the mental health and wellness needs of Canadians, and to catalyze collaborative solutions to mental health system challenges" (Mental Health Commission of Canada, 2016).

The Structure and Organization of Canada's Health Care Services

Since this book focuses on *Canada's* approach to mental health, we have asked ourselves: What is distinctive about Canada and its services? In his poem "We are

More," delivered at the opening ceremonies of the 2010 Winter Olympics held in Vancouver, British Columbia, Shane Koyczan (2010) offers the following image:

> And some say what defines us
> Is something as simple as "please" and "thank you"
> And as for "you're welcome," well, we say that, too
> But we are more than genteel or civilized
> We are an idea in the process of being realized
> We are young, we are cultures strung together then woven into a tapestry
> And the design is what makes us more than the sum total of our history
> We are an experiment going right for a change

Canada has a national health care insurance scheme that aims to support egalitarian principles, which means that efforts are made to ensure that all Canadian residents are able to obtain good quality health care, regardless of their social or economic status. Historically, Canadians have been proud of this commitment, often considering our approach to be more humane than that taken in many other countries where only those with financial means can access quality health care services.

Canada Health Act

To some degree, health care services in Canada are shaped by the **Canada Health Act**, a piece of federal legislation that stipulates key characteristics of the health care insurance coverage provided by Canada's provinces and territories (Minister of Justice, 2009). The five principles of the *Canada Health Act* are universality, accessibility, portability, comprehensiveness, and public administration, each described below. If a province or territory does not comply with these principles, the federal government may impose a penalty by withholding funds that would otherwise have been transferred to the province or territory for health care services.

The principle of universality stipulates that *all* Canadian residents are entitled to receive coverage for health care services—a principle that, as mentioned above, has been a source of pride for many Canadians.

The principle of accessibility indicates that all Canadians should have access to services, regardless of their geographical location. Of course, with Canada's vast size and dispersed population, there are enormous challenges in providing services to people living in rural and remote areas. Nevertheless, it is expected that mechanisms will be in place to arrange access to health care services for all residents, including emergency and ambulance responses serving all corners of a province or territory.

The principle of portability stipulates that health care insurance coverage should remain intact when a Canadian travels or moves from one province or territory to another (or requires urgent health care when travelling in another country).

The principle of comprehensiveness refers to coverage of all "medically necessary" health care services. However, there is substantial dispute as to which health care

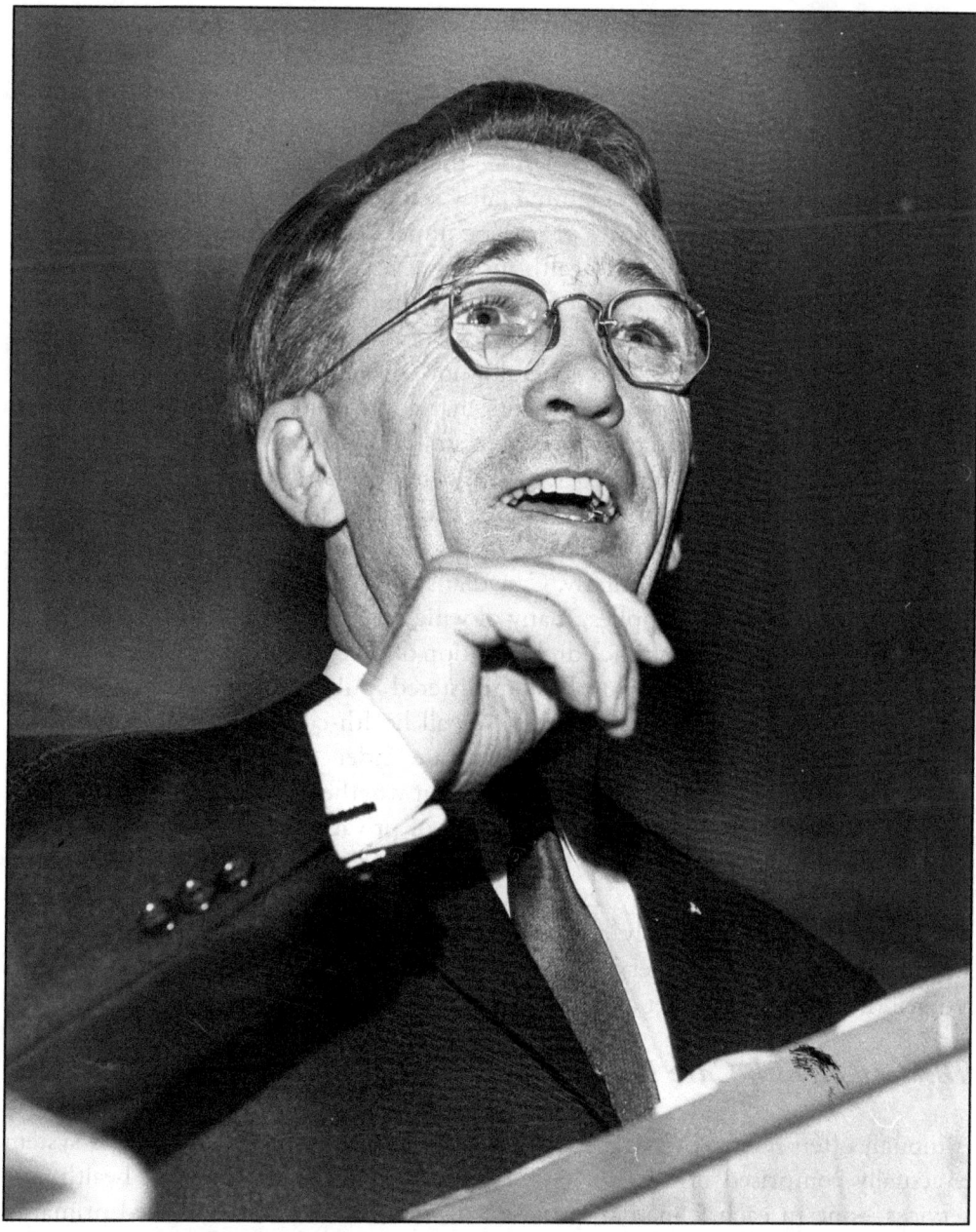

Figure 15.1: Tommy Douglas is credited as the "founding father of Medicare" (our national health insurance program).

Source: GetStock/Barry Philp

services are included or excluded from this definition. There is a common misconception that, in Canada, all health care services are covered by the national health insurance scheme. In fact, it is estimated that approximately 30 percent of health care services received in Canada are not covered by government. This 70/30 public/private split has been fairly consistent since the early 2000s, with the public-sector share of total health spending remaining fairly stable at around 70 percent, covering hospitals, medications, health care provider compensation, and other spending. The private sector includes extended health insurance expenditure and "out of pocket" spending, which currently averages $994 per individual in Canada (Canadian Institute for Health Information, 2021). As one example of private sector health care expenses, dental services are generally not covered by the government. Some Canadians have jobs with private benefits that cover some portion of their dental bills (and their employers may also provide similar benefits that cover other health care bills for individuals, their partners, and dependents). However, a person without a private health care plan and without the means to pay for dental care may have to go without treatment for even serious dental problems, such as infections, cavities, and broken teeth. Similarly, Canadians will often have to cover the costs of medications and medical supplies, many of which are very expensive.

Finally, the principle of public administration denotes that the provincial/territorial health care insurance plan must be administered "publicly," that is, as a non-profit enterprise undertaken by governments. Not all health care services in Canada are publicly administered, and some services operate under "private" administration for profit. There is substantial ongoing debate about whether governments should relax some of the restrictions against the operation of private, for-profit health care services in Canada. Those in favour argue that these could improve the quality and availability of services (Babony, 2019). Those who are opposed warn that increased privatization would inevitably advantage wealthy Canadians and reduce access to and quality of health care services for those who have lower socioeconomic status (Angell, 2008; Armstrong et al., 2016).

Thirteen Health Care Insurance Plans and Delivery Systems

Although often referred to as a "national" health insurance plan, Canada's system is actually comprised of 13 different schemes that cover the costs of health care services—one in each Canadian province or territory. These are funded primarily through taxes that our governments collect each year. In fact, the health care portion is by far the largest portion of the government budget covered by our taxes. We are each issued a health care card that identifies us as having insurance coverage, and we each have a unique personal health care number that is recorded for billing purposes, such as when we obtain services at a hospital, doctor's office, or other setting.

Health care services in Canada are structured differently than those in most other countries, with responsibility for these services primarily residing with each individual province or territory. Consequently, decisions about most activities, policies, and priorities are made at this level. The strong role of provincial and territorial governments in Canadian health care services can make it difficult to implement national initiatives or policies. To some extent, each province or territory is likely to "march to its own drum," pursuing different goals and initiatives.

Responsibility for the delivery of services within a province or territory is often further divided among a number of smaller administrative regions, known as Health Authorities in British Columbia, Local Health Integration Networks in Ontario, and Health and Social Services Institutions in Quebec, for example. Regardless of their name, these authorities are generally responsible for the delivery of health care services within a defined geographical region of the province or territory, including all inpatient and outpatient hospital care, diagnostic laboratories, emergency services, various clinics, long-term care facilities, and home care services. These health authorities are often headed by chief executive officers and groups of executive managers. Although they may vary considerably in the size of the population they serve, many are very large enterprises with annual operating budgets in the billions of dollars. Indeed, they often employ more people than any other business or company within a region.

Another feature of Canadian health care services is that the administration of physician services operates independently from the direct control of health authorities, through agreements negotiated by physician associations directly with provincial or territorial governments. Because physicians are generally not employed or managed by health authorities, there can be challenges in coordinating physician practice with policies and procedures undertaken by health authorities.

While the provinces and territories play a key role in the organization and provision of Canada's health care services, there are also a number of federally funded components. These include national agencies with responsibility for health research, evaluation, and public health activities. Table 15.1 provides a brief description of the roles of a number of these agencies. At times, the federal and provincial/territorial governments and agencies may disagree on policies and activities, and it is sometimes difficult to achieve effective and harmonious cooperation of these different health care components. Later in this chapter, we will return to a discussion of the Mental Health Commission of Canada and its unique role in catalyzing improvements to mental health services in Canada.

The federal government also holds responsibility for delivery of health services for specific groups in Canada, including inmates of federal correctional facilities. Health care for Indigenous peoples in Canada is complex, with funding and service delivery the responsibility of different federal, provincial/territorial, and Indigenous jurisdictions. In 2013, British Columbia established the First Nations Health Authority (FNHA), the first province-wide health authority of its kind in Canada. FNHA is responsible for the delivery of services for First Nations communities in British Columbia and supports BC First Nations individuals, families, and communities to achieve and enjoy the highest level of health and wellness (FNHA, 2016).

Table 15.1: Select list of federally funded health-related agencies in Canada

Name of Agency	Mission And Purpose
Public Health Agency of Canada (PHAC)	Goal: To promote health, prevent, and control chronic diseases and injuries, prevent and control infectious diseases, prepare for and respond to public health emergencies, and strengthen public health capacity
Canadian Institutes for Health Research (CIHR)	Responsible for funding health research in Canada with goals to fund more research on targeted priority areas; build research capacity in underdeveloped areas such as population health and health services research; train the next generation of health researchers; and focus on knowledge translation, so that the results of research are transformed into policies, practices, procedures, products, and services
Health Canada	Federal department responsible for helping the people of Canada maintain and improve their health
Statistics Canada	Produces statistics about many issues that help Canadians better understand their country—its population, resources, economy, society, and culture; health statistics are one of many sets of statistics that are produced regularly
Canadian Centre on Substance Abuse (CCSA)	Goal: To provide national leadership and evidence-informed analysis and advice to mobilize collaborative efforts to reduce alcohol- and other drug-related harms
Mental Health Commission of Canada	Goal: To help bring into being an integrated mental health system that places people living with mental illness at its centre

Many mental health services in Canada are covered by our national health insurance plans, including treatment delivered in hospitals, emergency services, and outpatient treatment provided by family physicians and psychiatrists. In addition, some community-based treatment services delivered by various other health professionals are available for people who meet certain diagnostic criteria for mental illnesses. However, these services are generally reserved for people with the most serious and acute (i.e., urgent) mental illnesses. People with less severe mental health challenges often have great difficulty obtaining access to appropriate treatment through the public health care system. Numerous mental health services in Canada require people to pay out of pocket and may be too expensive for many people to afford. These include many psychological treatments for depression, anxiety, and other common mental health challenges, couples or family therapy, and specialized treatment for substance use challenges.

Delivery of Mental Health Care Services

A broad spectrum of service providers is called into play to comprehensively address mental health challenges. These include primary care providers, nurses, psychiatrists,

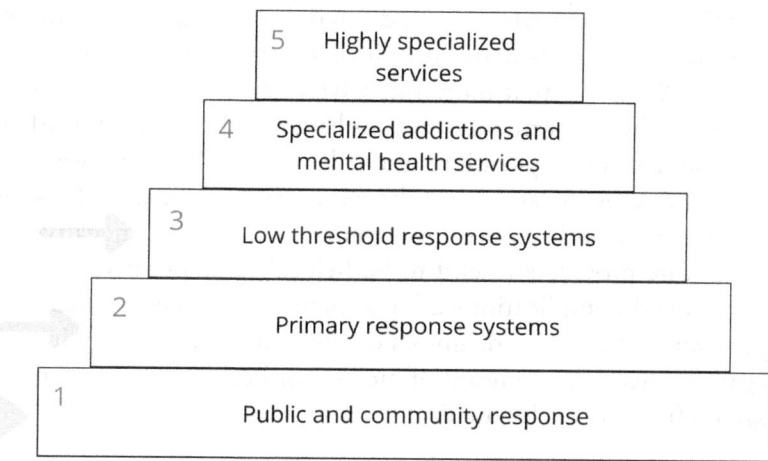

Figure 15.2: The stepped-care model showing that large numbers of people are served by "lower steps" (involving less resource-intensive services). Individuals who require more intensive levels of care may move up (and later back down) these steps, accessing the minimally intensive level of care required. This preserves resources for people who need them most and avoids imposing more invasive care upon those who do not require it.

and other medical specialists, psychologists, social workers, occupational therapists, counsellors, couples and family therapists, peer support workers, pharmacists, dieticians, and housing and employment support workers. Figure 15.2 depicts how mental health services operate at various levels. Services at the bottom of the figure are low-intensity interventions, are more readily available, and are accessed by a large number of individuals. In contrast, services at the top of the triangle are high-intensity interventions suited to a much smaller number of people who require this more specialized treatment. An example of a low-intensity service would be group sessions delivered by a nurse to help individuals to manage symptoms of depression. An example of a high-intensity intervention would be inpatient hospital treatment programs for people with severe depression or who are at risk of self-harm or suicide. Such programs may include a combination of medications or other biologically oriented treatments, psychotherapy, or other psychosocial supports delivered by a team of health care professionals.

Stepped-Care

When mental health care systems are well designed, they ensure that the high-intensity treatments are reserved for those people who truly need them by applying a **stepped-care approach** (see Figure 15.2). This means that the system generally aims to provide low-intensity treatment for most people and will *step up* the intensity of treatments if needed (Richards et al., 2012; van Straten et al., 2015). Since many people will respond well to the low-intensity intervention, it would be a mistake to provide more intensive treatments when not indicated. Indeed, limited money and resources must be utilized to help as many people as possible. Further, intrusiveness should be minimized. We know that more intensive interventions, such as hospitalization, during which individuals may receive multiple medications and other treatments, come with the risk of complications and side effects. Therefore, we should avoid intruding with this type of care unless there is a strong imperative for doing so. In the delivery of mental health services, interventions can have a negative impact—even when health care providers intend to be helpful. This negative impact can be due to side effects and complications of treatments, and other indirect effects, such as self-stigmatization following diagnosis or difficulty reintegrating into everyday life. Such negative outcomes as a result of medical or health care intervention are known as **iatrogenic** (i.e., caused by medical care).

Early Intervention

One approach to enhancing the effectiveness of mental health care is to provide intervention at an early stage in the course of the mental health condition. By intervening early, it is hoped that symptoms will be effectively addressed and functional impairment prevented. An exemplar of this approach is the provision of early psychosis intervention (EPI). EPI is ideally implemented when individuals experience "first-episode psychosis" related to diagnoses such as schizophrenia, schizoeffective disorder, bipolar disorder, and depression with psychotic features. The treatment approach generally involves the use of medication, cognitive behavioural therapy (CBT), and/or family therapy, specifically tailored to individuals experiencing symptoms of psychosis. A CBT approach to this early intervention might include education about the condition, approaches to improving social function and self-esteem, coping strategies for managing symptoms, and methods for relapse prevention (Drake et al., 2014). A family therapy intervention, delivered to the individual with psychosis as well as their family members, might incorporate education about the condition, communication strategies to reduce criticism and negative affect, problem-solving techniques, and methods for expanding social support. A 2018 systematic review and meta-analysis concluded that "in early-phase psychosis, early intervention services were associated with superior outcomes compared with treatment as usual, which supports the need for funding and use of early intervention services in patients with early-phase psychosis" (Correll et al., 2018).

Primary, Secondary, and Tertiary Health Care

Primary health care services refer to the initial, entry-level services that one receives when accessing health care. In Canada, this level of care is generally provided by primary care providers (i.e., family physicians and nurse practitioners) and other general health care professionals. As the first point of contact for a health challenge, primary health care services are designed to provide an initial diagnosis and treatment and, ideally, will be able to resolve the problem without the need for further intervention. However, in many cases, primary health care services may be the start of a referral pathway to other services. When it comes to mental health care, primary care providers have limited time, and due to a lack of available specialists, can experience barriers to patient referral.

Another step in accessing health care consists of low-barrier services, that is, services that require little in the way of formal referral procedures. Low-barrier services are found to be important in facilitating access to care, particularly for those who may not otherwise receive them. For example, the availability of low-barrier services for people who are homeless and experiencing substance use challenges increases the likelihood that treatment will be utilized (Kerman et al., 2019). In Canada, various low-barrier services are often provided by non-governmental organizations (NGOs) and non-profit agencies. Such organizations often deliver important components of care to people with mental health and substance use challenges. A description of such an agency is provided later in this chapter.

Secondary health care comprises the services provided by specialists, such as outpatient treatment by psychiatrists and hospital care by teams of health care professionals. **Tertiary health care** includes specialized long-term treatment services, such as the ones provided in a residential mental health facility, as well as highly specialized care for rare, complex, or treatment-resistant conditions. Generally, tertiary services are delivered by teams with special expertise and staffing levels to meet the specific needs of their clientele. Assertive Community Treatment (ACT) is an example of tertiary mental health care that is widely used in Canada and many other countries. ACT provides intensive care to individuals living with severe mental illnesses in a community setting. The client-centred approach includes a multidisciplinary team to facilitate community living, psychosocial rehabilitation, and recovery for clients who have not benefitted from traditional outpatient programs due to their complex presentation. Historically, ACT success is measured by reducing hospitalizations, decreasing incarcerations, improving housing stability, decreasing psychiatric symptoms and substance use, and increasing medication use, engagement with services, and employment. The key "ingredients" for ACT include small, shared caseloads (maximum client-to-staff ratio of 10:1), individualized care, 24-hour crisis response, regular team meetings, a team approach, and no discharge policies.

Another example of tertiary health care services is residential treatment for substance use disorders. Residential treatment centres provide intensive individual and group therapy, psychosocial education, and 24-hour support from health care providers and centre staff in a live-in environment. While residential treatment may be beneficial for many individuals seeking treatment for problematic substance use, these centres are predominantly abstinence-based, meaning that any use of substances can lead to removal from the program—an approach that has been critiqued as contrary to a harm reduction philosophy (see Chapter 14). Additionally, residential treatment is largely private, which means it tends not to be covered under Canada's universal health care system, which may present an insurmountable challenge for many seeking treatment.

Virtual Services

The vast expansion of the internet and other digital technologies in the past decade has created unprecedented opportunities for virtual services to support individuals experiencing mental health challenges. Some virtual services connect people directly with a mental health care professional via videoconferencing, phone, or messaging platforms. These services build on technology that most of us already use and remove many of the barriers that may affect those seeking mental health care, including travel, limited service availability in rural and remote communities, or discomfort with in-person communication. Other virtual services are described as "asynchronous" and do not involve real-time communication with a health care provider. For example, the BounceBack online program was developed in partnership with the Canadian Mental Health Association (CMHA) to help adults and youth aged 15+ to cope with low mood, stress, anxiety, and mild to moderate symptoms of depression. The program offers 20 different workbooks, including "Changing Extreme and Unhelpful Thinking" and "Understanding Worry and Stress," and optionally integrates phone calls with a coach to support progress through the online workshops. While BounceBack and many other Canadian programs are based in research evidence, it is important to recognize that there are hundreds of online programs and smartphone apps that are not (Neary & Schueller, 2018), which can lead to potential harms or lack of treatment response. Additionally, virtual services may not be appropriate for managing symptoms of severe mental illness.

Use of Existing Treatment Services

Figure 15.3 provides information compiled by the Public Health Agency of Canada about the use of formal health services (i.e., those provided by the publicly funded services, such as primary care providers, psychiatrists, and hospitals) for mental illnesses in Canada across the lifespan. Note that for individuals 15 years of age and older, females use mental health services more frequently than males. You may remember the discussion in Chapter 7 describing that men generally experience greater challenges in requesting assistance when they experience mental health issues such as depression (Johnson et al., 2012; Oliffe et al., 2019). Many men also report that they view help-seeking behaviour as a "feminine" characteristic that exposes personal weakness and vulnerability (Chambers & Murphy, 2011; Cole & Ingram, 2020). Men often ignore or deny serious symptoms, may have limited knowledge about their bodies and health care, and consider it necessary to endure high degrees of pain and conceal mental health challenges (Clark et al., 2018).

In contrast, Figure 15.3 shows that males in the younger age groups are more likely than females to receive health services for mental health challenges. This is likely due, in part, to higher rates of various childhood mental health challenges, such as conduct disorder and attention deficit disorder, among boys (Public Health Agency of Canada, 2015).

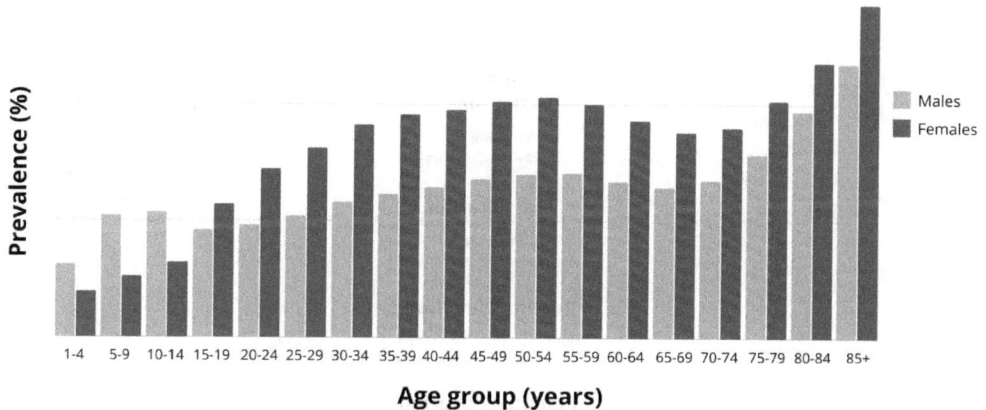

Figure 15.3: Age-specific annual prevalence (%) of the use of health services for mental illnesses among people aged one year and older by sex, Canada, 2009–10.

Source: Adapted from Public Health Agency of Canada. (2015). *Report from the Canadian chronic disease surveillance system: Mental Illness in Canada, 2015 (No. 140526)*. https://www.canada.ca/content/dam/canada/health-canada/migration/healthy-canadians/publications/diseases-conditions-maladies-affections/mental-illness-2015-maladies-mentales/alt/mental-illness-2015-maladies-mentales-eng.pdf

Services and Involvement of Patients, Peers, and Caregivers

It is widely accepted that people with lived experience of mental illnesses and their family members and caregivers should be involved in the development, planning, delivery, and evaluation of mental health services. There are many different forms of involvement for people with lived experiences. Peer interventions, for example, include self-help groups and peer-run organizations and services, either delivered alone or as a complement to clinical care. As discussed in Chapter 14, the general benefits of social and peer support, as well as the widespread availability, have led to recommendations for peer interventions as a complementary treatment for many mental health challenges, including depression (Parikh et al., 2016).

As noted by the Mental Health Commission of Canada, for Canadians living with mental health challenges, caregivers are critical to recovery. Caregivers are individuals who provide unpaid support and may be relatives (i.e., parents, adult children, partners, etc.) or other significant people drawn from broader circles. Yet, despite caregivers' pivotal role and important contributions, the effects of caregiving can take a toll. Provision of mental health support for caregivers *themselves* is also critical. The Mental Health Commission of Canada's (2013) *National Guidelines for a Comprehensive Service System to Support Family Caregivers of Adults with Mental Health Problems and Illnesses* identifies five levels of tasks for meeting the support needs of family caregivers (see Figure 15.4). While fewer families may require Levels 4 (Consultation) and 5 (Family Therapy), the Guidelines state that Levels 1

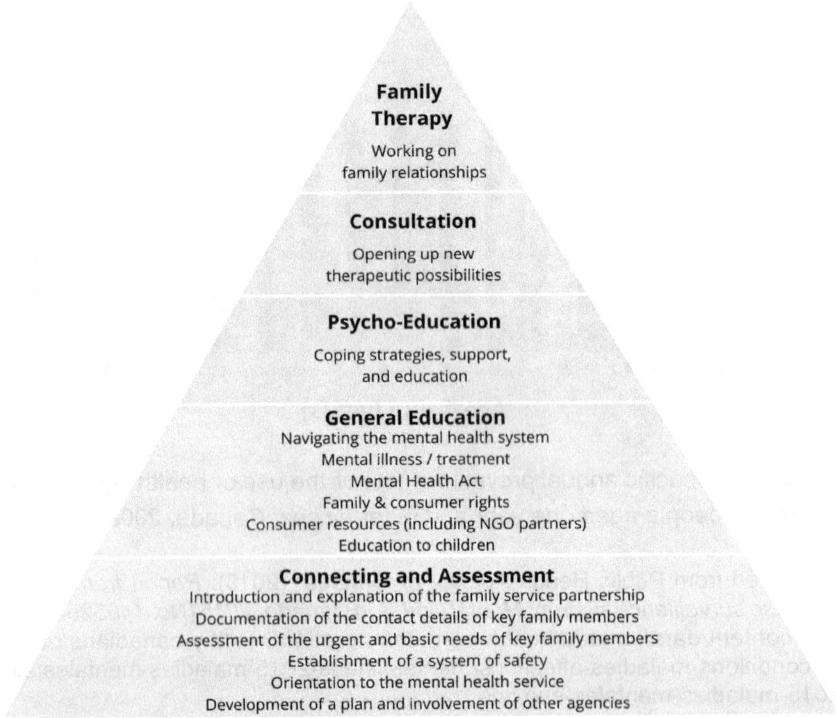

Figure 15.4: The pyramid of family care framework illustrates five levels of support needs for caregivers of people with mental health challenges.

Source: Adapted from MacCourt, P. (2013). *National guidelines for a comprehensive service system to support family caregivers of adults with mental health problems and illnesses.* Family Caregivers Advisory Committee, Mental Health Commission of Canada. https://www.mentalhealthcommission.ca/sites/default/files/Caregiving_MHCC_Family_Caregivers_Guidelines_ENG_0.pdf

(Connecting and Assessment) and 2 (General Education) should be reassessed at each point of contact with the mental health system to ensure that caregivers' support needs are being adequately met. Given the high levels of stress associated with caregiving, many caregivers are likely to require Level 3 (Psycho-Education) support, including assistance with developing and maintaining coping strategies.

Establishment of a Mental Health Strategy for Canada

The 2006 Canadian Senate Report *Out of the Shadows at Last* recommended the creation of the Mental Health Commission of Canada, noting that the

> whole complex, pervasive problem of mental illness and addiction in Canadian society continues to be neglected. The Canadian Mental Health Commission

will provide a much needed national (*not federal*) focal point that will keep mental health issues in the mainstream of public policy debates in Canada and accelerate the development and implementation of effective solutions to the long-standing problems of this sector. (Kirby & Keon, 2006)

The Mental Health Commission of Canada was subsequently established in 2008 to enable a national approach to mental health issues and serve as a catalyst for reforming mental health policies and improvements in service delivery. In keeping with the vision of mental health and wellness for all, the mission of the Mental Health Commission of Canada is to "raise awareness of the mental health and wellness needs of Canadians, and to catalyze collaborative solutions to mental health system challenges."

A significant achievement of the Mental Health Commission of Canada was development of the first mental health strategy for Canada: *Changing Directions, Changing Lives: The Mental Health Strategy for Canada*. The strategic directions of the strategy are reproduced in Box 15.2 and were developed alongside extensive public consultation across the country. Importantly, the strategy recognizes that all Canadians, and individuals with mental illnesses and their caregivers in particular, play a role in improving the mental health system as a whole. It also acknowledges that the mental health and well-being of individuals and communities is not the concern of the health sector alone. Rather, the policies and practices of many sectors (including education, corrections, social services, etc.) have a major impact on people's mental health. Additionally, workplaces, non-government organizations, the media, and many others all have a role to play in supporting mental health.

Box 15.1: Changing Directions, Changing Lives: The Mental Health Strategy for Canada

Drawing on the best available evidence and on input from thousands of people across Canada, *Changing Directions, Changing Lives* translates this vision into recommendations for action. The scope of the strategy is broad, and its recommendations are grouped into six key Strategic Directions. Each Strategic Direction focuses on one critical dimension, and together they combine to provide a comprehensive blueprint for change. The six Strategic Directions are as follows:

1. *Promote mental health across the lifespan in homes, schools, and workplaces, and prevent mental illness and suicide wherever possible.* Reducing the impact of mental health problems and illnesses and improving the mental health of the population require promotion and prevention efforts in everyday settings where the potential impact is greatest.

2. *Foster recovery and well-being for people of all ages living with mental health problems and illnesses and uphold their rights.* The key to recovery is helping people to find the right combination of services, treatments, and supports and eliminating discrimination by removing barriers to full participation in work, education, and community life.
3. *Provide access to the right combination of services, treatments, and supports, when and where people need them.* A full range of services, treatments and supports includes primary health care, community-based and specialized mental health services, peer support, and supported housing, education, and employment.
4. *Reduce disparities in risk factors and access to mental health services and strengthen the response to the needs of diverse communities and Northerners.* Mental health should be taken into account when acting to improve overall living conditions and addressing the specific needs of groups such as new Canadians and people in northern and remote communities.
5. *Work with First Nations, Inuit, and Métis to address their mental health needs, acknowledging their distinct circumstances, rights, and cultures.* By calling for access to a full continuum of culturally safe mental health services, the *Mental Health Strategy for Canada* can contribute to truth, reconciliation and healing from intergenerational trauma.
6. *Mobilize leadership, improve knowledge, and foster collaboration at all levels.* Change will not be possible without a whole-of-government approach to mental health policy, without fostering the leadership roles of people living with mental health problems and illnesses, and their families, and without building strong infrastructure to support data collection, research, and human resource development.

It will take time to implement the recommendations in this strategy, and it will take sustained commitment and leadership at many levels. The strategy calls for:

- people living with mental health problems and illnesses and their families to become more engaged in the planning, organization, delivery, and evaluation of mental health services, treatments, and supports
- mental health service providers to work with planners, funders, and users of the system to examine what changes are required in the way that they work in order to create a system that is better integrated around people's needs and fosters recovery
- governments to take a comprehensive approach to addressing mental health needs, to re-focus spending on improving outcomes, and to correct years of underfunding of mental health
- senior executives in both the public and private sectors to create workplaces that are as mentally healthy as possible, and to actively support the broader movement for improved mental health
- all Canadians to promote mental health in everyday settings and reduce stigma by recognizing how much we all have in common—there is no "us" and "them" when it comes to mental health and well-being.

Conclusion

The unique structure and organization of health services in Canada affects many features of service delivery. A consequence of the prominent role given to provinces and territories in governing health care is a system that varies across the country's 13 geographical jurisdictions, despite a number of common principles guided by the *Canada Health Act*.

Mental health services in Canada are delivered by a wide variety of health professionals and are ideally implemented using a stepped-care model that reserves costlier and more intensive services for those who require them. In addition to formal health care services delivered through hospitals and various community-based programs, many non-health care services and supports contribute to the recovery of people with mental health challenges. Services supplied with peer and caregiver support are also critical components of a comprehensive mental health system.

In Canada, the mental health sector has undergone a significant shift and finds itself at a critical crossroad, with mental health increasingly seen as a priority. The Mental Health Commission of Canada provides a national voice on mental health and serves as a catalyst for system and service delivery improvements.

Glossary

Canada Health Act: Federal legislation that stipulates key characteristics of the health care insurance coverage provided by Canada's provinces and territories.

iatrogenic: Negative outcomes as a result of medical or health care intervention.

primary health care: Initial, entry-level services that one receives when accessing health care, designed to provide an initial diagnosis and treatment, and may be the start of a referral pathway to other services.

secondary health care: Services provided by specialists who generally do not have first contact with patients, such as outpatient treatment by psychiatrists and hospital care by teams of health care professionals.

stepped-care approach: An approach where the system generally aims to provide low-intensity treatment for most people and will step up the intensity of treatments as needed.

tertiary health care: Specialized long-term treatment services, such as a long-stay mental health facility, including highly specialized treatment for rare, complex, or treatment-resistant conditions.

Critical Thinking Questions

1. Briefly describe each of the five principles of the *Canada Health Act*.
2. How is the Canadian health care system structured?

3. What is a stepped-care model, and why is it important to mental health services?
4. What role do peers and caregivers play in the delivery of mental health services?
5. Briefly describe the six strategic directions of the *Mental Health Strategy for Canada* developed by the Mental Health Commission of Canada. How do these strategic directions aim to improve the mental health of Canadians?

Recommended Readings

Cornish, P. (2020). *Stepped care 2.0: A paradigm shift in mental health.* Springer.
Fierlbeck, K. (2011). *Health care in Canada: A citizen's guide to policy and politics.* University of Toronto Press.
Marchildon, G. P. (2013). *Health systems in transition: Canada* (2nd ed.). University of Toronto Press.

Recommended Websites

BounceBack. www.bouncebackbc.ca
The Canadian Association for Health Services and Policy Research. www.cahspr.ca
Canadian Institute for Health Information. www.cihi.ca
Health Canada—Health Care System. www.canada.ca/en/health-canada/topics/health-care-systems.html
The Mental Health Commission of Canada. www.mentalhealthcommission.ca
World Health Organization—Health System Governance. www.who.int/health-topics/health-systems-governance

References

Angell, M. (2008). Privatizing health care is not the answer: Lessons from the United States. *Canadian Medical Association Journal, 179*(9), 916–919. https://doi.org/10.1503/cmaj.081177
Armstrong, P., Armstrong, H., & MacLeod, K. K. (2016). The threats of privatization to security in long-term residential care. *Ageing International, 41*, 99–116. https://doi.org/10.1007/s12126-015-9228-0
Babony, A. (2019). Privatization and the future of Canadian healthcare. *Global Health: Annual Review, 1*(4).
Canadian Institute for Health Information. (2021). *National health expenditure trends, 2020.* https://www.cihi.ca/sites/default/files/document/nhex-trends-2020-narrative-report-en.pdf
Chambers, D., & Murphy, F. (2011). *Learning to reach out: Young people, mental health literacy and the internet.* Inspire Ireland Foundation.

Clark, L. H., Hudson, J. L., Dunstan, D. A., & Clark, G. I. (2018). Barriers and facilitating factors to help-seeking for symptoms of clinical anxiety in adolescent males. *Australian Journal of Psychology, 70*(3), 225–234. https://doi.org/10.1111/ajpy.12191

Cole, B. P., & Ingram, P. B. (2020). Where do I turn for help? Gender role conflict, self-stigma, and college men's help-seeking for depression. *Psychology of Men & Masculinities, 21*(3), 441–452. https://doi.org/10.1037/men0000245

Correll, C. U., Galling, B., Pawar, A., Krivko, A., Bonetto, C., Ruggeri, M., Craig, T. J., Nordentoft, M., Srihari, V. H., Guloksuz, S., Hui, C. L. M., Chen, E. Y. H., Valencia, M., Juarez, F., Robinson, D. G., Schooler, N. R., Brunette, M. F., Mueser, K. T., Rosenheck, R. A., ... & Kane, J. M. (2018). Comparison of early intervention services vs treatment as usual for early-phase psychosis: A systematic review, meta-analysis, and meta-regression. *JAMA Psychiatry, 75*(6), 555–565. https://doi.org/10.1001/jamapsychiatry.2018.0623

Drake, R., Day, C., Picucci, R., Warburton, J., Larkin, W., Husain, N., Reeder, C., Wykes, T., & Marshall, M. (2014). A naturalistic, randomized, controlled trial combining cognitive remediation with cognitive-behavioural therapy after first-episode non-affective psychosis. *Psychological Medicine, 44*(9), 1889–1899. https://doi.org/10.1017/S0033291713002559

First Nations Health Authority. (2016). *2016/2017 FNHA summary service plan.* https://www.fnha.ca/Documents/FNHA-Summary-Service-Plan-2016-2017.pdf

Johnson, J. L., Oliffe, J. L., Kelly, M. T., Galdas, P., & Ogrodniczuk, J. S. (2012). Men's discourses of help-seeking in the context of depression. *Sociology of Health & Illness, 34*(3), 345–361. https://doi.org/10.1111/j.1467-9566.2011.01372.x

Kerman, N., Gran-Ruaz, S., Lawrence, M., & Sylvestre, J. (2019). Perceptions of service use among currently and formerly homeless adults with mental health problems. *Community Mental Health Journal, 55*, 777–783. https://doi.org/10.1007/s10597-019-00382-z

Kirby, M. J. L., & Keon, W. J. (2006). *Out of the shadows at last: Transforming mental health, mental illness and addiction services in Canada.* The Standing Senate Committee on Social Affairs, Science and Technology. https://parl.gc.ca/39/1/parlbus/commbus/senate/Com-e/SOCI-E/rep-e/pdf/rep02may06part1-e.pdf

Koyczan, S. (2010). We are more. *Vancouver Is Awesome.* www.vancouverisawesome.com/2010/02/12/shane-koyczans-we-are-more/

MacCourt P. (2013). *National guidelines for a comprehensive service system to support family caregivers of adults with mental health problems and illnesses.* Family Caregivers Advisory Committee, Mental Health Commission of Canada. https://www.mentalhealthcommission.ca/sites/default/files/Caregiving_MHCC_Family_Caregivers_Guidelines_ENG_0.pdf

Mental Health Commission of Canada. (2013). *National guidelines for a comprehensive service system to support family caregivers of adults with mental health problems and illnesses*. https://www.mentalhealthcommission.ca/wp-content/uploads/drupal/Caregiving_MHCC_Family_Caregivers_Guidelines_ENG_0.pdf

Mental Health Commission of Canada. (2016). *Mental Health Commission of Canada—Strategic Plan 2017–2022*. https://www.mentalhealthcommission.ca/English/who-we-are/annual-report/mhcc-strategic-plan-2017-2022

Minister of Justice. (2009). *Consolidation: Canada Health Act—Chapter C-6*. https://laws-lois.justice.gc.ca/PDF/C-6.pdf

Neary, M., & Schueller, S. M. (2018). State of the field of mental health apps. *Cognitive and Behavioral Practice, 25*(4), 531–537.

Olliffe, J. L., & Phillips, M. J. (2008). Men, depression and masculinities: A review and recommendations. *Journal of Men's Health, 5*(9), 194–202. https://doi.org/10.1016/j.cbpra.2018.01.002

Oliffe, J. L., Rossnagel, E., Seidler, Z. E., Kealy, D., Ogrodniczuk, J. S., & Rice, S. M. (2019). Men's depression and suicide. *Current Psychiatry Reports, 21*, Article 103. https://doi.org/10.1007/s11920-019-1088-y

Parikh, S. V., Quilty, L. C., Ravitz, P., Rosenbluth, M., Pavlova, B., Grigoriadis, S., Velyvis, V., Kennedy, S. H., Lam, R. W., MacQueen, G. M., Milev, R. V., Ravindran, A. V., Uher, R., & the CANMAT Depression Work Group. (2016). Canadian Network for Mood and Anxiety Treatments (CANMAT) 2016 clinical guidelines for the management of major depressive disorder: Section 2. Psychological treatments. *Canadian Journal of Psychiatry, 61*(9), 524–539. https://doi.org/10.1177%2F0706743716659418

Public Health Agency of Canada. (2015). *Report from the Canadian chronic disease surveillance system: Mental illness in Canada, 2015 (No. 140526)*. https://www.canada.ca/content/dam/canada/health-canada/migration/healthy-canadians/publications/diseases-conditions-maladies-affections/mental-illness-2015-maladies-mentales/alt/mental-illness-2015-maladies-mentales-eng.pdf

Richards, D. A., Bower, P., Pagel, C., Weaver, A., Utley, M., Cape, J., Pilling, S., Lovell, K., Gilbody, S., Leibowitz, J., Owens, L., Paxton, R., Hennessy, S., Simpson, A., Gallivan, S., Tomson, D., & Vasilakis, C. (2012). Delivering stepped care: An analysis of implementation in routine practice. *Implementation Science, 7*(3). https://doi.org/10.1186/1748-5908-7-3

van Straten, A., Hill, J., Richards, D. A., & Cuijpers, P. (2015). Stepped care treatment delivery for depression: A systematic review and meta-analysis. *Psychological Medicine, 45*(2), 231–246. https://doi.org/10.1017/S0033291714000701

Chapter 16

Canada's Role in Global Mental Health

Jill Murphy and Leena Chau

No one can say, with the image of the blue and green Earth floating in their heads, that others don't count as much as "we" do, that others don't hold the same status as we do, are not as significant as us, are ultimately just not as human as us.
—Roméo Dallaire (Canadian humanitarian, retired lieutenant-general, and senator)

Introduction

Canada is a multicultural nation with a diverse and dynamic population. Our country is shaped by this diversity, its global connections, and international outlook. Canada also has a rich history of leadership and investment in international development and global health research. The Government of Canada has collaborated with various other countries—particularly those classified as *low- and middle-income*—to promote investment and research in global health. Indeed, Canadian researchers have made substantial contributions in global health fields such as nutrition, HIV/AIDS, and infectious disease (Nixon et al., 2018). In the last decade, Canada has been at the forefront of the emerging field of **global mental health**, providing leadership in funding, research, capacity development, and international partnerships. Canada's engagement in global mental health enables us to contribute resources and knowledge about mental health around the world. Our country also benefits by learning from international innovation, which may ultimately improve the lives of our diverse populations.

In this chapter, we provide an overview of mental health in the global context, including addressing the significant gaps in mental health and mental health care in many of the world's nations. We then discuss key priorities in global mental health that aim to improve mental health promotion, prevention, and treatment. Finally, we present a series of case studies that illustrate Canada's role in global mental health in four core areas: funding, research, capacity development, and international policy. In doing so, we highlight how the knowledge and resources shared between Canada and many low- and middle-income countries has contributed benefits to mental health worldwide.

Mental Health in the Global Context

The global toll of mental ill health is profound, accounting for an estimated 13 percent of the global burden of disease (Vigo et al., 2016). Of the various mental illnesses, depression results in the most disability adjusted life years (DALYs) for both men and women, followed by anxiety and problematic drug and alcohol use (Rehm & Shield, 2019). While beliefs and understandings about mental illnesses vary across cultures, they are experienced in every part of the world (Kleinman, 1988; Murphy et al., 2018) and, often, with significant impacts to quality of life.

Despite the high global burden of mental illnesses, many of the world's populations lack access to evidence-based mental health care. In **low- and middle-income countries (LMICs)** (i.e., countries with less than $3,995 gross national income per person), these gaps in care are particularly acute. In these nations, an estimated 76–85 percent of people living with severe mental illnesses receive no treatment at all, compared to 35–50 percent in high-income countries (World Health Organization [WHO], 2013). Contributing to these challenges is a low level of investment in mental health by various national governments and overseas development agencies (Gilbert et al., 2015). Many countries are also faced with a shortage of **mental health human resources**—that is, health professionals and other personnel with mental health training, including psychiatrists, psychologists, and nurses (Kakuma et al., 2011).

Mental health has historically been neglected in the global health field. A particularly poignant example was its omission from the United Nations' 2000–2015 Millennium Development Goals. This oversight meant that mental health was not addressed through the many global development initiatives during this time, such as those that led to substantial deteriorations in child and maternal mortality and in HIV/AIDS. The exclusion of mental health from the global development agenda has been described by some as a moral failure (Kleinman, 2009). Fortunately, over the last decade or so, several advances have been achieved. The World Health Organization (WHO) established the mhGap program—now implemented in over 100 countries—to support the broad scale-up (i.e., expansion) of mental health care. The United Nations' Sustainable Development Goals now include mental health priorities and, in 2013, the WHO initiated the *Mental Health Action Plan*, which has since been renewed until 2030 (WHO, 2013). While there is still a long way to go in terms of meeting the mental health needs of our global populations, these and other initiatives offer hope and the investments needed to make advances.

Key Priorities in Global Mental Health

The overall mandate of the global mental health field is to improve mental health promotion, prevention, and treatment in low- and middle-income countries. Below, we identify and describe key priorities in the field.

Cross-Cultural Approaches to Mental Health

While mental health challenges and mental illnesses affect all cultures and populations, the *experience* of these conditions is often culturally bound—or shaped by local beliefs, practices, and norms. Understanding these variations in symptom manifestation and experience is fundamental to providing appropriate and effective mental health care (Gopalkrishnan, 2018). Indeed, a criticism of the global mental health field is that it has largely neglected the role of culture in its efforts to scale-up mental health care and related services (Summerfield et al., 2008). For example, historically, many of the mental health interventions that have been scaled-up in low- and middle-income countries have been developed in other—often Western—contexts. There is now growing understanding that efforts must be made to ensure that the interventions developed are valid and appropriate for the ways in which people in these settings understand and experience mental health and illness (Murphy et al., 2018).

Mental Health in Emergency Settings

At any given time, there are emergency situations and settings across the globe. Examples include areas affected by conflict—such as regions afflicted by war, genocide, and other armed combat. The current climate crisis has also led to an increase in emergency settings as a result of natural disasters such as hurricanes and typhoons, floods, wildfires, and extreme heat. The COVID-19 pandemic, which began in 2020, called attention to the widespread mental health impact of global health emergencies. In these settings and circumstances, there are often urgent and unmet mental health care needs (Charlson et al., 2019). Indeed, such circumstances and events have both immediate and long-term psychological effects, including post-traumatic stress, depression, anxiety, and substance use (Hayes et al., 2018). In these settings, vulnerable and marginalized communities, including Indigenous populations, children, people with disabilities, and seniors, experience compounded risk (Hayes et al., 2018). While emergency situations demand urgent access to mental health interventions, it is also critical for these to be integrated into existing services in local communities. This helps to ensure that the needs of people who experience long-term mental health consequences will continue to be met after the immediate emergency has resolved (Ventevogel et al., 2015). In areas where mental health systems are weak, emergencies may actually serve as an opportunity to bring awareness to existing gaps in order to "build back better"—that is, to strengthen mental health care delivery systems beyond what previously existed (Epping-Jordan et al., 2015).

Child and Youth Mental Health

Up to 90 percent of the world's children live in low- and middle-income countries. In these regions, mental, developmental, and intellectual disorders contribute to a significant proportion of the burden of disease, affecting between 20–30 percent of children and adolescents (Kieling et al., 2011). Anxiety and depression are among the most prevalent mental health conditions for children under 10 years of age (Patel, Kieling et al., 2013). Among adolescents, suicide is the third leading cause of death (Remschmidt & Belfer, 2005). A large proportion of adult mental illnesses originate earlier in life, with 50 percent emerging by age 14 (Bruha et al., 2018; Kessler et al., 2005). This means that prevention and early intervention for mental health challenges among children and youth in these regions is essential. Children living in the most vulnerable circumstances are particularly at risk, including those who are affected by conflict and disaster, those who are victims of exploitation and forced labour, and those living on the streets.

Access to mental health care for children and youth in low- and middle-income countries remains a significant challenge. Patel, Kieling, and colleagues (2013) identify three main barriers: (1) limited research evidence conducted in low- and

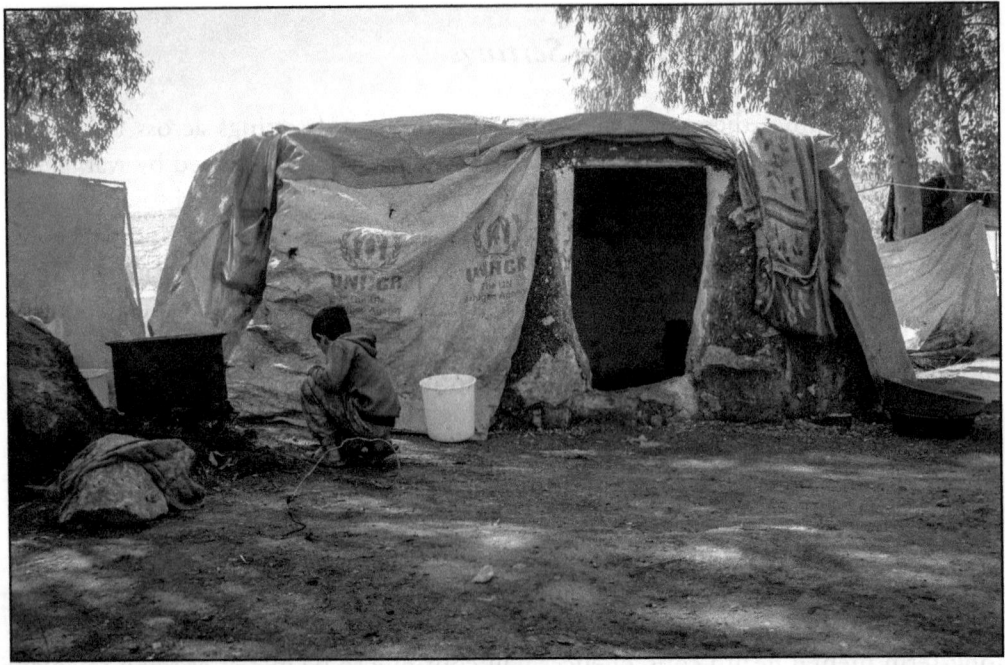

Figure 16.1: Children living in vulnerable circumstances—including those affected by conflict and disaster—are particularly at risk for mental health challenges.

Source: Pexels/Ahmed akacha

middle-income countries on child and youth mental health; (2) limitations of diagnostic measures for children's mental health, which may not be valid for use in certain cultural contexts and are often utilized infrequently (if at all); and (3) a shortage of skilled health human resources. Innovations to address these barriers are emerging, including promising approaches that integrate mental health services into routine health care and non–health care settings, such as schools. For example, Farm Radio, a Canadian non-profit organization, has been working in partnership with Canadian mental health researchers to implement a multi-pronged initiative

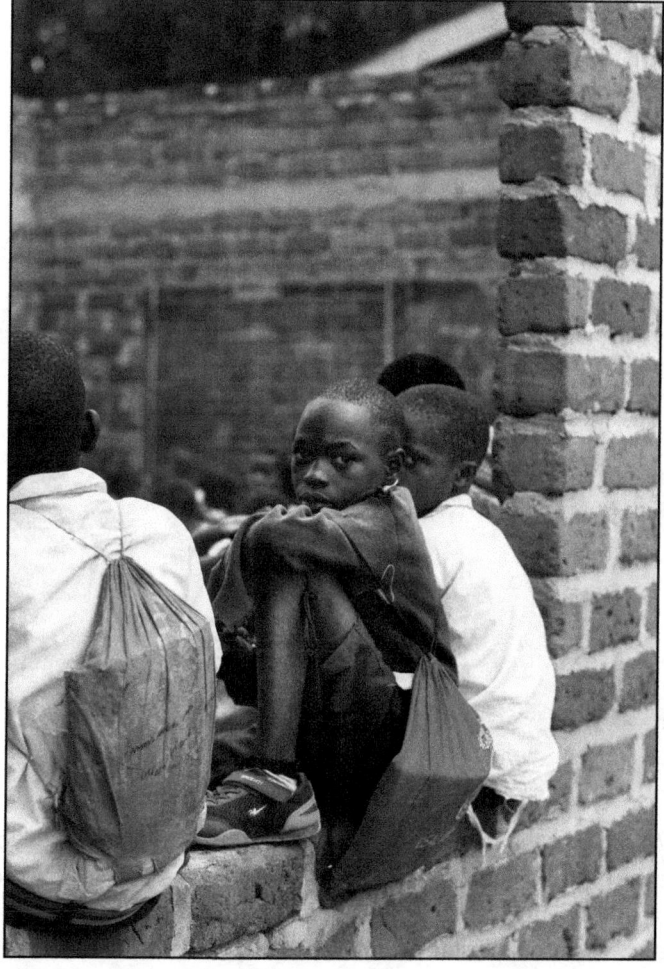

Figure 16.2: School children in Tanzania. A Canadian non-profit organization is currently working to implement a school-based mental health education program in Tanzania to address depression among adolescents.

Source: Unsplash/CLEMENT MABULA

to address adolescent depression in Malawi and Tanzania. The program includes school-based mental health education, radio-based awareness raising campaigns, and training of primary care providers. As attention to child and youth mental health in low- and middle-income countries increases, further steps will be taken to address this priority area of the global mental health field.

Integration of Mental Health into Primary Care and Community-Based Settings

Primary care is typically a person's first point of contact with the health care system and serves to integrate and direct the care provided by other providers, including mental health specialists. Indeed, the majority of people who seek treatment for mental health challenges do so from their primary care provider, who is often a family physician or nurse practitioner. However, many continue to encounter

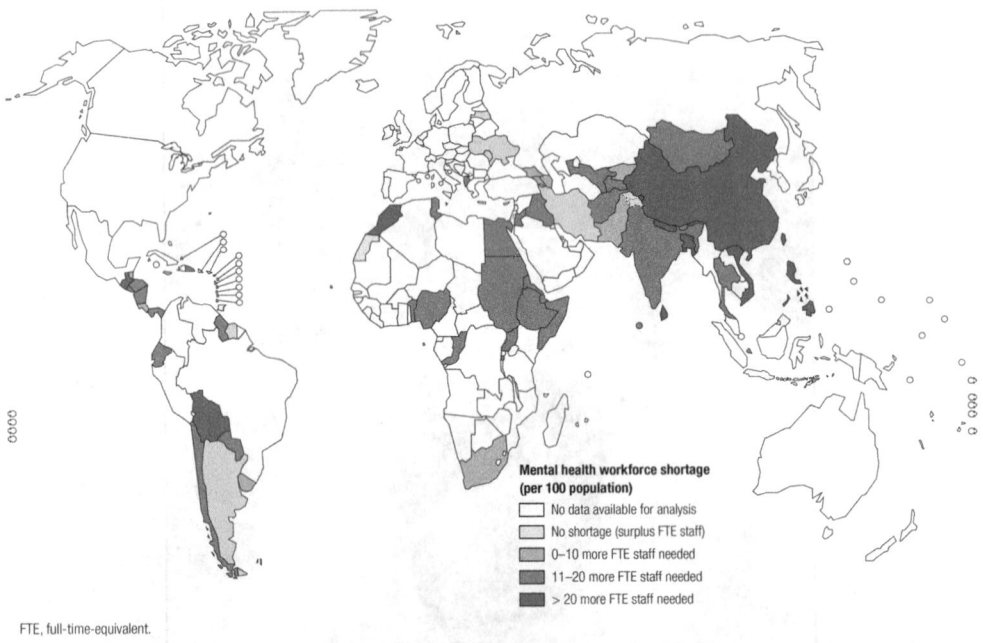

Figure 16.3: Within low- and middle-income countries, there is a critical shortage of mental health care professionals. This world map illustrates that all low-income countries and over half of middle-income countries have insufficient mental health human resources to deliver a core set of mental health interventions for priority challenges, including depression, schizophrenia, suicide, and problematic substance use.

Source: Bruckner, T. A., Scheffler, R. M., Shen, G., Yoon, J., Chisholm, D., Morris, J., Fulton, B. D., Dal Poz, M. R., & Saxena, S. (2011). The mental health workforce gap in low- and middle-income countries: A needs-based approach. *Bulletin of the World Health Organization, 89*(3), 184–194.

barriers to mental treatment in these settings, including long wait times and limited availability of mental health specialists (Goldner et al., 2011; Skosireva et al., 2014).

In low- and middle-income countries, mental health human resources are even more limited. For example, in research by Bruckner and colleagues (2011), it was identified that within the 58 low- and middle-income countries included in their study, an additional 362,000 health professionals were needed to fill the gaps in care. One strategy for increasing the mental health human resources available, particularly in low- and middle-income countries, is through **task-sharing**, where non-specialist providers, such as primary care practitioners or community health workers, deliver mental health care services (Patel et al., 2007). In fact, strengthening the primary health care system to better include the provision of mental health services is identified as key to addressing mental health care shortfalls. Primary care services and programs can effectively support people experiencing mild to moderate symptoms of mental illnesses (WHO and World Organization of Family Doctors, 2008). Moreover, it allows for care in the familiarity of one's environment, can empower communities to develop strategies that incorporate their unique values and needs, and supports links between services and institutions (Kirby & Keon, 2006). While many recognize that mental health care should be a core component of primary care (Patel, Belkin et al., 2013), further work is needed to support effective integration globally.

Box 16.1: Buena Semilla Project in Guatemala

Buena Semilla (Good Seed) is a community-based psychosocial intervention led by a researcher at McGill University in Montreal, Quebec. It is an example of task-sharing, where non-specialist providers deliver integrated mental health care to marginalized new mothers in Guatemala (Chomat et al., 2019). This innovation consists of group sessions involving education, various skill-developing activities (e.g., problem solving), cognitive behavioural therapy, and Indigenous practices. Sessions are delivered in the community and facilitated by trained women peers, traditional midwives, and community health workers. Among women who have participated in the sessions, 93 percent report improved self-esteem, and 89 percent identify improved emotional health and enhanced relationships with their children (Buena Semilla, 2019). Buena Semilla reflects a promising strategy to improve the mental well-being of new mothers in Guatemala and has reached nearly 30 communities to date.

Promotion and Prevention in Low- and Middle-Income Countries

To effectively reduce the global burden associated with mental illnesses, greater attention must be given to the full spectrum of mental health intervention, including promotion and prevention, in addition to treatment. **Mental health promotion**, which will be detailed further in Chapter 17, is the process of empowering individuals and communities to take control over their mental health, enhancing individual and community resilience, and promoting supportive social environments and policies (Barry et al., 2019; WHO, 1986). Mental health promotion strategies focus on activities targeting the social determinants of health, such as income, social status, and physical environments, to improve quality of life and maximize good mental health (Tol, 2015). Mental health promotion is often focused on initiatives at the community level to build strengths and capacity. In contrast, **prevention** is usually targeted towards risk factors for poor mental health, with the goal of avoiding or reducing the severity of mental illnesses (WHO, 2002). Prevention and treatment differ in that treatment is solely focused on helping people who have a diagnosed mental illness (Tol, 2015). Importantly, promotion and prevention are part of a spectrum of interventions that aim to achieve positive mental health outcomes and to reduce the incidence of mental ill health.

In recent years, there has been a growing emphasis on promotion and prevention in the global mental health context. A major advancement was when mental health promotion and prevention were added as priorities to the United Nations' Sustainable Development Goals. In recognition of the importance of promotion and prevention, the WHO included an objective in their 2013–2020 Global Action Plan for mental health that focused specifically on promotion and prevention strategies (WHO, 2013). In 2018, the Government of Canada's Health Minister, along with the United Kingdom's Secretary of State for Health and Social Care, and Australia's Minister for Health, co-founded the Alliance of Champions for Mental Health and Well-being with the aim of promoting positive mental health through collective action and leadership (Public Health Agency of Canada, 2018). The Government of Canada has reaffirmed its commitment to leadership in global mental health by promising to continue engaging with political leaders internationally to promote mental health and prevent mental ill health. Despite these advancements, further attention is needed to target the broader social determinants of mental health.

Technology and Digital Health

Given the gaps in accessible mental health care, globally, there are efforts underway to establish innovative treatment modalities to overcome existing barriers. With the increasing use of electronic devices such as computers and mobile phones worldwide, many countries are recognizing the potential for harnessing the capabilities and functionality of these technologies in the interdisciplinary field of **digital health**. In the context of mental health, digital health services can include the use of text messages, applications (apps), and videoconferencing to deliver services and supports ranging from education to psychotherapy (Stawarz et al., 2018). Digital health allows individuals, even those in remote communities, to readily receive care in their own setting. In doing so, it improves access, allows people to track and self-monitor symptoms and also helps to overcome barriers to treatment that often

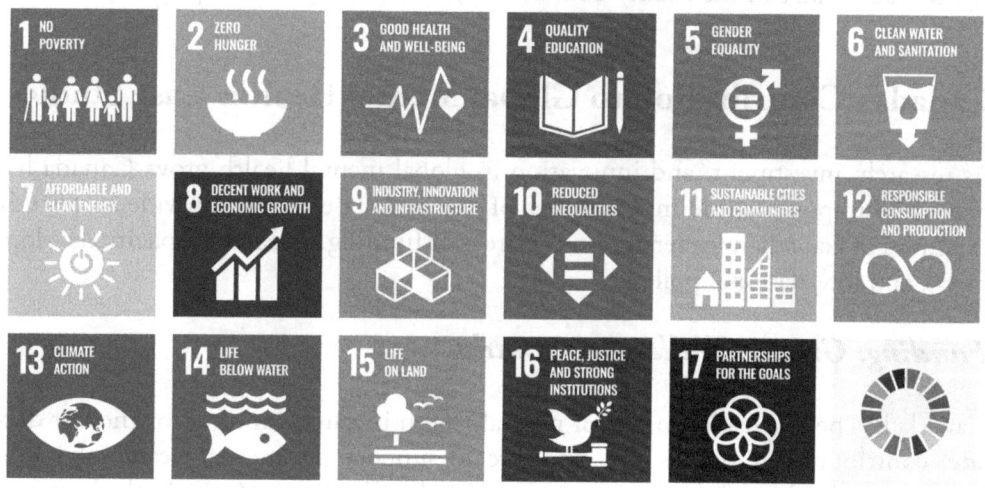

Figure 16.4: The United Nations' Sustainable Development Goals include mental health promotion and prevention as key global priorities.

Source: United Nations. (n.d.). *Sustainable development goals*. https://www.un.org/sustainable development/sustainable-development-goals/

stem from mental health stigma, which remains entrenched in many global contexts (Brian & Ben-Zeev, 2014; Van Ameringen et al., 2017). At the health systems level, digital health is cost-effective for depression (Massoudi et al., 2019), one of the most common mental illnesses—an important consideration, particularly in low- and middle-income countries where resources are extremely limited.

With the widespread use of smartphones, there has been a recent explosion in smartphone apps created for mental health. According to Aitken and Lyle (2015), there were 165,000 mobile health apps released in 2015 for Android and iOS platforms, with approximately 7 percent addressing mental health. These apps include functions that facilitate assessment, include journaling or mood-tracking, support symptom monitoring, and assist in treatment (Van Ameringen et al., 2017). An example is *Step-by-Step*, which is a technology-based self-help intervention for depression that utilizes behavioural activation, a cognitive behavioural therapy skill (Carswell et al., 2018). Users are guided through illustrated and informative narrative stories followed by interactive components where individuals practise the various skills they have been introduced to. Users are also provided guidance from "e-helpers"—non-specialist university graduates, through telephone, online messaging, or email. Further research is needed to build better understandings of the impacts of digital mental health resources—including whether they are effective as a standalone treatment or whether they are better when integrated into standard mental health care. Moreover, there are various challenges that remain underexplored, including network infrastructure access and quality, language and technology literacy, data confidentiality and security, and overall user acceptability.

Canada's Contribution to Global Mental Health: Case Studies

As research, investment, and innovation in global mental health grow, Canada has played an important role in a number of key areas. Below, we provide case study examples of Canadian leadership in the areas of funding, research, capacity development, and international policy.

Funding: Grand Challenges Canada

Canada has been a leader in global mental health research funding for the last decade, contributing resources and evidence to support the mental health of populations worldwide. While there are many funding bodies in Canada that support research addressing global mental health, Grand Challenges Canada has been at the forefront. Grand Challenges Canada is a national funding agency that includes a specific program for mental health research. This program has a mandate to fund innovations that can enhance the lives of vulnerable individuals and populations both in Canada and in low- and middle-income countries by improving treatment and access to care and by developing local capacity. Grand Challenges Canada (n.d.) advocates for *flipping the treatment gap*. That is, instead of only 10 percent of people with mental illnesses having access to care—as is the case currently—they aim for projects that would contribute to 90 percent (or more) of people being able to receive the care they need. From 2012 through 2017, Grand Challenges Canada's global mental health program invested over $42 million to fund 85 innovative research projects based in 31 different countries, most of which are low- and middle-income countries. An example of a highly successful Grand Challenges Canada-funded project is the Friendship Bench, a low-cost therapy using task-sharing approaches to alleviate symptoms of mental illnesses among individuals with HIV/AIDS in Zimbabwe (Chibanda, 2017). With support from the Zimbabwean Government, the Friendship Bench program can potentially expand to reach 14,000 individuals across primary care facilities nationwide. This and other projects have improved access to mental health treatment for nearly 160,000 individuals who experience mental illnesses around the world.

Research: Improving Mental Health in Vietnam

Strong research evidence is essential to the development and scale-up of evidence-based mental health care in low- and middle-income countries. An example of a Canadian contribution is the Mental Health in Adults & Children—Frugal Interventions

(MAC-FI) study, which seeks to enhance access to care for those experiencing depression in Vietnam. Indeed, like many people living in low- and middle-income countries, people living in Vietnam have very limited access to treatment for depression. Funded by Grand Challenges Canada, this randomized controlled trial examines the effectiveness of Supported-Self Management (SSM) for treating mild to moderate depression among adults in community-based settings across eight provinces of Vietnam. This low-cost intervention is based on principles of cognitive behavioural therapy and involves guiding users through a series of activities to address illness symptoms. This is combined with supportive coaching (i.e., frequent check-ins and goal setting with a lay health worker). Preliminary results suggest that the SSM intervention is effective, indicating the potential benefits of task-sharing for the treatment of depression in community-based settings. The team has since received funding for follow-up research to explore factors influencing the implementation and scale-up of the intervention to support sustainability. While these studies are based in Vietnam, they will contribute knowledge that can be used to inform the scale-up of similar mental health initiatives, globally.

Capacity Development: The Toronto Addis Ababa Psychiatry Project

One of the biggest contributors to the gaps in access to mental health care in low- and middle-income countries is the critical shortage of trained mental health professionals (Kakuma et al., 2011). To address this, there has been an emphasis in global mental health on task-sharing, as described above. However, to support the quality and sustainability of this approach, there remains a need for a trained mental health workforce who can provide support and supervision to non-specialist providers (Kemp et al., 2019). A Canadian partnership and capacity building initiative—the Toronto Addis Ababa Psychiatry Project (TAAPP)—is doing just this, through building psychiatric expertise in Ethiopia, with wide reaching implications.

Ethiopia is one of Africa's most populous and diverse countries, with over 109 million people speaking more than 80 different languages (Alem et al., 2010; World Bank, 2018). Though Ethiopia has seen substantial growth in economic and social indicators in the last two decades, 30 percent of the population live on less than US $2 per day (World Bank, 2018), and over 90 percent of people with severe mental illnesses lack access to care (Fekadu & Thornicroft, 2014). Indeed, there has been extremely limited mental health care expertise in the country and significant "brain drain" of those who have more advanced levels of education. In 2003, for example, there were only 11 psychiatrists for a population of 70 million (Alem et al., 2010).

Three of these psychiatrists were faculty members in the Addis Ababa University's Department of Psychiatry and recognized the need for a mental health training program based in and tailored to the context of Ethiopia. Connections between faculty at this university and the University of Toronto led to the development of TAAPP (Alem et al., 2010).

The project supports a three-year psychiatric training program that initially involved two Toronto faculty and one resident visiting Ethiopia for one month, three times a year, to teach and supervise the first Ethiopian psychiatric residents. Since its conception in 2003, TAAPP has helped graduate over 80 psychiatrists in Ethiopia; of these, 95 percent have chosen to remain in the country. Mental health services have since extended into eight general hospitals in Addis Ababa. TAAPP has produced an effective and workable framework for accelerating the training of medical specialists in Ethiopia and has been embraced as a model capacity building collaboration. TAAPP's impact is not limited to Ethiopia. Learnings from the partnership about the essential role of culture in psychiatric diagnosis and care has led the University of Toronto's Department of Psychiatry to expand its training in cultural competency and trans-cultural mental health.

International Policy: The APEC Digital Hub for Mental Health

Essential to improving mental health in a global context and promoting mental health equity (i.e., reducing unjust disparities in access to care between nations) is a commitment by policy makers—both nationally and internationally—to prioritize mental health. An initiative that is working to address this need in the Asia Pacific region is housed right here in Canada.

Asia Pacific is a diverse region that is home to 39 percent of the world's population. Though mental illnesses account for 20 percent of years lost to disability and 9.3 percent of disability adjusted life years (DALYs) in the region, less than half of these people have access to care (Ng, 2018). The Asia Pacific Economic Cooperation (APEC) is an intergovernmental organization dedicated to promoting development, trade, growth, and investment in the Asia Pacific region. APEC is made up of 21 member economies, ranging from high to low- and middle-income countries. In 2014, APEC recognized the critical importance of mental health to economic development. This led to the adoption of the APEC Roadmap to Promote Mental Wellness in a Healthy Asia Pacific (2014–2020; Asia Pacific Economic Cooperation, 2014). The Roadmap called for the creation of a Hub for best practices and innovation in mental health. A new 2021–2030 Roadmap was endorsed by APEC in 2021 and has renewed the mandate of the APEC Digital Hub for Mental Health.

In 2016, the APEC Digital Hub for Mental Health was created and is hosted in Canada as a partnership between the University of British Columbia, the University of Alberta, the Mood Disorders Society of Canada, and the Canadian Network for Mood and Anxiety Treatments. The Digital Hub is a coordinating centre for mental health in the Asia Pacific region. The Digital Hub has identified several priority foci under the 2021–2030 Roadmap, including child and youth mental health, integration with primary care, data metrics, Indigenous communities, workplace wellness, substance use disorders, disaster resilience, and suicide and self-harm. The activities of the Digital Hub include research, policy advocacy, capacity building, and international collaboration for the sharing of best practices. Though the Digital Hub is hosted in Canada, its leadership and membership are representative of the diverse Asia Pacific region.

Conclusion

Though it has been neglected until relatively recently, mental health has emerged as a global health priority. Through investment in funding, innovative research, capacity building initiatives, and leadership in international mental health policy, Canada has been at the forefront of this important field. Given Canada's diverse population and global ties, understanding mental health from a global perspective and investing in measures to improve mental health equity worldwide are imperative to our country. Canada also has much to learn and gain from the initiatives taking place around the world and from the collaborative partnerships that are fundamental to working in the global mental health arena.

Glossary

digital health: Use of text messages, applications (apps), videoconferencing, and other technologies to deliver services and supports, allowing individuals to readily receive care in their own setting.

global mental health (GMH): The contribution of funding, research, capacity development, and international partnerships related to mental health around the world.

low- and middle-income countries (LMICs): Countries with less than $3,995 gross national income per person.

mental health human resources: Health professionals and other personnel with mental health training, including psychiatrists, psychologists, and nurses.

mental health promotion: The process of empowering individuals and communities to take control over their mental health, enhancing individual and community resilience, and promoting supportive social environments and policy.

prevention: Targets risk factors for poor mental health with the goal of reducing the incidence and severity of mental illnesses.

task-sharing: A practice in which non-specialist providers, such as primary care practitioners or community health workers, deliver mental health care services.

Critical Thinking Questions

1. What are some of the barriers that limit good mental health in low- and middle-income countries?
2. Describe the rationale for integrating mental health care into primary care and community-based settings.
3. Define task-sharing as it relates to mental health care and describe some benefits and challenges with this practice.

4. Describe how international partnerships in global mental health can have positive impacts for the "provider" of knowledge and resources (i.e., Canada and other high-income countries).

Recommended Readings

Kohrt, B. A., & Mendenhall, E. (Eds). (2015). *Global mental health: Anthropological Perspectives.* Taylor & Francis.
Mills, C. (2014). *Decolonizing global mental health: The psychiatrization of the majority world.* Routledge.
Patel, V., Prince, M., Cohen, A., & Minas, H. (Eds). (2013). *Global mental health: Principles and practice.* Oxford University Press.

Recommended Websites

Doctors Without Borders—Mental Health. www.doctorswithoutborders.ca/mental-health
Farm Radio. https://farmradio.org
Grand Challenges Canada—Global Mental Health. www.grandchallenges.ca/programs/global-mental-health
World Health Organization—Mental Health Action Plan 2013–2030. www.who.int/initiatives/mental-health-action-plan-2013-2030
World Health Organization—Mental Health Gap Action Programme (mhGAP). www.who.int/teams/mental-health-and-substance-use/mental-health-gap-action-programme

References

Aitken, M., & Lyle, J. (2015). *Patient adoption of mHealth: Use, evidence and remaining barriers to mainstream acceptance.* IMS Institute for Health Informatics. https://www.iqvia.com/-/media/iqvia/pdfs/institute-reports/patient-adoption-of-mhealth.pdf
Alem, A., Pain, C., Araya, M., & Hodges, B. D. (2010). Co-creating a psychiatric resident program with Ethiopians, for Ethiopians, in Ethiopia: The Toronto Addis Ababa Psychiatry Project (TAAPP). *Academic Psychiatry, 34*(6), 424–432. https://doi.org/10.1176/appi.ap.34.6.424
Asia Pacific Economic Cooperation. (2014). *APEC roadmap to promote mental wellness in a healthy Asia Pacific (2014–2020).* https://mentalhealth.apec.org/sites/default/files/APEC_Roadmap_to_Promote_Mental_Wellness_in_a_Healthy_Asia_Pacific_2014-2020_1.pdf

Barry, M. M., Clarke, A. M., Petersen, I., & Jenkins, R. (Eds.). (2019). *Implementing mental health promotion* (2nd ed.). Springer.

Brian, R. M., & Ben-Zeev, D. (2014). Mobile health (mHealth) for mental health in Asia: Objectives, strategies, and limitations. *Asian Journal of Psychiatry, 10*, 96–100. https://doi.org/10.1016/j.ajp.2014.04.006

Bruckner, T. A., Scheffler, R. M., Shen, G., Yoon, J., Chisholm, D., Morris, J., Fulton, B. D., Dal Poz, M. R., & Saxena, S. (2011). The mental health workforce gap in low- and middle-income countries: A needs-based approach. *Bulletin of the World Health Organization, 89*(3), 184–194.

Bruha, L., Spyridou, V., Forth, G., & Ougrin, D. (2018). Global child and adolescent mental health: Challenges and advances. *London Journal of Primary Care, 10*(4), 108–109. https://doi.org/10.1080/17571472.2018.1484332

Buena Semilla. (2019). *Women's circles.* https://buena-semilla.org/womens-circles/

Carswell, K., Harper-Shehadeh, M., Watts, S., van't Hof, E., Abi Ramia, J., Heim, E., Wenger, A., & van Ommeren, M. (2018). Step-by-step: A new WHO digital mental health intervention for depression. *mHealth, 4*, 34–34. https://doi.org/10.21037/mhealth.2018.08.01

Charlson, F., van Ommeren, M., Flaxman, A., Cornett, J., Whiteford, H., & Saxena, S. (2019). New WHO prevalence estimates of mental disorders in conflict settings: A systematic review and meta-analysis. *The Lancet, 394*(10194), 240–248. https://doi.org/10.1016/S0140-6736(19)30934-1

Chibanda, D. (2017). Reducing the treatment gap for mental, neurological and substance use disorders in Africa: Lessons from the Friendship Bench in Zimbabwe. *Epidemiology and Psychiatric Sciences, 26*(4), 342–347. https://doi.org/10.1017/S2045796016001128

Chomat, A. M., Menchú, A. I., Andersson, N., Ramirez-Zea, M., Pedersen, D., Bleile, A., Letona, P., & Araya, R. (2019). Women's circles as a culturally safe psychosocial intervention in Guatemalan indigenous communities: A community-led pilot randomised trial. *BMC Women's Health, 19*(1), Article 53. https://doi.org/10.1186/s12905-019-0744-z

Epping-Jordan, J. E., van Ommeren, M., Ashour, H. N., Maramis, A. Marini, A., Mohanraj, A., Noori, A., Rizwan, H., Saeed, K., Silove, D., Suveendran, T., Urbina, L., Ventevogel, P., & Saxena, S. (2015). Beyond the crisis: Building back better mental health care in 10 emergency-affected areas using a longer-term perspective. *International Journal of Mental Health Systems, 9*, Article 15. https://doi.org/10.1186/s13033-015-0007-9

Fekadu, A., & Thornicroft, G. (2014). Global mental health: Perspectives from Ethiopia. *Global Health Action, 7*, Article 25447. https://doi.org/10.3402/gha.v7.25447

Gilbert, B. J., Patel, V., Farmer, P. E., & Lu, C. (2015). Assessing development assistance for mental health in developing countries: 2007–2013. *PLoS Medicine, 12*(6), e1001834.

Goldner, E. M., Jones, W., & Fang, M. L. (2011). Access to and waiting time for psychiatrist services in a Canadian urban area: A study in real time. *The Canadian Journal of Psychiatry, 56*(8), 474–480. https://doi.org/10.1177%2F070674371105600805

Gopalkrishnan, N. (2018). Cultural diversity and mental health: Considerations for policy and practice. *Frontiers in Public Health, 6*, Article 179. https://doi.org/10.3389/fpubh.2018.00179

Grand Challenges Canada. (n.d.). *Grand Challenges Canada: Global mental health*. https://www.grandchallenges.ca/programs/global-mental-health/

Hayes, K., Blashki, G., Wiseman, J., Burke S., & Reifels, L. (2018). Climate change and mental health: Risks, impacts and priority actions. *International Journal of Mental Health Systems, 12*, Article 28. https://doi.org/10.1186/s13033-018-0210-6

Kakuma, R., Minas, H., Ginneken, N., Dal Poz, M. R., Desiraju, K., Morris, J. E., Saxena, S., & Scheffler, R. M. (2011). Human resources for mental health care: Current situation and strategies for action. *The Lancet, 378*(9803), 1654–1663. https://doi.org/10.1016/S0140-6736(11)61093-3

Kemp, C. G., Petersen, I., Bhana, A., & Rao, D. (2019). Supervision of task-shared mental health care in low-resource settings: A commentary on programmatic experience. *Global Health: Science and Practice, 7*(2), 150–159. https://doi.org/10.9745/GHSP-D-18-00337

Kessler, R. C., Berglund, P., Demler, O., Jin, R., Merikangas, K. R., & Walters, E. E. (2005). Lifetime prevalence and age-of-onset distributions of DSM-IV disorders in the National Comorbidity Survey Replication. *Archives of General Psychiatry, 62*(6), 593–602. https://doi.org/10.1001/archpsyc.62.6.593

Kieling, C., Baker-Henningham, H., Belfer, M., Conti, G., Ertem, I., Omigbodun, O., Rohde, L. A., Srinath, S., Ulkuer, N., & Rahman, A. (2011). Child and adolescent mental health worldwide: Evidence for action. *The Lancet, 378*(9801), 1515–1525. https://doi.org/10.1016/S0140-6736(11)60827-1

Kirby, M. J. L., & Keon, W. J. (2006). *Out of the shadows at last: Transforming mental health, mental illness and addiction services in Canada*. Standing Senate Committee on Social Affairs, Science and Technology. http://www.parl.gc.ca/content/sen/committee/391/soci/rep/rep02may06-e.htm.

Kleinman, A. (1988). *Rethinking psychiatry: From cultural category to personal experience*. The Free Press.

Kleinman, A. (2009). Global mental health: A failure of humanity. *The Lancet, 374*(9690), 603–604. https://doi.org/10.1016/S0140-6736(09)61510-5

Massoudi, B., Holvast, F., Bockting, C. L. H., Burger, H., & Blanker, M. H. (2019). The effectiveness and cost-effectiveness of e-health interventions for depression and anxiety in primary care: A systematic review and meta-analysis. *Journal of Affective Disorders, 245*, 728–743. https://doi.org/10.1016/j.jad.2018.11.050

Murphy, J., Goldner, E. M., Corbett, K. K., Morrow, M., Nguyen, V. C., Linh, D. T., & Oanh, P. T. (2018). Conceptualizing depression in Vietnam: Primary health care providers' explanatory models of depression. *Transcultural Psychiatry, 55*(2), 219–241. https://doi.org/10.1177%2F1363461517748846

Ng, C. H. (2018). Mental health and integration in Asia Pacific. *BJPsych international, 15*(4), 76–79. https://doi.org/10.1192/bji.2017.28

Nixon, S. A., Lee, K., Bhutta, Z. A., Blanchard, J., Haddad, S., Hoffman, S. J., & Tugwell, P. (2018). Canada's global health role: Supporting equity and global citizenship as a middle power. *The Lancet, 391*(10131), 1736–1748. https://doi.org/10.1016/S0140-6736(18)30322-2

Patel, V., Araya, R., Chatterjee, S., Chisholm, D., Cohen, A., De Silva, M., Hosman, C., McGuire, H., Rojas, G., & van Ommeren, M. (2007). Treatment and prevention of mental disorders in low-income and middle-income countries. *The Lancet, 370*(9591), 991–1005. https://doi.org/10.1016/S0140-6736(07)61240-9

Patel, V., Belkin, G. S., Chockalingam, A., Cooper, J., Saxena, S., & Unutzer, J. (2013). Grand challenges: Integrating mental health services into priority health care platforms. *PloS Med, 10*(5): e1001448. https://doi.org/10.1371/journal.pmed.1001448

Patel, V., Kieling, C., Maulik, P. K., & Divan, G. (2013). Improving access to care for children with mental disorders: A global perspective. *Archives of Disease in Childhood, 98*(5), 323–327. http://dx.doi.org/10.1136/archdischild-2012-302079

Public Health Agency of Canada. (2018). *Government of Canada co-founds Alliance of Champions for Mental Health and Well-Being*. https://www.canada.ca/en/public-health/news/2018/05/government-of-canada-co-founds-alliance-of-champions-for-mental-health-and-wellbeing.html

Rehm, J., & Shield, K. D. (2019). Global burden of disease and the impact of mental and addictive disorders. *Current Psychiatry Reports, 21*, Article 10. https://doi.org/10.1007/s11920-019-0997-0

Remschmidt, H., & Belfer, M. (2005). Mental health care for children and adolescents worldwide: A review. *World Psychiatry: Official Journal of the World Psychiatric Association, 4*(3), 147–153.

Skosireva, A., O'Campo, P., Zerger, S., Chambers, C., Gapka, S., & Stergiopoulos, V. (2014). Different faces of discrimination: Perceived discrimination among homeless adults with mental illness in healthcare settings. *BMC Health Services Research, 14*, Article 376. https://doi.org/10.1186/1472-6963-14-376

Stawarz, K., Preist, C., Tallon, D., Wiles, N., & Coyle, D. (2018). User experience of cognitive behavioral therapy apps for depression: An analysis of app functionality and user reviews. *Journal of Medical Internet Research, 20*(6), e10120. https://doi.org/10.2196/10120

Summerfield, D. (2008). How scientifically valid is the knowledge base of global mental health. *BMJ, 336*(7651), 992–994. https://doi.org/10.1136/bmj.39513.441030.AD

Tol, W. A. (2015). Stemming the tide: Promoting mental health and preventing mental disorders in low- and middle-income countries. *Global Mental Health, 2*, e11. https://doi.org/10.1017/gmh.2015.9

United Nations. (n.d.). *Sustainable development goals.* https://www.un.org/sustainabledevelopment/sustainable-development-goals/

Van Ameringen, M., Turna, J., Khalesi, Z., Pullia, K., & Patterson, B. (2017). There is an app for that! The current state of mobile applications (apps) for DSM-5 obsessive-compulsive disorder, posttraumatic stress disorder, anxiety and mood disorders. *Depression & Anxiety, 34*(6), 526–539. https://doi.org/10.1002/da.22657

Ventevogel, P., van Ommeren, M., Schilperoord, M., & Saxena, S. (2015). Improving mental health care in humanitarian emergencies. *Bulletin of the World Health Organization, 93*(10), 666. https://doi.org/10.2471/BLT.15.156919

Vigo, D., Thornicroft, G., & Atun, R. (2016). Estimating the true global burden of mental illness. *The Lancet Psychiatry, 3*(2), 171–178. https://doi.org/10.1016/S2215-0366(15)00505-2

World Bank. (2018). *Ethiopia country profile.* https://databank.worldbank.org/views/reports/reportwidget.aspx?Report_Name=CountryProfile&Id=b450fd57&tbar=y&dd=y&inf=n&zm=n&country=ETH

World Health Organization. (1986). *Ottawa Charter for Health Promotion: 1st International Conference on Health Promotion.* https://www.who.int/teams/health-promotion/enhanced-wellbeing/first-global-conference

World Health Organization. (2002). *Prevention and promotion in mental health.* https://www.who.int/mental_health/media/en/545.pdf

World Health Organization. (2013). *Mental Health Action Plan 2013–2020.* https://www.who.int/publications/i/item/9789241506021

World Health Organization and World Organization of Family Doctors. (2008). *Integrating mental health care into primary care: A global perspective.* http://apps.who.int/iris/bitstream/handle/10665/43935/9789241563680_eng.pdf;jsessionid=6A162769074BB8A63CE48A7BB05D7803?sequence=1

Chapter 17

Population Perspectives on Mental Health and Substance Use

> Health care is vital to all of us some of the time, but public health is vital to all of us all the time.
>
> —C. Everett Koop (American Paediatric Surgeon and Public Health Administrator)

Introduction

In this chapter, we draw together many of the elements discussed throughout the book and address the question: "How can we improve the mental health of our populations?" This turns out to be a question of critical importance because good mental health is strongly associated with so many key characteristics that are desirable in human society: happiness, productivity, good physical health, and satisfaction with life. Indeed, it has been pointed out that there can be "no *health* without *mental health*" (Prince et al., 2007) because of the intricate relationship between mental and physical health and well-being.

In this chapter, we discuss opportunities to bring about meaningful improvements in mental health and we hope to inspire you to participate in actions that will enhance the mental health of our society. We begin the chapter by describing a population and public health approach and then discussing the application of this paradigm to mental health in Canada.

The Population and Public Health Paradigm

Within Canada, the field of **public health** (i.e., organized efforts aimed at keeping societies healthy and preventing disease and early death) has been combined with a more recent **population health** approach (i.e., coordinated initiatives aimed at enhancing the health of populations and minimizing inequities) to create the population and public health paradigm. Public health dates back many centuries and initially addressed sanitation conditions, including efforts to provide clean water, adequate waste control, and other measures to prevent and control the spread of infectious disease—measures that resulted in better health outcomes for populations. In modern times, one of the most significant contributions to public health has been the development of vaccines to prevent and virtually eradicate some of the deadliest infectious diseases that, in earlier times, ravaged human life. The public health approach emphasizes promotion of health and prevention of illness. A public health approach is now applied far more broadly and is just as important to mental health and substance use as it is to infectious disease.

The population health approach emphasizes social and structural determinants, such as income, education, and housing, as key factors influencing the health of populations (see Chapter 3). This paradigm brings attention to the social gradient in health; that is, the consistent finding that the health of populations is highly associated with socioeconomic status—those who are poor also tend to have poor health.

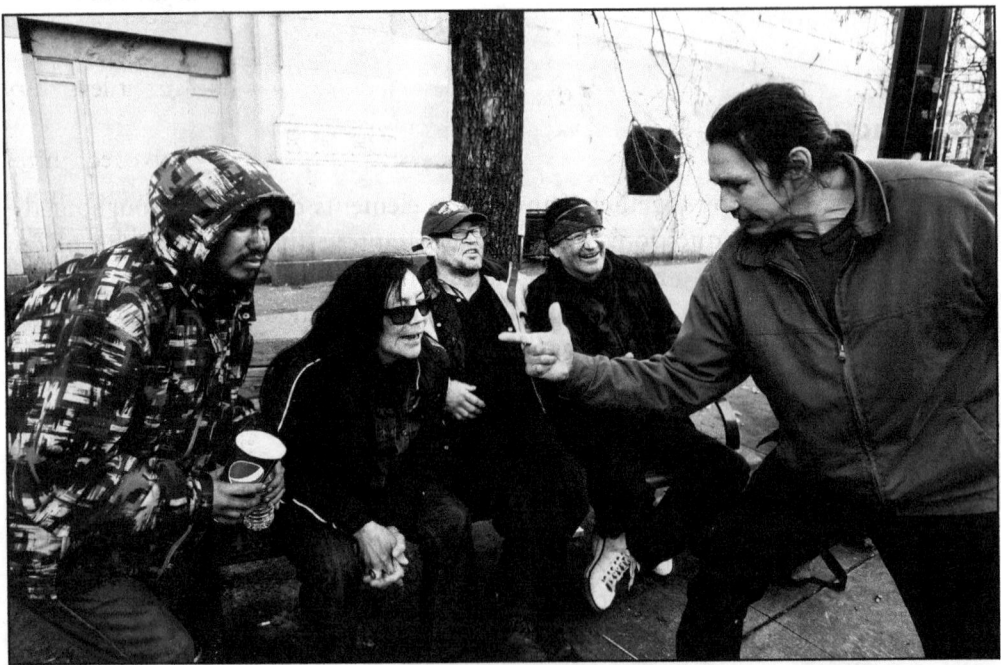

Figure 17.1: Socioeconomic status is one of the key social determinants of health. Vancouver's Downtown Eastside community is one of the most impoverished neighbourhoods in North America and many of its residents experience significant challenges to their mental and physical health.

Source: Chris Sang Yeob Park, Photographer

This is certainly true with regard to mental health. Although mental illnesses can affect all people, irrespective of their wealth, people who have low socioeconomic status or who lack access to the social and structural determinants of good health are far more likely to have mental health challenges at a population level (Meyer et al., 2014; Reiss, 2013).

The relationship between poverty and mental ill health is bi-directional. Those who live below the poverty line are likely to experience increased stresses and have fewer resources and supports, often leading to increased levels of anxiety, depression, and substance use. Conversely, people with mental health challenges often encounter barriers to employment, housing, and income security due to both disability and the resultant stigma and discrimination. Consequently, they are less likely to be able to escape poverty.

In combining the traditions of public and population health to create the population and public health paradigm, a number of principles have emerged as central features.

1. *An emphasis on health promotion.* This focuses efforts on resilience and capacity-building activities as well as efforts to redress issues of inequity to strengthen a population's resistance and diminish susceptibility to health challenges.
2. *An emphasis on illness prevention.* This principle centres attention on the benefits of stopping the development of illnesses before they start, or at least very early in their course.
3. *A focus on the population rather than the individual.* This perspective recognizes the importance of understanding the characteristics of populations (since a focus on individuals may "miss the big picture"), fostering actions that will benefit a large proportion of society.
4. *An effort to address health equity.* Social and structural determinants are recognized as key factors influencing the health of populations and an effort is made to improve the health of populations disproportionately impacted by the social gradient.

Historically, population and public health efforts have largely neglected mental health. However, an increasing awareness that positive mental health contributes to both individual and societal well-being has led to an increased emphasis on achieving improvements to mental health at a population level. One implication of this is heightened attention to the laws and public policies made by governments and society that will have a broad impact on the mental health of Canada's populations.

Laws and Public Policies Addressing Mental Health and Substance Use

Laws and public policies are developed and implemented to prevent harm, to promote health and safety of our populations, and to facilitate the smooth functioning of society. Laws are binding rules of conduct meant to enforce justice in society, carrying penalties for those who refuse or fail to obey. Public policies can be defined as the decisions or rules enacted by governments to solve particular issues and problems or to guide actions. Ultimately, laws and public policies seek to enact ideas about how to best address key issues we face and common goals we seek as a society. A good law or public policy can transform knowledge, values, and ideals into adopted practices and social structures that benefit many people. However, a bad law or public policy can lead to great harms. We empower governments and legislators to create laws and public policies that are in the best interests of our citizens. In democratic societies, complex electoral processes have been put in place to determine which political parties and leaders will be given the authority (and heavy responsibility) to steer public policy and enact legislation.

Canadian governments engage in a great deal of legislative and public policy efforts, including those directed towards health. Laws and public policies are often debated when complex health issues surface or manage to capture government or public interest. In the following sections, we discuss laws and public policies that relate to mental health and substance use in Canada, topics that are often surrounded by great controversy. We also describe efforts that focus on mental health promotion and mental illness prevention, as these are critical facets of a population and public health approach to improving mental health in Canada.

Mental Health Law and Public Policy

Laws, acts, and statutes that are relevant to mental health may govern key decisions about detainment and involuntary hospitalization, responsibility for criminal acts and incarceration, penalties for substance use, and other issues. They also direct certain actions of health professionals, police, judges, and others who may have a substantial impact on people who experience mental health challenges. In Chapter 13, we discussed the Mental Health Act, provincial legislation that stipulates how individuals who are thought to have a mental illness may be detained in hospital on an involuntary basis. Existing legislation also governs how people are treated when they commit criminal acts and their capacity for rational behaviour has been impaired by a mental illness (see Chapter 12).

A key issue is one of human rights. Particular care and attention is required to ensure that the rights of people with mental health challenges are upheld and respected. Some people with mental illnesses are vulnerable due to limitations in their capacity for decision making as a result of their condition and the stigma they face within society.

In addition to the laws that have been passed to define the rights of people with mental illnesses, there are many relevant public policies that influence the health and quality of life of people with mental health challenges and their families. The World

Health Organization (WHO) has highlighted the following three recommendations for policy related to the organization of mental health services: (1) deinstitutionalize mental health care; (2) integrate mental health into general health care; and (3) develop community mental health services (WHO, 2008). In addition to government policies that address the delivery of mental health services, there are many other essential policy issues that influence mental health. Public policy addressing social determinants of mental health, such as income, housing, education, and early childhood development, are of critical importance.

> **Box 17.1: Headlines Theatre's *after homelessness***
>
> Working to influence policy can be hard work, but not all of it needs to be tedious and boring. In 2009, Vancouver-based Theatre for Living (formerly Headlines Theatre) began its production of *after homelessness*, a show that featured actors who had personal experience with homelessness and mental illnesses. This production, like others produced by Theatre for Living, was crafted to influence policy. Unlike traditional theatre performances, *after homelessness* staged two shows every night. The first showcased the screenplay written by the participating actors, while the second allowed members of the audience to "interject" and join the stage to model how they would like to see the issues handled. This unique process allowed for collaboration between actors with lived experience, citizens, advocates, local government officials, health care professionals, and others to help shape strategies to address important issues. At the conclusion of the production, audience suggestions were compiled and presented to local officials to incorporate into future policy development.

Substance Use Laws and Public Policies

The most extreme substance use control policies are those of **prohibition**, in which the possession, selling, or marketing of a substance is criminalized—that is, made illegal. In Canada, heroin, opium, cocaine, amphetamines, and various other drugs are prohibited through the Controlled Drugs and Substances Act. This legislation includes maximum penalties for possession, trafficking, exportation, and production of different groups of drugs. However, prohibition has not achieved its intended goal of eliminating drug use; even when severe punishments are in place, the use of illegal drugs continues. Canada is one of a number of countries that attempted to prohibit alcohol use but later abandoned such efforts when this proved to be unsuccessful.

Box 17.2: Prohibition in Canada

In the early 20th century, most regions of Canada instituted prohibition, under which the use and sale of alcohol was illegal. To a large degree, prohibitionist policies were brought about through efforts to assert social control over racialized and Indigenous communities. However, prohibition of alcohol was short-lived in Canada, and most provinces repealed the legislation soon after it was initiated. In the United States, prohibition lasted for a longer period and was not repealed until 1933. What was the outcome of this experiment? Prohibition was intended to diminish alcohol use and, as a result, reduce crime, solve social problems, and improve the health of citizens. Instead, alcohol use became more popular under prohibition and created a huge black market for alcohol sales. Canada became the source of much of the alcohol smuggled into the United States and a thriving underground economy of booze smuggling became prominent. Most considered prohibition in North America to be a profound policy failure (Asbury, 2018). Despite acknowledgment of this policy failure, the prohibition of other currently illegal substances continues—with grave consequences. Indeed, as outlined by the Canadian Drug Policy Coalition, "Modern drug policies are based on prohibition … Although drug laws today have changed somewhat, they continue to disenfranchise and adversely affect the health and well-being of marginalized populations." Further, these policies contribute to fuelling the drug poisoning crisis, described as one of the worst public health crises Canada has faced in the past century.

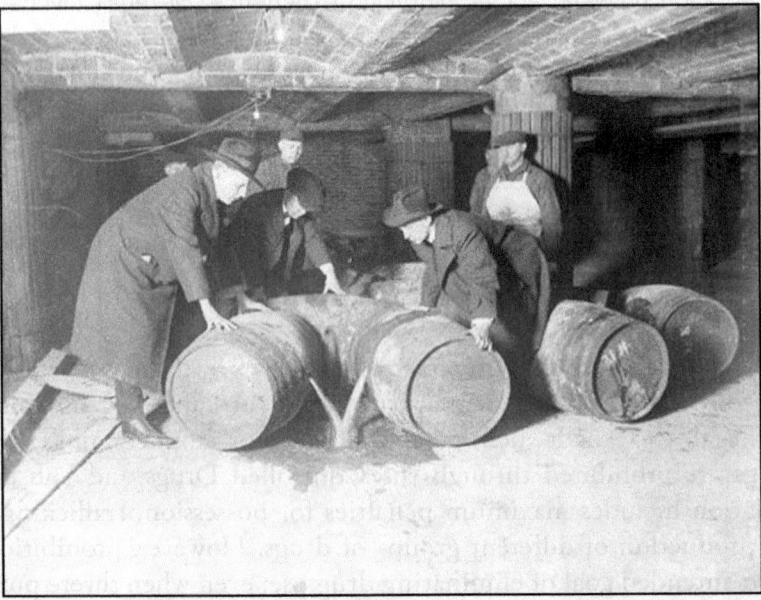

Figure 17.2: The prohibition of alcohol in the early 20th century was a short-lived policy in Canada; however, continued prohibition of a variety of other substances continues.

Source: United Church of Canada Archives

Currently, extreme control policies related to alcohol, such as prohibition, have been replaced with more moderate policies to diminish harms caused by alcohol use in Canada. These include limits on the minimum age for the purchase and consumption of alcohol, laws governing alcohol use and operation of motor vehicles, restrictions on the hours during which alcohol can be sold, and liquor taxes. There is now very good scientific evidence showing that such policy and legislation is effective at diminishing alcohol-related harms (Benny et al., 2019; Giesbrecht et al., 2013). Among the most successful targeted interventions are deterrence-based policies directed at drinking and driving. The imposition of blood alcohol concentration limits for drivers, strongly enforced through highly visible sobriety checkpoints and breath testing by police, can have a sustained effect on reducing alcohol-related motor vehicle accidents, injuries, and deaths (Blais et al., 2015).

The policies that have been enacted to address substance use vary dramatically around the world. In some countries, use of certain substances is prohibited under criminal law and draws serious punishment. In others, use of these substances may be tolerated or accepted. The degree to which control policies are adopted in a country is often related to its type of government (e.g., countries with authoritarian governments are more likely to impose strict and extreme prohibitory policies, laws, and practices).

A useful classification of substance use policies makes use of the notion that there is both a demand for and a supply of drugs. **Supply reduction** efforts are those that aim to decrease the availability of drugs through means such as seizures of illegal drug shipments and arrest and prosecution of drug suppliers. **Demand reduction** refers to efforts to reduce the desire and preparedness to obtain and use drugs by potential consumers, including education, prevention, treatment programming, and social pressures and deterrents.

Cannabis is one of the most widely used substances in Canada, and debate about laws and policies to address the use of cannabis has been prominent. Many health care providers, policy makers, and government officials long advocated for the legalization of adult cannabis use along the lines of tobacco and alcohol, arguing that its status as an illegal drug caused more harm to Canadian citizens (through criminalization and black market trade) than access to the drug itself. In 2018, Canada became the second country (after Uruguay) to legalize non-medicinal cannabis possession and use, with the public health goals of minimizing use among youth and reducing criminality associated with illegal cannabis market. How have rates of cannabis use changed since legalization? The short answer is very little. Despite fears that legalization would lead to increased use among young people, rates of recent cannabis use (within the past three months) have actually decreased among 15- to 17-year-olds, from 19.8 percent to 10.4 percent (Rotermann, 2020). Past three-month use of cannabis increased slightly for Canadians 25 years and older (13.1 percent to 15.5 percent), but the proportion of the population that uses cannabis daily has remained consistent.

Box 17.3: Vancouver's Insite Program

The Downtown Eastside of Vancouver is home to high rates of substance use. Some of the consequences include significant infectious disease transmission (e.g., it is estimated that most people who live in Vancouver's Downtown Eastside and use drugs have been infected with the hepatitis C virus), overdose and death, and drug-related crime. Among residents of this neighbourhood, violence, poverty, homelessness, and mental health challenges are widespread and people living in this neighbourhood experience considerable stigma, discrimination, and other forms of structural violence. However, these challenges are accompanied by a strong sense of community and mutual support. Insite, Vancouver's supervised injection site, is a service that operates within the Downtown Eastside, providing clean needles, syringes, water, and other items needed to inject drugs, and nurses who are available to help monitor and intervene in emergencies, such as overdose. This service, which is provided free to people who meet certain criteria, has been operating since 2003, despite being highly controversial and politically inflammatory. It operates through a constitutional exception to the *Controlled Drugs and Substances Act*. Canada's federal Minister of Health previously refused to renew the program's exemption, which would have forced its closure, but this decision was overturned by a Supreme Court of Canada, ruling that application of the act would be unconstitutional. Hence, Insite has been permitted to continue its operations.

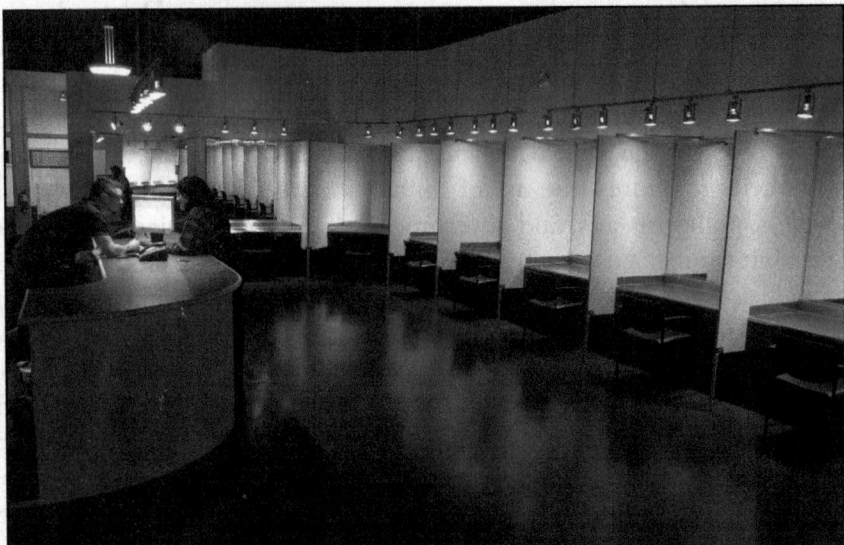

Figure 17.3: Inside the injection room at Insite—Vancouver's supervised injection site.

Source: Vancouver Coastal Health

Harm reduction policies, as discussed in Chapter 5, aim to reduce the harms that can result from drug use. The federal government provides funding to support harm reduction programs across the country and affords exemptions to the *Controlled Drugs and Substance Act* for particular harm reduction programs, such as overdose prevention sites. However, harm reduction policies are largely determined at the provincial government level, resulting in considerable disparities in access to harm reduction services across jurisdictions (Hyshka et al., 2017). Harm reduction policies and programs have been implemented to address the potential risks associated with both injection and non-injection drug use. For example, needle exchange programs are a common harm reduction strategy used to reduce the spread of communicable disease resulting from shared injection equipment. Encouragement of the use of vaporizers for cannabis and free ride programs for people who have been drinking are examples of harm reduction activities focused on minimizing the harms of non-injection drug use.

Mental Health Promotion

Efforts to bring attention to the importance of mental health promotion have become more prominent in recent years, particularly as the COVID-19 pandemic has contributed to a deterioration in population mental health and illustrated the profound mental health inequities experienced by certain subgroups of society. Mental health promotion follows the general tenants of health promotion, recognizing that opportunities to build strong foundations for good health can be sound investments, resulting in less illness and a healthier society in the long term. Mental health promotion is focused on strengths—as opposed to deficits—and represents an evidence-based approach to enhancing positive mental health for *all* people, including those experiencing mental health challenges or "risk." It comprises initiatives to strengthen individuals and communities and to mitigate structural barriers (e.g., poverty, discrimination, racism). Through these efforts, populations build competencies and resources to improve their mental health and well-being. Mental health promotion is described as "upstream" as it aims to alter the "causes of causes" or the social and structural determinants of mental health.

Leveraging the need for action on mental health in the context of the COVID-19 pandemic, the International Union for Health Promotion and Education released a Position Paper in 2021—*Critical Actions for Mental Health Promotion*—advocating for countries globally to adopt a population and public health approach to mental health, inclusive of mental health promotion. In this paper, eight evidence-based priority areas for mental health promotion are presented: (1) promote infant and maternal mental health, (2) cultivate child and adolescent mental health and well-being, (3) implement parenting and family strengthening programs, (4) support mentally healthy workplaces, (5) initiate community empowerment programs, (6) incorporate mental health promotion within health services, (7) enhance public awareness of ways of promoting positive mental health and reducing stigma associated with mental ill health, and (8) adopt a "mental health in all policies" approach. Examples of mental health promotion activities mentioned earlier in this text include programming geared to building empathy in schoolchildren through regular contact with infants (Chapter 9) and programs that pair older adults with children to foster well-being (Chapter 10).

8 Priority Areas for Mental Health Promotion

- **Promote infant and maternal mental health** through integrating a focus on social and emotional development and positive mental health into early child development services including prenatal care, home visiting, and parenting programs.
- **Cultivate child and adolescent mental health and well-being** through school education initiatives and whole-school approaches, including social and emotional learning programmes in preschool, school, and youth settings.
- **Implement parenting and family strengthening programmes** that promote the emotional and behavioural functioning of school-going children and their parents.
- **Support mentally healthy workplaces** by integrating mental health promotion into workplace health and safety policies and practices, including organizational change.
- **Initiate community empowerment programs** (e.g., community participation, volunteering, youth action, community microfinance and debt management paired with life skills training, and violence prevention/promotion of healthy relationships) to enhance social capital and environments that promote mental health and well-being across the life course.
- **Incorporate mental health promotion within health services** through a focus on service users' mental health and well-being as part of routine primary health care and mental health services.
- **Enhance public awareness of ways of promoting positive mental health and reducing stigma associated with mental ill health** through mental health literacy programming, campaigns, and local community actions.
- **Adopt a "mental health in all policies" approach** to promote multi- and inter-sectoral policies and actions that create supportive environments for mental health and enhance equity and social justice.

Figure 17.4: There is a growing evidence-base informing mental health promotion. The International Union for Health Promotion and Education has identified eight priority areas for action.

Source: Adapted from International Union for Health Promotion and Education. (2021). *Critical actions for mental health promotion.* https://www.iuhpe.org/images/IUHPE/Advocacy/IUHPE_Mental-Health_PositionStatement.pdf

> **Box 17.4: Physical Activity as Mental Health Promotion**
>
> Physical activity is one of the most effective mental health promotion activities a person can do. Regular physical activity—whether it is yoga, hockey, swimming, cycling, hiking, or some other activity—has been found to reduce stress, anxiety, and depression and bring about many mental health benefits. Various explanations have been proposed, including neurotransmitter release, elevated blood flow to the brain, release and distraction from unpleasant thoughts or preoccupations, and increased social contact. Although it is recommended that Canadians should engage in at least 150 minutes per week of moderate-to-vigorous physical activity, accumulated in bouts lasting at least 10 minutes, only a small proportion of Canadians do so. A Statistics Canada survey found that only 15 percent of adults (17 percent of men and 14 percent of women) meet that minimum—most of us are far too sedentary. How about you? Do you meet this minimum recommended standard? If not, see if there are ways that you could fit in some type of regular physical activity every week. It will improve both your physical and mental health!

As discussed in Chapter 9, Peterson and Seligman (2004) identified six main groups of core virtues that are consistently valued across cultures and across time: wisdom, courage, humanity, justice, temperance, and transcendence. Though Peterson and Seligman's virtues emerged as part of a new field of positive psychology, the shift in the mental health field to a focus on strengths has occurred in other clinical disciplines, such as social work and nursing. It is consistent with a population and public health paradigm in which efforts work towards the development of resistance and resilience, building long-standing capacity for protection against key risk factors. Resistance refers to the ability of individuals (or communities) to withstand very stressful events or ongoing stressful situations. Resilience refers to the ability of these individuals or populations to rebound from very stressful events.

The term "mental capital" has been used to refer to "a person's cognitive and emotional resources. It includes their cognitive ability, how flexible and efficient they are at learning, and their 'emotional intelligence,' such as their social skills and resilience in the face of stress. It therefore conditions how well an individual is able to contribute effectively to society, and also to experience a high personal quality of life" (Foresight Mental Capital and Well-being Project, 2008). Use of the word "capital" is used to denote a similarity with financial assets, which can either be squandered or invested wisely. Beyond this individual notion of mental capital, researchers and advocates are now encouraging governments to finance population level mental capital through "well-being budgets." Such investments would "put well-being at the centre of economic and fiscal policies" (National Collaborating Centre for Healthy Public Policy, 2021), and move beyond Gross Domestic Product (a measure of economic growth and welfare) as a way to propel health, social, and economic recovery post-pandemic.

Prevention of Mental Health and Substance Use Challenges

Efforts to prevent mental health and substance use challenges aim at reducing their incidence, prevalence, and recurrence as well as associated harms. Some preventive strategies focus on addressing physiological risk factors for developing mental illnesses. For example, the use of folic acid supplements (also known as "vitamin B9") by women who are planning to become pregnant can prevent problems in fetal brain development. Consequently, the Government of Canada recommends that all women who could become pregnant take a multivitamin daily that contains 0.4 mg of folic acid and continue to do so throughout their entire pregnancy (Government of Canada, 2018). The addition of iodine to table salt in many countries (including Canada) has effectively prevented iodine deficiency, the leading preventable cause of developmental disability (Vanderpas & Moreno-Reyes, 2017). Prevention and early treatment of infectious diseases, such as syphilis, has greatly reduced neuro-psychiatric conditions that were once much more common (Willeford & Bachmann, 2016).

Effective prevention of mental illnesses has also been accomplished by fostering changes in behaviour through laws and policies and by introducing education and social programming in schools and other venues. For example, laws requiring the wearing of seat belts and helmets have decreased brain injuries (Mbarga et al., 2018; Sethi et al., 2015), and school-based mental health interventions—including mindfulness and cognitive behavioural therapy programs as well as anti-bullying initiatives—have been found to be effective at decreasing anxiety, depression, and other mental health challenges (Šouláková et al., 2019).

Prevention strategies have been classified according to the group of people being targeted. **Universal prevention** strategies aim to impact entire populations; for example, a school-based program that is designed for all students and provides information about substance use and how to minimize harms. **Selective prevention** targets subgroups of the population whose risk of developing a mental illness is significantly higher than average. Higher risk may be determined on the basis of a variety of factors, such as family history, socioeconomic status, age, or exposure to trauma. An example of selective prevention would be a program that aims to prevent the development of depression and other mental health challenges in children who have experienced family violence. **Indicated prevention** strategies are those targeted at high-risk individuals who do not meet diagnostic criteria for a mental illness or substance use disorder but are identified as having minimal but detectable signs or symptoms. For example, the Fast Track program was developed to help young children at risk for anti-social behaviour and includes a classroom-wide educational component, social skills training, tutoring, and parenting and home training (Conduct Problems Prevention Research Group, 2020).

Table 17.1 lists examples of various risk factors and protective factors that are relevant to the prevention of mental illnesses and substance use disorders.

Table 17.1: Risk factors and protective factors for mental health and substance use challenges

Risk Factors	Protective Factors
Maternal malnutrition during pregnancy	Social and conflict management skills
Child abuse and neglect	Adaptability
Chronic pain	Self-esteem
Academic failure	Skills for life
Elder abuse	Literacy
Excessive substance use	Good parenting
Loneliness	Exercise
Low social class	Feelings of security
Low birth weight	Feelings of mastery and control
Poor work skills and habits	Positive parent-child interaction
Social incompetence	Socio-emotional growth
Stressful life events	Stress management
Emotional immaturity	Social support of family and friends
Family conflict	Early cognitive stimulation
Medical illness	Stable housing
Personal loss—bereavement	Good quality education
Reading disabilities	Positive relationships with peers

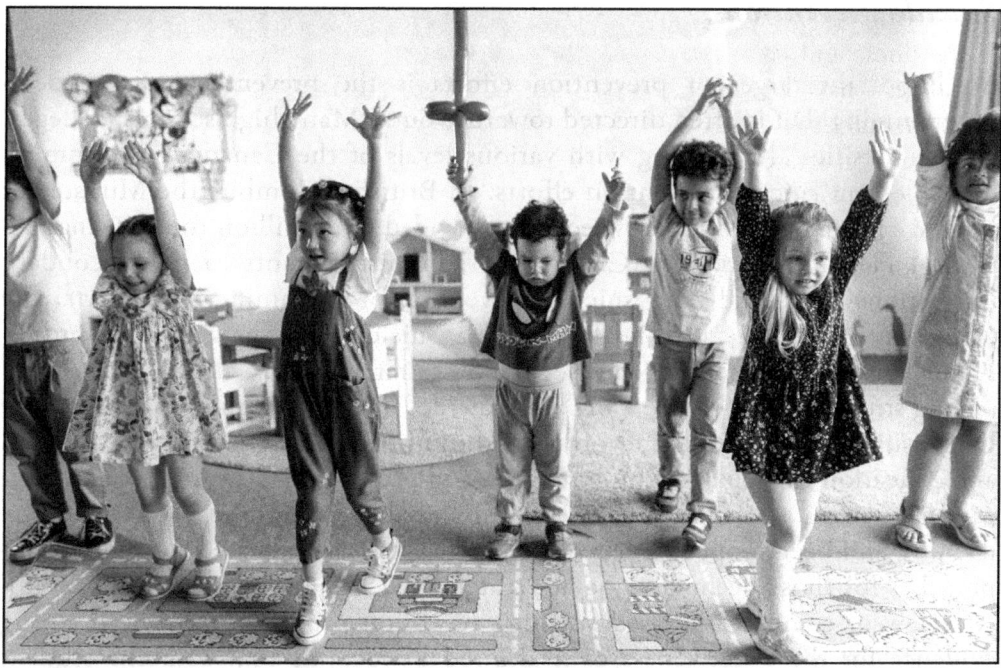

Figure 17.5: Early in human life, there is great opportunity to shape health and social outcomes throughout the life course. At the community level, it is crucial to invest in early childhood education and to support children and their parents and caregivers through addressing the social determinants of mental health.

Source: Pexels/Pavel Danilyuk

Although efforts to promote good mental health and to prevent mental illnesses and substance use disorders are valuable at *all* stages of life, it is particularly important to implement policies and strategies aimed at helping children and youth. Early in human life, there is great opportunity to shape the course for the lifetime. An important value for our society calls on us to recognize the importance of the mental health and well-being of our children and youth and invest great efforts in support of parenting, education, and policies that protect children against poverty, homelessness, and other negative experiences that increase risk for adverse mental health outcomes.

In Chapter 9, we discussed the many pressures faced by teens and the potential for these challenges to result in negative mental health impacts, including depression, problematic substance use, and suicidal thoughts. Indeed, given that adolescence is a stage of development during which many mental health challenges first arise, it is an opportune time for prevention efforts. The provision of supports to adolescents and their families can help them effectively traverse this period and build capacity to cope well with stressors. There are many other opportunities for the prevention of mental illnesses that can contribute to better lives for our younger generations.

Suicide Prevention

An important target of prevention efforts is the prevention of suicide—programming that is often directed towards youth. Many high schools, colleges, and universities are working with various levels of the Canadian government to implement suicide prevention efforts. In British Columbia, the Ministry of Mental Health and Addictions recently provided $1.3 million to the Canadian Mental Health Association (CMHA) to administer grants to post-secondary institutions to expand their suicide prevention programming. In Alberta, the University of Calgary (2021) developed a Suicide Awareness and Prevention Framework, which focuses on seven key strategies for suicide prevention among students, with the goal of "zero suicide." Most programs—including the University of Calgary's Framework—tend to utilize a combination of awareness and education curricula, training referral, and peer support. Awareness and education curricula are usually delivered as universal interventions, whereas referral training and peer support are designed as selected or indicated prevention approaches for those deemed to be at greater risk (Wolitzky-Taylor et al., 2018). A review of community-based suicide prevention programs has found strong evidence for the effectiveness of multimodal programs that combine student education in school settings, screening, and referral training (Robinson et al., 2018). However, other research has raised concerns, suggesting that more data is needed to determine the safety and effectiveness of this programming (Kutcher et al., 2017).

> **Box 17.5: Preventing Suicide in Inuit Communities**
>
> As mentioned in Chapter 8, suicide is a public health issue that disproportionately affects certain Indigenous communities in Canada, with astonishingly high rates occurring in Nunavut. The suicide rate in Nunavut, a territory that has a predominately Inuit population, is 13.5 times higher than the average suicide rate in Canada and is amongst the highest suicide rates in the world. This distressingly high statistic prompted the territory of Nunavut to declare suicide a public health emergency in 2015. The high suicide rate among the Inuit peoples is partially due to socio-economic conditions driven by policies of colonization. This has resulted in inadequate funding and resources, which has led to high rates of poverty, low levels of education, housing issues, and significant unemployment. Intergenerational trauma resulting from historical and ongoing colonial policies that affect the community has also been identified as a key contributing factor. For example, beginning in the 1950s, Inuit peoples were displaced from their family-based land camps and forcibly moved to overcrowded land settlements. Their children were removed and sent to residential schools. These policies shifted parenting, increased the prevalence of domestic violence, and led to loss of language and culture. To prevent suicide within the Inuit community, programs and strategies must be culturally relevant, and responsive to the specific and diverse needs of this population. Research examining suicide prevention in Inuit communities has found that successful programming involves connection to elders, land-based activities (e.g., travelling on river ice as a family), and talking to friends and family. Importantly, the community must be directly involved in developing and implementing such efforts—"a form of sovereignty on the ground" (Kral, 2016).

Science and Research

Science and research provide us with the important means to create and test new knowledge, including the identification and understanding of effective approaches to build resilience, prevent and treat illness, reduce harm, and use our societal resources in the most effective and efficient ways possible. Neuroscientists study the brain and the many fascinating mental functions (discussed in Chapter 2), including wakefulness/arousal, sensation and perception, thought, memory, and so forth. Despite the daunting challenge of making sense of what may be the most complex and elegant apparatus in existence, neuroscientists continue to make strides in revealing the fascinating mysteries of the human brain. A host of scientists work to expand our understanding of the intricate biological mechanisms that are involved in mental function and physiological responses to psychoactive substances, focusing on anatomy, physiology, chemistry, pharmacology, molecular biology, genetics, and other biological sciences. However, scientific research relevant to mental health and substance use goes beyond laboratory studies done by scientists in white coats using microscopes and test tubes. Social scientists, applying many approaches and disciplinary traditions, such as psychology, sociology, anthropology, criminology, and others, also contribute important knowledge; only a brief survey of some of the more prominent findings by social scientists relevant to mental health were presented in Chapter 3.

The Canadian Institutes of Health Research, which is the Government of Canada agency responsible for funding health research in Canada, recognizes four pillars of research. Table 17.2 lists these pillars and notes examples of the type of research that may be conducted within each. Biomedical research produces findings about the fundamental mechanisms that are involved in mental function. Although most biomedical research studies are incremental, slowly adding small pieces of information to solve a large jigsaw puzzle, such research does occasionally create breakthroughs with the potential to eliminate disease and create radical improvements. Clinical research is needed to make advances in treatment and often focuses on the development and evaluation of new therapeutics for various conditions, such as depression, anxiety, psychosis, dementia, and so on. In recent decades, clinical research in mental health has tended to focus largely on pharmacotherapy. Health systems and policy research produces knowledge about improved approaches to the delivery of services and the advancement of practices and policies that guide our collective efforts. Population health research addresses the determinants of health and provides understandings of how various social systems relate to health, often drawing on social science, public health, and epidemiological research traditions.

An important advancement in mental health research has been the utilization of participatory research approaches and the inclusion of people with lived experience as a key source of knowledge in understanding mental health and illness. In the past, research tended to be undertaken on "subjects" who played a passive role and

Table 17.2: The four pillars of research

Research Pillar	Examples of Type of Research
Basic Science/Biomedical	Molecular studies Neuropharmacological studies
Clinical	Clinical trials Clinical conceptual studies
Health Services and Policy	Examination of costs and outcomes of service Evaluation of efforts to improve access to and delivery of services
Population Health	Social and cultural impacts on the health of the population Preventive strategies

had no opportunity to contribute meaningfully to the design of research studies or the analysis or interpretation of research findings. Today, more researchers are conducting community-based research activities and patient-oriented research, both of which emphasize the importance of including people with lived experience of mental health and/or substance use challenges in the creation of new knowledge.

Scientific research provides valuable evidence to inform good policy decisions and improvements that governments and health care systems might adopt. In addition, researchers are continually providing new findings that can help clinicians to provide better treatment, and inform people with mental health challenges, and their family members, about how to optimize recovery.

Knowledge Translation and Mobilization

Knowledge translation and mobilization can be defined as "closing the gap between what we know and what we do" (Graham & Tetroe, 2009). The concepts of "push" and "pull" initiatives are important in understanding knowledge translation and mobilization. "Push" initiatives are those efforts directed at enhancing the movement of knowledge from those who generate it outward to those who may be able to benefit from its utilization. It involves gathering, synthesizing, and funnelling high quality information. Push strategies can take various forms, including scientific publications, reports, systematic reviews, guidelines, online materials, conference presentations, courses, webinars, educational outreach, prompts, social marketing efforts, financial incentives, and media campaigns. Knowledge is "pulled" when health care providers, policy makers, patients, or communities seek out the knowledge that is needed to guide their actions. Such efforts can be facilitated by effective search tools that can locate high quality information, access to knowledge syntheses and databases, training in the identification and application of research findings in decision making, critical appraisal skill development, and creation of rapid response units and government-university liaisons and partnerships (Goldner, 2014). In recent years, the concept of *integrated* knowledge translation and mobilization has emerged. Such approaches are grounded in participatory research paradigms and move beyond the push and pull of research findings between knowledge producers and knowledge users to instead involve the co-creation of knowledge to enhance research applicability and uptake.

An important aspect of knowledge translation and mobilization involves fostering health literacy, that is, the ability of individuals to access and use information to make informed decisions to maintain good health. This has been identified as a critical factor for improved health outcomes (Guzys et al., 2015) and is consistent with the Recovery Model that has been identified as a valuable framework for mental health (see Chapter 14).

Advocacy and Involvement

A critical strategy for improving mental health and related systems in Canada and globally is through advocacy. The Canadian Nurses Association's (CNA) Code of Ethics for Registered Nurses provides a helpful definition: "Advocacy refers to the act of supporting or recommending a cause or course of action, undertaken on behalf of persons or issues. It relates to the need to improve systems and societal structures to create greater equity and better health for all" (CNA, 2017). There are ample opportunities to play a part in creating needed change; however, many people will need to participate. Each of us has unique strengths and abilities to contribute, regardless of our age, education, experience, or background. In the following, we list a series of opportunities for advocacy; these represent some of the various ways in which you might become involved. You may even be interested in supporting more than one of these activities.

1. *Help address the social determinants of mental health—poverty, housing, education, and so on.* Despite Canada's status as a relatively wealthy country, there are many groups of people who are marginalized and experiencing barriers to the social determinants of good mental health. Recognizing the social gradient that exists within Canadian society in regard to mental health, we need to advocate for stronger support systems that minimize or prevent these inequities in income, housing, and education. Since, as a whole, we are a relatively fortunate group of people in Canada, we also have a social responsibility as global citizens to contribute to knowledge production as well as promotion, prevention, and treatment efforts within less resourced countries. Canadians have a social responsibility to share the considerable expertise we have gained in research, education, and other service delivery.
2. *Contribute to public policy activities related to mental health and substance use.* This can be accomplished either through political activities and advocacy efforts, including lobbying decision makers, or by working or volunteering within government or other organizations that contribute to policy development and implementation.
3. *Help address human rights and other legal issues relevant to mental health and substance use.* Opportunities exist to become involved in legal societies and human rights activities that are geared to help people who may be marginalized on the basis of a mental illness or substance use.
4. *Contribute to mental health promotion, prevention, or treatment.* There are various ways to become involved in such activities, either as part of the formal health care work force or through more informal or volunteer efforts. A wide range of skills and talents can be put to use, with particular roles drawing on certain strengths and virtues.

5. *Contribute to research endeavours.* A wide range of research activities are underway and there are many contributions to be made by people with various skills, whether these are related to expanding knowledge through biological, social, or other scientific traditions or through research that applies lived experience.
6. *Become active in knowledge translation and mobilization.* There are unlimited opportunities to exchange valuable knowledge about mental health and to move knowledge to action that results in improvements to mental health. Once again, such activities can be done as part of formal organizational initiatives or undertaken in more informal, individual efforts.

We hope you will find some areas that excite your interest and enthusiasm and that you will become engaged in action to enhance mental health outcomes in Canada or beyond. Various organizations, including the Canadian Mental Health Association (CMHA) and the Mental Health Commission of Canada, intend to expand opportunities for people across Canada to become involved—we hope you will do so!

Conclusion

In Chapter 1, we signalled the value of a broad approach to mental health in Canada, one that goes "from synapse to society" and avoids the reductionism that often undermines successful collaborative efforts. The population and public health paradigm focuses on opportunities to make improvements to mental health at the population level, including those that focus on policies, laws, and government-supported initiatives. A strengths-based approach is consistent with a mental health promotion perspective; such an approach constitutes a significant shift to the delivery of mental health programming that, in the past, has tended to focus on pathology and illness. We have described opportunities to foster improvements in Canada's mental health system by addressing social determinants of mental health; contributing to public policy activities; addressing human rights and other legal issues; participating in mental health promotion, prevention, and treatment activities; and becoming involved in knowledge exchange and mobilization.

Glossary

demand reduction: Efforts to reduce the desire and preparedness to obtain and use drugs by potential consumers, including education, prevention and treatment programs, social pressures, and deterrents.
indicated prevention: Prevention strategies targeted at high-risk individuals who are identified as having minimal but detectable signs or symptoms.

knowledge translation and mobilization: Refers to the processes involved in reducing the gap between what is known from the scientific evidence and what is done in practice.

population health: Coordinated initiatives aimed at enhancing the health of populations and minimizing inequities.

prohibition: Policy in which the possession, selling, or marketing of a substance is made illegal.

public health: The science and art of preventing disease, prolonging life, and promoting health through the organized efforts and informed choices of society, organizations, communities, and individuals.

selective prevention: Prevention strategies that target subgroups of the population whose risk of developing mental illnesses is significantly higher than average.

supply reduction: Efforts to decrease the availability of drugs through means such as the arrest and prosecution of drug suppliers.

universal prevention: Prevention strategies that target entire populations.

Critical Thinking Questions

1. Identify ways in which public policy can address mental health and substance use.
2. What is harm reduction, and why has it been a controversial approach?
3. Using the classified prevention strategies discussed in this chapter, highlight ways in which mental illnesses and substance use can be prevented.
4. Citing specific examples, explain why science and research is important in improving mental health systems and service delivery.
5. Explain some of the various strategies that can be used to improve the mental health of our populations?

Recommended Readings

Barry, M. M., Clarke, A. M., Petersen, I., & Jenkins, R. (Eds.). (2019). *Implementing mental health promotion* (2nd ed.). Springer.

Chandler, J. A., & Flood, C. M. (2016). *Law and mind: Mental health law and policy in Canada*. LexisNexis Canada.

Jenkins, E., Chartier, M., Fox, C., Fanslow, J., Rickwood, D., Ardiles, P., Fleury, J., Verins, I., Dadaczynski, K., Clarke, A., Stansfield, J., Novak, M., Okan, O., Tamminen, N., & Barry, M. M. (2021). *Critical actions for mental health promotion*. International Union for Health Promotion and Education. https://www.iuhpe.org/images/IUHPE/Advocacy/IUHPE_Mental-Health_PositionStatement.pdf

Katz, J. (2018). *Ensouling our schools: A universally designed framework for mental health, well-being, and reconciliation*. Portage & Main Press.

Recommended Websites

CMHA—Public Policy. www.cmha.ca/document-category/public-policy
Centre for Addiction and Mental Health—Inspiring Hope through Science & Research. www.camh.ca/en/science-and-research
Canadian Public Health Association. www.cpha.ca/public-health-approach-population-mental-wellness
Centre for Suicide Prevention. www.suicideinfo.ca
Government of Canada—Promoting Positive Mental Health. www.canada.ca/en/public-health/services/promoting-positive-mental-health.html
Mental Health Commission of Canada. www.mentalhealthcommission.ca

References

Asbury, H. (2018). *The great illusion: An informal history of prohibition.* Dover Publications, Inc.

Benny, C., Gatley, J. M., Sanches, M., & Callaghan, R. C. (2019). Assessing the impacts of minimum legal drinking age laws on police-reported violent victimization in Canada from 2009 to 2013. *Drug and Alcohol Dependence, 197,* 65–72. https://doi.org/10.1016/j.drugalcdep.2018.12.025

Blais, É., Bellavance, F., Marcil, A., & Carnis, L. (2015). Effects of introducing an administrative .05% blood alcohol concentration limit on law enforcement patterns and alcohol-related collisions in Canada. *Accident Analysis & Prevention, 82,* 101–111. https://doi.org/10.1016/j.aap.2015.04.038

Canadian Nurses Association. (2017). *Code of ethics for Registered Nurses.* https://www.cna-aiic.ca/en/nursing/regulated-nursing-in-canada/nursing-ethics

Conduct Problems Prevention Research Group. (2020). *The Fast Track Program for children at risk: Preventing antisocial behavior.* The Guilford Press.

Foresight Mental Capital and Wellbeing Project. (2008). *Final Project report—Executive summary.* The Government Office for Science. https://assets.publishing.service.gov.uk/government/uploads/system/uploads/attachment_data/file/292453/mental-capital-wellbeing-summary.pdf

Giesbrecht, N., Wettlaufer, A., April, N., Asbridge, M., Cukier, S., Mann, R., McAllister, J., Murie, A., Pauley, C., Plamondon, L., Stockwell, T., Thomas, G., Thompson, K., & Vallance, K. (2013). *Strategies to reduce alcohol-related harms and costs in Canada: A comparison of provincial policies.* Centre for Addiction and Mental Health. http://madd.ca/media/docs/Strategies-to-reduce-alcohol-related-harms-and-costs_ENG_FINALrevised.pdf

Goldner, E. M. (2014). Knowledge translation. In K. L. Bassil & D. M. Zabkiewicz (Eds.), *Health research methods: A Canadian perspective* (pp. 251–278). Oxford University Press.

Government of Canada. (2018). *Folic acid and neural tube defects*. https://www.canada.ca/en/public-health/services/pregnancy/folic-acid.html

Graham, I. D., & Tetroe, J. M. (2009). Getting evidence into policy and practice: Perspective of a health research funder. *Journal of the Canadian Academy of Child and Adolescent Psychiatry, 18*(1), 46–50.

Guzys, D., Kenny, A., Dickson-Swift, V., & Threlkeld, G. (2015). A critical review of population health literacy assessment. *BMC Public Health, 15*(1), Article 215. https://doi.org/10.1186/s12889-015-1551-6

Hyshka, E., Anderson-Baron, J., Karekezi, K., Belle-Isle, L., Elliott, R., Pauly, B., Strike, C., Asbridge, M., Dell, C., McBride, K., Hathaway, A., & Wild, C. (2017). Harm reduction in name, but not substance: A comparative analysis of current Canadian provincial and territorial policy frameworks. *Harm Reduction Journal, 14*, Article 50. https://doi.org/10.1186/s12954-017-0177-7

International Union for Health Promotion and Education (2021). Critical Actions for Mental Health Promotion. Paris: IUHPE.

Kral, M. J. (2016). Suicide and suicide prevention among Inuit in Canada. *The Canadian Journal of Psychiatry, 61*(11), 688–695. https://doi.org/10.1177%2F0706743716661329

Kutcher, S., Wei, Y., & Behzadi, P. (2017). School-and community-based youth suicide prevention interventions: Hot idea, hot air, or sham? *The Canadian Journal of Psychiatry, 62*(6), 381–387. https://doi.org/10.1177%2F0706743716659245

Mbarga, N. F., Abubakari, A. R., Aminde, L. N., & Morgan, A. R. (2018). Seatbelt use and risk of major injuries sustained by vehicle occupants during motor-vehicle crashes: A systematic review and meta-analysis of cohort studies. *BMC Public Health, 18*, Article 1413. https://doi.org/10.1186/s12889-018-6280-1

Meyer, O. L., Castro-Schilo, L., & Aguilar-Gaxiola, S. (2014). Determinants of mental health and self-rated health: A model of socioeconomic status, neighborhood safety, and physical activity. *American Journal of Public Health, 104*(9), 1734–1741.

National Collaborating Centre for Healthy Public Policy. (2021). *Build back better: Wellbeing budgets for a post COVID-19 recovery?* http://www.ncchpp.ca/docs/2021-Population-Mental-Health-Wellbeing-Budgets-Post-Covid-19.pdf

Peterson, C., & Seligman, M. (2004). *Character strengths and virtues: A handbook and classification*. Oxford University Press.

Prince, M., Patel, V., Saxena, S., Maj, M., Maselko, J., Phillips, M. R., & Raham, A. (2007). No health without mental health. *The Lancet, 370*(9590), 859–877. https://doi.org/10.1016/S0140-6736(07)61238-0

Reiss, F. (2013). Socioeconomic inequalities and mental health problems in children and adolescents: A systematic review. *Social Science & Medicine, 90*, 24–31. https://doi.org/10.1016/j.socscimed.2013.04.026

Robinson, J., Bailey, E., Witt, K., Stefanac, N., Milner, A., Currier, D., Pirkis, J., Condron, P., & Hetnick, S. (2018). What works with youth suicide prevention?

A systematic review and meta-analysis. *EClinicalMedicine, 4,* 52–91. https://doi.org/10.1016/j.eclinm.2018.10.004

Rotermann, M. (2020). *What has changed since cannabis was legalized?* Statistics Canada—Health Reports. https://www150.statcan.gc.ca/n1/pub/82-003-x/2020002/article/00002-eng.htm

Sethi, M., Heidenberg, J., Wall, S. P., Ayoung-Chee, P., Slaughter, D., Levine, D. A., Jacko, S., Wilson, C., Marshall, G., Pachter, H. L., & Frangos, S. G. (2015). Bicycle helmets are highly protective against traumatic brain injury within a dense urban setting. *Injury, 46*(12), 2483–2490. https://doi.org/10.1016/j.injury.2015.07.030

Šouláková, B., Kasal, A., Butzer, B., & Winkler, P. (2019). Meta-review on the effectiveness of classroom-based psychological interventions aimed at improving student mental health and well-being, and preventing mental illness. *The Journal of Primary Prevention, 40,* 255–278. https://doi.org/10.1007/s10935-019-00552-5

University of Calgary. (2021). *Suicide awareness and prevention framework.* https://www.ucalgary.ca/wellness-services/suicide-awareness-and-prevention-framework

Vanderpas, J. B., & Moreno-Reyes, R. (2017). Historical aspects of iodine deficiency control. *Minerva Medica, 108*(2), 124–135. https://doi.org/10.23736/s0026-4806.17.04884-4

Willeford, W. G., & Bachmann, L. H. (2016). Syphilis ascendant: A brief history and modern trends. *Tropical Diseases, Travel Medicine and Vaccines, 2*(1), Article 20. https://doi.org/10.1186/s40794-016-0039-4

Wolitzky-Taylor, K., LeBeau, R. T., Perez, M., Gong-Guy, E., & Fong, T. (2018). Suicide prevention on college campuses: What works and what are the existing gaps? A systematic review. *Journal of American College Health, 68*(4), 419–429. https://doi.org/10.1080/07448481.2019.1577861

World Health Organization. (2008). Integrating mental health into primary care: a global perspective. Retrieved from: https://apps.who.int/iris/bitstream/handle/10665/43935/9789241563680_eng.pdf?sequence=1&isAllowed=y

Copyright Acknowledgements

Figures

Figure 1.1: Adapted from the Canadian Mental Health Association
Figure 1.2: Adapted from the Government of Canada
Figure 1.3: APS Healthcare
Figure 1.4: GetStock/Judy Waytiuk
Figure 1.5: GetStock/Charline Xia
Figure 1.6: GetStock/topham Picture Point
Figure 1.7: Adapted from Lesage, A.D., Morissette, R., Fortier, L., Reinharz, D., & Contandriopoulos, A.-P. (2000). Downsizing psychiatric hospitals: Needs for care and services of current and discharged long-stay inpatients. *Canadian Journal of Psychiatry*, 45(6), 526–531.
Figure 1.8: Adapted from Statistics Canada. (2021b). *Perceived mental health, by age group (Table 13-10-0096-03)*. https://www150.statcan.gc.ca/t1/tbl1/en/tv.action?pid=1310009603.
Figure 1.9: Adapted from Mental Health Commission of Canada. (2013a). *Making the case for investing in mental health in Canada*. https://www.mentalhealthcommission.ca/sites/default/files/2016-06/Investing_in_Mental_Health_FINAL_Version_ENG.pdf
Figure 1.10: Adapted from Mental Health Commission of Canada. (2013a). *Making the case for investing in mental health in Canada*. https://www.mentalhealthcommission.ca/sites/default/files/2016-06/Investing_in_Mental_Health_FINAL_Version_ENG.pdf
Figure 1.11: Adapted from Mental Health Commission of Canada. (2013a). *Making the case for investing in mental health in Canada*. https://www.mentalhealthcommission.ca/sites/default/files/2016-06/Investing_in_Mental_Health_FINAL_Version_ENG.pdf
Figure 2.1: iStockphoto/Xiaofeng Luo
Figure 2.2: iStockphoto/ktsimage
Figure 2.3: Alamy Stock Photo/Science History Images
Figure 2.4: Daniel Wierzbicki

Figure 2.5: iStockphoto/artisteer
Figure 2.6: Brenden Westman
Figure 3.1: iStockphoto/Nicole S. Young
Figure 3.2: Unsplash/Julie Ricard
Figure 3.3: Adapted from Kahneman, D., & Deaton, A. (2010). High income improves evaluation of life but not emotional well-being. *Proceedings of the National Academy of Sciences of the United States of America, 107*(38), 16489–16493. doi:10.1073/pnas.1011492107
Figure 3.4: iStockphoto/Steve Geer
Figure 3.5: Adapted from Urban Matters CCC & BC Non-Profit Housing Association. (2018). *Vancouver homeless count 2018.* https://vancouver.ca/files/cov/vancouver-homeless-count-2018-final-report.pdf
Figure 4.1: Wikimedia Commons/gruntzooki
Figure 4.2: First Nations Health Authority
Figure 4.3: Pexels/Kindel Media
Figure 5.1: Adapted from the Centre for Innovation in Campus Mental Health. (n.d.). *Understanding substance use.* https://campusmentalhealth.ca/toolkits/cannabis/cannabis-substance-use/understanding
Figure 5.2: iStockphoto/Martin McCarthy
Figure 5.3: iStockphoto/Stephanie Horrocks
Figure 5.4: Chris Sang Yeob Park
Figure 5.5: Adapted from Fischer, B., Russell, C., Sabioni, P., van den Brink, W., Le Foll, B., Hall, W., Rehm, J., & Room, R. (2017). Lower-Risk Cannabis Use Guidelines: A comprehensive update of evidence and recommendations. *American Journal of Public Health, 107*(8), e1–e12. doi:10.2105/AJPH.2017.303818
Figure 5.6: iStockphoto/Brasil2
Figure 5.7: iStockphoto/KarenMower
Figure 5.8: Shutterstock/Tomas Nevesely
Figure 5.9: ANKORS Harm Reduction Project
Figure 6.1: Pexels/Life Matters
Figure 6.2: Unsplash/The New York Public Library
Figure 6.3: Adapted from the Centers for Disease Control and Prevention
Figure 6.4: Pexels/Loifotos
Figure 7.1: Unsplash/Sandy Millar
Figure 7.2: Unsplash/Toni Reed
Figure 7.3: Adapted from Public Health Agency of Canada. (2019). *Suicide in Canada: Key statistics.* https://www.canada.ca/en/public-health/services/publications/healthy-living/suicide-canada-key-statistics-infographic.html
Figure 8.1: Jessica Kumar
Figure 8.2: Gina Kim
Figure 8.3: iStockphoto/Miranda1066
Figure 8.4: Sean Kilpatrick/Canadian Press
Figure 8.5: Library and Archives Canada

Figure 8.6: Chris Sang Yeob Park
Figure 9.1: Feryal Almazni
Figure 9.2: iStockphoto/YsaL
Figure 9.3: Unsplash/Annie Spratt
Figure 9.4: Cassidy Jones
Figure 9.5: Pexels/RODNAE Productions
Figure 10.1: Adapted from the World Health Organization. (2021). Life expectancy at birth (years). https://www.who.int/data/gho/data/indicators/indicator-details/GHO/life-expectancy-at-birth-(years)
Figure 10.2: Pexels/RODNAE Productions
Figure 10.3: Daman Pabla
Figure 10.4: Jeanelle Aldaba
Figure 10.5: iStockphoto/alwekelo
Figure 11.3: Shutterstock/EdmontonMartin
Figure 11.4: Shutterstock/CSDigitalMedia
Figure 12.1: Unsplash/Scott Webb
Figure 12.2: Unsplash/Matt Collamer
Figure 12.3: Adapted from Substance Abuse and Mental Health Services Administration (SAMHSA). (2021). *The Sequential Intercept Model (SIM)*. https://www.samhsa.gov/criminal-juvenile-justice/sim-overview
Figure 12.4: Pexels/Kindel Media
Figure 13.1: iStockphoto/ilbusca
Figure 13.2: Library of Congress
Figure 14.1: GetStock
Figure 14.2: GetStock/AMELIE-BENOIST/BSIP
Figure 14.3: iStockphoto/GeorgeBurba
Figure 14.4: Unsplash/Ashley Batz
Figure 14.5: GetStock/Rick Madonik
Figure 14.6: Adapted from Substance Abuse and Mental Health Services Administration. (n.d.) *National consensus statement on mental health recovery.* http://store.samhsa.gov/shin/content/SMA05-4129/SMA05-4129.pdf
Figure 15.1: GetStock/Barry Philp
Figure 15.3: Adapted from Public Health Agency of Canada. (2015). *Report from the Canadian chronic disease surveillance system: Mental illness in Canada, 2015 (No. 140526).* https://www.canada.ca/content/dam/canada/health-canada/migration/healthy-canadians/publications/diseases-conditions-maladies-affections/mental-illness-2015-maladies-mentales/alt/mental-illness-2015-maladies-mentales-eng.pdf
Figure 15.4: Adapted from MacCourt P. (2013). *National guidelines for a comprehensive service system to support family caregivers of adults with mental health problems and illnesses.* Family Caregivers Advisory Committee, Mental Health Commission of Canada. https://www.mentalhealthcommission.ca/sites/default/files/Caregiving_MHCC_Family_Caregivers_Guidelines_ENG_0.pdf

Figure 16.1: Pexels/Ahmed akacha
Figure 16.2: Unsplash/CLEMENT MABULA
Figure 16.3: Reproduced from *The mental health workforce gap in low- and middle-income countries: A needs-based approach*. Bulletin of the World Health Organization, 89(3), Bruckner, T. A. et al. "Mental health worforce shortage," 190, 2011
Figure 16.4: United Nations. https://www.un.org/sustainabledevelopment/sustainable-development-goals/
Figure 17.1: Chris Sang Yeob Park
Figure 17.2: United Church of Canada Archives
Figure 17.3: Vancouver Coastal Health
Figure 17.4: Adapted from International Union for Health Promotion and Education. (2021). *Critical actions for mental health promotion*. https://www.iuhpe.org/images/IUHPE/Advocacy/IUHPE_Mental-Health_PositionStatement.pdf
Figure 17.5: Pexels/Pavel Danilyuk

Tables

Table 3.1: Cramer, C., Flynn, B., & LaFave, A. (1997). *Erik Erikson's 8 Stages of psychosocial development: Summary chart*. web.cortland.edu/andersmd/ERIK/sum.HTML
Table 3.3: Sareen, J., Afifi, T.O., McMillan, K.A., & Asmundson, G.J.G. (2011). Relationship between household income and mental disorders: Findings from a population-based longitudinal study. *Archives of General Psychiatry, 68*(4), 419–426. doi:10.1001/archgenpsychiatry.2011.15
Table 4.1: Adapted from World Health Organization. (2018). *ICD-11 for mortality and morbidity statistics (ICD-11 MMS): 2018 version*. https://icd.who.int/browse11/l-m/en
Table 5.1: Adapted from Csiernik, R. (2016). Substance use and abuse: Everything matters (2nd ed.). Canadian Scholars.
Table 6.1: Adapted from Defense Centers of Excellence for Psychological Health & Traumatic Brain Injury. (2013). *Posttraumatic stress disorder pocket guide: To accompany the 2010 VA/DoD clinical practice guideline for the management of post-traumatic stress*. https://www.healthquality.va.gov/guidelines/MH/ptsd/PTSDPocketGuide23May2013v1.pdf
Table 6.2: Adapted from EQUIP Health Care. *Principles of TVIC—Organizational and individual provider levels*. https://equiphealthcare.ca/resources/tvic-workshop/
Table 9.1: Gardner, H., & Hatch, T. (1989). Multiple intelligences go to school: Educational implications of the theory of multiple intelligences. *Educational Researcher, 18*(8), 4–10.
Table 9.2: Peterson, C., & Seligman, M. (2004). *Character strengths and virtues: A handbook and classification*. Oxford University Press.

Boxes

Box 4.2: Anderssen, E. (2008, June 20). The son who vanished... *The Globe and Mail*. http://www.theglobeandmail.com/life/health-and-fitness/the-son-who-vanished/article560793/

Box 4.3: Bess, G. (2016, January 6). Why picky eating could be a sign of an eating disorder. *Vice*. https://www.vice.com/en_us/article/mgmzga/some-picky-eaters-eating-disorder-arfid

Box 9.6: Adapted from Roots of Empathy. (2021). *About our program.* https://rootsofempathy.org

Index

bold page numbers indicate photos

Abbass, Andrew, 302
acculturation, 168–170
acculturative stress, 168–169
acute hospitalization, 240–241
adaptive learning, 51
addiction, 100, 152
adenosine diphosphate (ADP), 39
adenosine triphosphate (ATP), 39–40
adjustment disorders, 86
Adler, Alfred, 50, 166
adrenaline, 41
adult neurogenesis, 44
adverse childhood experiences (ACE), 130–131
advocacy for mental health, 392–393
affect regulation, 132
after homelessness (play), 379
ageism, 219
aggressive behaviour, 199, 244, 256, 319
Albert (relative of involuntary patient), 301
alcohol use
    in Canada, 102–103, 116
    effect on brain of, 96–97
    and health problems from, 100
    by Indigenous Peoples, 102. 179
    laws enforcing limits on, 379–380, 381
    by men, 155
    moral model for explaining, 114
    treatments for, 111, 313
Alzheimer's disease, 224, 225, 228
ANKORS Harm Reduction Services, 112–113
anomie, 56
anorexia nervosa, 40, 87, 88, 153, 206
anosognosia, 35, 82
antidepressants, 152, 229, 311–312
antipsychotic medications, 29, 310–311
anti-social behaviour, 55, 386
anxiety disorders
    and antidepressants, 311
    in children, 206–207, 360
    coping with, 56
    and crisis state, 237
    and personal mental health toolkit, 328–333
    psychedelics as treatment for, 111, 325
    and sexual dysfunction, 152
    treatments for, 317, 319, 323
    types of, 80–81
    and virtual services, 348
APEC Digital Hub for Mental Health, 368
APEC Roadmap to Promote Mental Wellness in a Healthy Asia Pacific, 368
Appelbaum, P. S., 289
Applied Behaviour Analysis (ABA), 207
asexuality, 148
Asia Pacific, 368
Asia Pacific Economic Cooperation (APEC), 368
Assertive Community Treatment (ACT), 274–275, 347
attachment theory, 198
attention deficit disorder, 79
attention deficit hyperactivity disorder (ADHD), 89, 206
atypical antipsychotics, 311
autism spectrum disorder, 89, 207
avoidant-restrictive food intake disorder (ARFID), 86, 87

B vitamins, 40
Back Alley, 116
behaviour therapy, 51
behavioural interventions, 207
behaviourism, 51–52
benzodiazepines, 110, 312
Bhutan, 63–64
Bigelow, Jesse, 82–84
binge eating disorder, 88

biological clocks, 42–43
biological embedding, 196
biomedical research, 390
bipolar disorder
    and antidepressants, 311
    and cognitive remediation therapy, 325–326
    described, 80
    and mood stabilizers, 312
    and psychotic emergencies, 243
birth cohorts, 57
Black Lives Matter, **128**
Blackstock, Cindy, **178**
blood-brain barrier, 40
borderline pattern, 88
borderline personality disorder, 318
BounceBack, 348
Bowlby, John, 198
brain
    and Alzheimer's disease, 224
    and biological embedding, 196
    cellular activity in, 39–40
    effect of alcohol on, 96–97
    effect of antidepressants on, 311
    effect of drugs on, 97, 107
    and hormones, 41–42
    how it differs from the mind, 7
    make up of and how it functions, 27–30, 37
    and neurostimulation, 315–316
    and physiological activity, 31–34
    plasticity of, 44
    research on, 389
    shock absorbers, 41
    and thought, emotion, and memory, 34–36
The BRAIN Initiative, 30
Breaking Bad (tv show), 107
Buena Semilla, 363
bulimia nervosa, 88, 318
bullying
    and acculturation, 169
    of children, 193, 201, **202**
    program for stopping, 386
burden of disease, 18–19

caffeine, 31, 106
Cameron, Ewen, 111
Canada Health Act, 340, 342
Canadian Institutes of Health Research, 390
Canadian Mental Health Association (CMHA), 348, 388, 393
cannabis, 104–106, 381
caregivers, 9, 349–350, 390–391, 393
cerebral hemispheres, 33, 34, 35

certification, 239, 287
Changing Directions, Changing Lives: The Mental Health Strategy for Canada (paper), 351–352
Charter of Rights and Freedoms, 298–300
child abuse, 199–200
child development
    adolescence, 203–204
    and the brain, 30, 40
    and childhood, 199–202
    and development of character, 204–205
    and education, 191–193, 201
    and Erikson's theory, 53–54
    and gender roles, 147–148
    and hormones, 42
    infancy, 197–199
    and prenatal development, 195–196
    transition to adulthood, 204
    why it takes as long as it does, 189
child poverty, 190–191
child sexual abuse, 200–201
children's mental health
    globally, 360–362
    and mental disorders, 205–207
    and mental health problem prevention, 387–388
    play therapy, 319–320
    programs for, 193, 194, 201
    and suicide prevention, 388
    and trauma, 130–131
    and use of prescription medications as stimulant, 114
chlorpromazine, 310
chronic pain, 105, 167, 218
cisgender, 146
classical conditioning, 51
clinical research, 390
clozapine, 83, 311
coca, 106
cocaine, 99, 106
cognitive behavioural therapy (CBT)
    as depression treatment, 318, 367
    described, 318
    and psychosis, 346
    replaces behaviour therapy, 51
    on smartphone app, 365
cognitive impairment, 222–223
cognitive remediation therapy, 325–326
cognitive-based therapies, 133
collective unconscious, 50
colonialism, 102, 147, 173, 389
committal, 238–239. *See also* involuntary hospitalization

Index

community-based care/treatment, 15–16, 274–275, 347
complex post-traumatic stress disorder (CPTSD), 132
compulsive sexual behaviour, 151–152
concurrent disorders, 86, 242, 256
conditional leave, 295–296
conversion therapy, 149
coping/coping styles, 56, 233–236
co-response triage, 264
Correctional Service of Canada (CSC), 270, 271–273
COVID-19 pandemic
    effect on mental health, 58, 246–247
    and global mental health, 359
    and long-term care facilities, 228
    and mental health promotion, 383
    and poverty, 61
    and school connectedness, 192
crack cocaine, 106
criminal justice system
    and corrections, 269–270
    and courts handling of mental illness, 252, 264–268
    and health promotion in prison, 273–274
    and how prisons impact mental health, 271–273
    intersections with mental health, 251
    overview of, 252–253
    police handling of mental illness, 238, 254, 257, 260–264
    and re-entry into society, 274–275
    and specialty courts, 268–269
criminal victimization, 16
Crisis Intervention Training (CIT), 263–264
crisis lines, 240
crisis state, 235–237
crowds, 51–52, 112
cultural safety, 167, 181–182
culture
    and alcohol use, 102
    and diagnosis of mental illness, 78–79
    effect on mental health, 163
    and identity, 164
    and improving global mental health, 359
    and patterns of behaviour, 36

DAREarts, 193
date rape drug, 110
de Grood, Matthew, 267
death and dying, 221, 223
Deborah (involuntary patient), 297
decolonization, 182–183

deep-brain stimulation (DBS), 315, 316
defund the police movement, 238, 261
deinstitutionalization, 15, 255, 293
dementia
    caring for people with, 227–228
    described, 223–225
    increasing rate of, 20, 21, 229
    therapy for, 224
dependence, 99–100. *See also* physiological dependence; psychological dependence
depression
    and antidepressants, 311
    care for, 348
    causes of, 42, 43, 169
    and CBT, 318, 367
    and child abuse, 200
    in children, 206, 360
    and crisis state, 237
    and digital health, 365
    and electroconvulsive therapy, 229, 315
    as leading contributor to disease, 19
    of LGBTQ2+, 150, 155
    and meditation, 323
    men diagnosed with, 154–155
    and neurostimulation treatment, 315
    in older adults, 218, 228–229
    postpartum, 154
    prevalence of women diagnosed with, 152–153
    problems diagnosing, 76
    and psychedelics, 111, 325
    psychotherapy treatment for, 322
    rate of years lived with, 18
    reductionistic thinking of, 8–9
    and sexual dysfunction, 152
    suffered by Indigenous Peoples, 179
    and supported self-management, 317
    treatment in Vietnam for, 367
depth psychology, 50
detoxification, 242, 247
developmental disability, 88–89
Diagnostic and Statistical Manual of Mental Disorders (DSM)
    and ARFID, 87
    described, 74
    and gender dysphoria, 146
    homosexuality removed from, 149
    Indigenous problem with, 79
    and prevalence, 80
dialectical behaviour therapy (DBT), 318–319
digital health, 364–366
digital phenotyping, 326
disability adjusted life years (DALY), 18–19

disaster response, 245–247
discrimination, 103, 127–128, 149–150, 156
dissocial disorders, 206
dissociality, 88
dissociative drugs, 112
Ditmars, Bryn, 296
diversion programs, 258, 269, 274, 275
Douglas, Tommy, **341**
Downtown Community Court (DCC), 269
drag queens, **145**
dreams, 31
drug checking, 117
drug poisoning crisis, 380
drug use
    and harm reduction sites, 112–113, 116–117, 382–383
    laws on, 381
    moral model for explaining, 114–115
    and motor activity, 34
    and prohibition, 380
    and withdrawal management, 241–242
DSM. *See Diagnostic and Statistical Manual of Mental Disorders* (DSM)
Durkheim, Emile, 56
Dziekanski, Robert, 261

Early Development Instrument (EDI), 191
early psychosis intervention (EPI), 346
eating disorders, 86–88, 317
Echaquan, Joyce, 166
economic conditions and mental health, 58–59, 61–62
ecstasy (MDMA), 107–108, 325
education and child development, 191–193, 201
Eidsvik, Kristine, 301
electric shock aversion therapy, 149
electroconvulsive therapy (ECT), 229, 315
Emiru, Erin Hawkes, 296
epidemiology, 17–19
epigenetics, 38–39
equity-oriented care practices, 167
erectile dysfunction, 151
Erikson, Erik
    and identity development theory, 53–54, 197–198, 199, 203, 208
    and older adults, 219
estrogen, 42
Ethan (involuntary patient), 297
Ethiopia, 367–368
ethnicity, 167–168
Exposure and Response Prevention, 319
exposure-based therapies, 133

externalizing disorders, 206
extrapyramidal symptoms, 310
eye movement desensitization and reprocessing (EMDR), 133

Facebook, 326
family members/caregivers, 9, 390–391, 393
family systems theory, 55–56
family therapy, 320, 346
Farm Radio, 361–362
Fast Track program, 386
feeding disorders, 86–88
fentanyl, 108, 117
fetal alcohol spectrum disorder (FASD), 197
First Nations, 174, 175, 180. *See also* Indigenous Peoples
first responders, 238, 246. *See also* police
Florence (involuntary patient), 301
Floyd, George, 261
flunitrazepam (Rohypnol), 110
folic acid supplements, 386
Forensic Assertive Community Treatment (FACT), 274
Freud, Sigmund, 13, **14,** 49–50
Friendship Bench, 366

gamma hydroxybutyrate (GHB), 110
Gardner, Howard, 193
gender, 143, 144
gender expression, 145
gender identity, 145
gender roles, 147–148
genetics, 37–39
glucose, 40
goal setting, 329
Grand Challenges Canada, 366
Granirer, David, **324**
Gray, John, 289
grief, five stages of, 221
gross national happiness, 63–64
grounding yourself, 329
Gulab, Manilal, 170
Gutheil, T. G., 289

hallucinations
    and dissociative drugs, 112
    and psychosis, 243
    and schizophrenia, 35, 82
    and severe mental disorders, 271
harm reduction, 112–113, 116–117, 167, 382–383
Harper, Stephen, 178
head trauma, 41

Index

health care services in Canada
    coverage of mental health services by, 344
    distinctiveness of, 339–340
    divided government responsibility for, 342–343
    and Indigenous Peoples, 103, 343
    what is covered under *Canada Health Act*, 340, 342
health literacy, 192, 257, 391
health promotion
    and older adults, 226–227
    population and public health paradigm, 377
    in prisons, 273–274
health systems and policy research, 390
herd behaviour, 52
heroin, 99
Hierarchy of Needs, 234
hippocampus, 44
hoarding disorder, 81
Hoffman, Albert, 111
homeless/homelessness
    described, 64–66
    and inhalants, 112
    and involvement with criminal justice system, 256
    and mental illness, 16
    as part of crisis state, 237
    and shelters, 240
    theatre production on, 379
    youth as, 190–191
homunculus, 33
hormones, 41–42
hospitalization, 240–241, 240–241. *See also* involuntary hospitalization
housing, 64–66. *See also* homeless/homelessness
Housing First model, 65–66
human rights
    advocacy, 392
    and C. Blackstock, 178
    and gender identity, 150
    and mental health law, 378
    and refugees, 59
    and social justice, 322
hydromorphone, 114
hypochondriasis, 81
hypomania, 80
hypothalamus, 42

iatrogenic outcomes, 346
ICD. *see International Classification of Diseases* (ICD)
identity formation, 53–54
illness prevention, 377
immigrants, 168–170
incidence, 18

Indian Act, 176–177
indicated prevention, 386
Indigenous Peoples
    and alcohol use, 102, 179
    brief descriptions of four First Nations, 175
    and cultural safety, 181–182
    diagnosis of mental disorders not relevant to, 79
    forced assimilation of, 176–177, 180–181
    groupings of, 174, 176
    health care of in Canada, 103, 343
    history of, 172–174
    mental health challenges of, 59–60, 179–181
    mental health methods of, 10–11
    and Missing and Murdered Indigenous Women and Girls, 128–129
    need of decolonization for, 182–183
    as part of national mental health strategy, 352
    racism experienced by, 103, 164, 165–166
    and residential school syndrome, 59–60
    and spiritual healing, 322–323
    and stimulants, 106
    and suicide, 179–180, 181, 389
    and Two-Spirit identity, 146–147
    use of psychedelics, 111, 325
    and use of term wellness, 163
infant psychiatry, 198, 199
inferiority complex, 50
inhalants, 112
Insite (supervised injection site), 382
instrumental conditioning, 51
integrated knowledge translation, 391
Integrated Youth Services (IYS), 193, 194
intellectual disability. *See* neurodevelopmental disorders
intelligence, components of, 193, 194
internalizing disorders, 206
International Classification of Diseases (ICD)
    and children's disorders, 207
    described, 73–74
    and dissocial disorders, 206
    and gender identity disorder, 146
    and Indigenous Peoples, 79
    list of neurodevelopmental disorders from Chapter VI of, 75
    and neurodevelopmental disorders, 88
    and obsessive-compulsive disorder, 81
    and personality disorders, 88
    and prevalence, 80
    and PTSD, 130, 132
    and removal of gender identity disorder, 146
    and sexual dysfunction, 151
    and stress, 86
    and substance use, 84–85

intersectionality, 60–61, 165
intersex, 144
intimate partner violence, 153
Inuit, 174, 176, 180, 389
involuntary hospitalization
 in Britain, 290–292
 in Canada, 287
 and *Charter of Rights and Freedoms*, 298–300
 civil libertarian approach v. human needs approach, 288–290
 criteria for across Canada, 293–295
 history in Canada, 293
 patients' experiences of, 287, 296–298, 300–302
 and procedural justice, 302–303
 through Mental Health Act, 238–239
 in US, 292–293
 and violations of patients' rights, 300–302
involuntary outpatient treatment, 295–296
iodine deficiency, 386
IV Feed, 116

Jasmine (involuntary patient), 297–298
JH (involuntary patient), 301–302
Jung, Carl, 50

Kainai, 175
Kaiser, H. Archibald, 288
ketamine therapy, 112–113, 325
knowledge translation and mobilization, 391, 393
Kohlberg, Lawrence, 8
Kohlberg's theory of moral development, 54–55, 201
Koyczan, Shane, 340

labelling theory, 77–78, 166
Laborit, Henri, 310
labyrinth walking, **323**
language rights, 300
learned helplessness, 237
LGBTQ2+
 defined, 148
 mental health problems and challenges of, 150, 155–156
 stigma and discrimination experienced by, 149–150, 156. *See also* transgender
life expectancy, 215, 216
light and darkness cycles, 42–43
limbic system, 34–35
lithium carbonate, 312
lived experience, 9, 390–391, 393
lobotomy, 292
long-term potentiation, 36

low-barrier services, 347
LSD (lysergic acid diethylamide), 111

magnetic seizure therapy, 315
maladaptive learning, 51
managed alcohol treatment, 313
mania, 80
MDMA (ecstasy), 107–108, 325
Medical Assistance in Dying (MAID), 222, 230
meditation, 32, 323, 330
memory, 36, 44, 228
memory loss, 222–223
meninges, 41
mental capital, 385
mental disorders/illnesses
 among refugees, 171
 and child abuse, 199–201
 in children and youth, 205–207
 combining treatments for, 324
 and committal through Mental Health Act, 238–239
 courts dealing with, 252, 264–269
 coverage for treatment of in Canada, 344
 and culture, 78–79
 definition of, 4
 and deinstitutionalization, 15, 255, 293
 and distorted perception, 33, 34
 due to substance use, 84–88
 electroconvulsive therapy for, 315
 emerging treatments for, 324–326
 experiences of involuntary hospitalization by people with, 287, 296–298, 300–302
 and genetics, 39
 and hippocampal function, 44
 history of treatment for in Britain, 290–292
 and homelessness, 16
 and hospital emergency departments, 239–240
 impact of crisis state on, 237
 and impaired memory, 36
 importance of careful evaluation of treatments for, 314, 333
 and lack of tie to social networks, 56
 LGBTQ2+ seen as, 146, 149
 and Medical Assistance in Dying, 222
 most common type of emergencies, 242–245
 neurostimulation therapy for, 315–316
 people in prison with, 16, 254, 255–258, 270, 271–273
 police intervention with, 238, 254, 257, 260–264
 prevention, 364, 386–388

Index

problems with reliability and validity of diagnosis, 76–77, 79
psychopharmacotherapy treatments for, 310–314
psychotherapy treatment for, 316–321
and re-entry to society from prison, 274–275
related to pregnancy, 153–154
religious/spiritual healing of, 322–323
research project on prevalence rates, 19–21
respecting rights of people with, 302–303
sexual dysfunctions, 151–152
social approaches to, 321–322
stigma of as threat, 289
top contributor to burden of disease, 18–19
two classification systems of, 73–74
variety of treatments for, 11–13, 309
and violence, 255–256. *See also* anxiety disorders; bipolar disorder; dementia; depression; post-traumatic stress disorder (PTSD); psychosis; schizophrenia

mental health
advocacy for, 392–393
Canada's global contribution to, 357, 366–368
characteristics of, 34, 375
and *Charter of Rights and Freedoms*, 298–300
concerns of diagnostic classification, 75–79
and culture, 163, 359
and dealing with challenges to, 37
definition, 3
and economic/political conditions, 58–59, 61–62
effect of COVID-19 on, 58, 246–247, 359
effect of prenatal development on, 195–196
and epidemiology, 17–21
as field of services and supports, 10
and genetics, 37–39
global state of, 358–366
how it intersects with criminal justice system, 251, 252, 264–270
how prisons impact, 271–273
indicators of, 4–5
Indigenous practices for, 10–11
and involuntary hospitalization law, 293–296, 302–303
its relation to mental illness, 2–3
knowledge translation and mobilization, 391
laws/policies effecting, 377–383
and memory, 36
and mood, 35
and motor activity, 33–34
national strategy for, 351–352
and pandemics, 246–247
and patients' rights, 298, 300–302
and personality characteristics, 36
promotion, 363–364, 383–385, 392
and Recovery Model, 326–328
science and research, 389–391
self-reporting on, 1
and social determinants of health, 321–322
of social groups, 52
socioecological perspective of, 3
stigma of, 155, 289, 348, 365
strategies for older adults, 226–227
survey of Canadians', 16–17
tests for evaluating, 5–7
and tie to social networks, 56
toolkit for, 328–333
view that it's socially constructed, 57
viewed through physical science/social science perspectives, 8–9. *See also* children's mental health; mental disorders/illnesses; mental health problems/challenges; mental health services; older adults

Mental Health Act, 238–239, 296, 297, 300–302
Mental Health Action Plan, 358
Mental Health Commission of Canada, 339, 350–351, 393
mental health courts, 268–269
Mental Health in Adults & Children—Frugal Interventions (MAC-FI), 366–367
mental health literacy, 171
mental health problems/challenges
and behaviour therapy, 51
from bullying, 201
definition of, 4
due to acculturation, 168–170
due to adverse childhood experiences, 131
due to political/economic conditions, 58–59, 61–62
due to racism, 166
homelessness, 64
of Indigenous Peoples, 59–60, 179–181
in infants, 199
of LGBTQ2+, 150, 155–156
men's reluctance to seek help for, 147, 348
of migrant workers, 172
and personal mental health toolkit, 328–333
prevalence of women diagnosed with, 152–153
prevention of, 364, 386–388, 392
and psychoanalysis, 13, 50
from public health emergencies, 246–247
of refugees, 171
and reliability/validity of diagnosis, 76–77, 79
tied to trauma, 132
violence experienced by people with, 132. *See also* homeless/homelessness; substance use; suicide; trauma

mental health services
- as accessible to trans population, 156
- for children, 193
- and committal, 238–239
- community care, 15–16, 274–275, 347
- components of for Indigenous Peoples, 181–183
- in corrections, 270, 273–274
- coverage for in Canadian health care system, 344
- digital health, 364–366
- for emergencies, 240–242
- and equity-oriented care practices, 167
- and harm reduction, 112–113, 116–117, 167, 382–383
- and help for caregivers, 349–350
- how emergency responders cope with providing, 246
- and impact of increasing numbers of older adults on, 229
- importance of compassionate treatment by, 242
- importance of early intervention of, 346
- for mental health emergencies, 240–242
- migrant workers/refugees difficulty accessing, 171
- and negative impacts of care, 346
- as patchwork of different programs, 339
- and peer interventions, 349
- and police response units, 238, 264
- possible results of handling crises badly, 232
- primary/secondary and tertiary care, 346–347
- providers experiences of trauma, 132–133
- and psychotic emergencies, 243–244
- and Recovery Model, 326–328
- and risk of violence by patients, 256
- and role in mental health courts, 268–269
- stepped-care approach to, 345–346
- for substance use emergencies, 244–245
- and suicide emergencies, 242–243
- Trauma and Violence Informed Practice, 125–126, 135–136, 167, 303
- underfunding of, 258, 260
- variety of providers of, 344–345
- virtual service, 348. *See also* involuntary hospitalization; psychiatric hospitals

mental status examination, 5, **6**
methamphetamines, 107
methylenedioxymethamphetamine (MDMA, ecstasy), 107–108, 325
Métis, 176, 180
mhGap program, 358
microaggressions, 127
migrant workers, 171–172
Mi'kmaq, 175
mind, 7, 50
mindfulness, 323
Minkowitz, Tina, 288
mobile services, 240
Moms Stop the Harm, 110
monoamine oxidase inhibitors (MAOIs), 311
mood, 35
mood disorders, 18, 80, 311
mood stabilizers, 312
Moose Cree, 175
moral distress, 133
moral model of substance use, 114–115
motivational interviewing, 320–321
multiculturalism, 164
music therapy, 224
Mussell, Bill, 182

naloxone, 109, 313
National Inquiry into Missing and Murdered Indigenous Women and Girls, 128–129
natural disasters, 126, 359
needle exchange programs, 117, 383
neurodevelopmental disorders, 88–89
neurostimulation, 315–316
neurotransmitters, 27–30, 99, 106
Not Criminally Responsible on account of Mental Disorder (NCRMD), 265, 266–268
Nurse-Family Partnership program, 198

obsessive-compulsive disorder, 81, 319, 325
older adults
- and dementia, 223–225
- and electroconvulsive therapy, 315
- experience and wisdom of, 216–217
- health of, 218
- health promotion strategies for, 226–227
- loneliness and isolation, 218–219, 221
- memory loss in, 222–223
- and polypharmacy, 220
- and preparation for death, 221, 223
- proportion of population in Canada, 215, 229
- and treatment of depression, 228–229

opioid agonist therapies (OATs), 313
opioids, 108–110, 312–313
opium, 97
O'Reilly, Richard, 289
oxycodone, 114

PACT (Police and Crisis Team), 264
palliative care, 222
pandemics, 246–247. *See also* COVID-19 pandemic

Index

panic attacks, 81, 318
pansexuality, 148
paraphilias, 151
Pavlov, Ivan, 51
PCP (phenylcyclohexyl piperidine), 112
peer support, 321, 349
personality, 36, 53–54
personality disorders, 36, 88
pharmaceutical industry, 79
pharmacotherapy, 134, 151, 222, 390
phobias, 81
physical activity and mental health, 385
physiological dependence, 103, 110
play, 200
play therapy, 319–320
police
    and diversion models for mentally ill, 260, 263–264
    and mental health interventions, 238, 254, 257, 260–261
    and mental health training, 260, 262–263
    as part of Vancouver ACT team, 274–275
political conditions and mental health, 58–59, 61–62, 79
polypharmacy, 220, 313
population and public health paradigm, 377–385
population health approach, 376–377
population health research, 390
postpartum depression, 154
post-traumatic stress disorder (PTSD)
    described, 86, 129–130
    historic events causing, 132
    and Indigenous Peoples, 59, 179
    in prisons, 271
    and public health emergencies, 246
    as result of racism, 166
    as result of violence against women, 153
    symptoms of, 132
    treatment for, 108, 111, 134
poverty, 58–59, 61–62, 376–377
pregnancy, 153–154, 386
prescription medications, 114
prevalence, 17–18
primary care, 362–363
problem solving, 331–332
procedural justice, 302–303
progesterone, 42
prohibition, 379–380
psilocybin (magic mushroom), 111, **134**, 325
psychedelics, 111, 134, 325
psychiatric hospitals, 13, 15, 77, 255
psychiatry program in Ethiopia, 367–368

psychoactive substances
    effect on brain of, 96–97, 118
    harm from, 98–99, 118
    used for therapeutic purposes, 98
psychoanalysis, 13, 49–50, 319
psychoanalytic theories, 319
psychological dependence, 99–100, 103–104, 108
psychological development, 53–56
psychological tests, 5
psychopharmacology, 14
psychopharmacotherapy, 310–314
psychosis
    and case of Frank the shaman, 58
    and child abuse, 200
    and cognitive remediation therapy, 325–326
    and early intervention, 346
    and pregnancy, 153
    psychopharmacotherapy for, 310–311
    and schizophrenia, 82
    and use of stimulants, 106
psychosocial stress, 62
psychosocial theories, 14
psychotherapy
    advent of, 14
    and conversion of homosexuals, 149
    and infant-parent, 199
    and psychedelics, 325
    in treatment of trauma, 133
    types of, 316–321
psychotic emergencies, 243–244
PTSD. *See* post-traumatic stress disorder (PTSD)
public health, 245–247, 359, 376
pull initiatives, 391
push initiatives, 391

race as biological construct, 164–165
racialization, 165
racism
    and ethnicity, 167, 168
    experienced by Indigenous Peoples, 103, 164, 165–166
Recovery Model, 326–328, 391
reductionistic thinking, 8–9
refugees, 59, 171
relative deprivation theory, 62
relaxation ideas, 329–330
religious/spiritual treatments, 322–323
residential asylums, 12–13
residential care, 13
residential school syndrome, 59–60
residential schools, 177–179, **180**, 389
residential treatment, 347

resilience, 385
resistance, 385
retraumatization, 125, 135
Right Living Units, 274
risky play, 200
Rohypnol, 110
romantic love, 152
Roots of Empathy, 201
Rosenhan, David, 77

schizoaffective disorder, 84
schizophrenia
    and anosognosia, 35
    and cannabis use, 105
    and cognitive remediation therapy, 325–326
    described, 81–84
    difficulty proving, 58
    and genetics, 39
    problems diagnosing, 76
    and psychotic emergencies, 243
    story of Jesse Bigelow, 82–84
schizotypal disorders, 84
school connectedness, 192
science and research, 389–391, 393
Seasonal Affective Disorder (SAD), 43
sedatives, 110, 312
selective mutism, 207
selective prevention, 386
selective serotonin reuptake inhibitors (SSRIs), 311
self-help resources, 317, 333
self-management, 317
self-stigmatization, 346
separation anxiety disorder, 207
Sequential Intercepts Model, 258, **259**
serotonin and norepinephrine reuptake inhibitors (SNRIs), 311
Sevels, Edwin, 289
sex, 143, 144
sex addiction, 152
sexual dysfunctions, 151–152
sexual orientation, 148–150
sexuality, 151, 152
Shambhala Music Festival, 112, 113
shell shock, 129
shelters, 240
Sinclair, Brian, 166
slow breathing method, 330
smartphone apps, 365
Smith, Ashley, 272
social approaches to mental health, 321–322
social constructionism, 56, 57, 58
social control, 302

social determinants of health
    and child development, 189, 190–193
    and criminal behaviour of mentally ill, 256–258, 275
    described, 60–66
    importance of incorporating into immigrant settlement, 169
    and mental health treatment, 321–322
    and promotion of mental health, 364
    and research, 390
    and substance use, 116
social determinants of mental health
    and advocacy, 392
    and child development, 387
    and mental health promotion, 364, 383–385
    and public policy, 379
    and social approaches, 321
    and social justice, 322
social justice, 322
social networks, 56
social prescriptions, 321–322
social sciences, 49
social service systems, 229
social support networks, 332–333
Spitzer, Robert, 149
Step-by-Step (smartphone app), 365
stepped-care approach, 345–346
stereotypes, 127–128, 147–148
stigma
    of being LGBTQ2+, 149–150, 156
    defined, 127
    and increased level of contact with criminal justice system, 257
    internalized, 166
    of men's mental health, 155, 348
    of mental health globally, 365
    of mental illness as a threat, 289
    and NCR defence in court, 267
stimulants, 106–108
Streetohome Foundation, 66
strengths-based approach, 393
stress, 235, 328–333, 348
stress disorders, 86
stressors, 235
strokes, 35
structural violence, 128, 129, 132, 166
structured problem solving, 331–332
substance use
    and advocacy, 392
    by baby boomers, 57
    in Canada, 102–114, 116
    and CBT, 318

disorders due to, 84–88
effect of alcohol on brain, 96–97
and harm reduction, 112–113, 116–117, 167, 382–383
and homeless, 64
by Indigenous Peoples, 179
laws and policies on, 379–383
and managed alcohol, 313
by men, 155
models used to explain, 114–116
and opium, 97
prevention of, 386, 387
and psychedelics, 325
and psychological dependence, 99–100
and residential treatment, 347
responding to emergency of, 244–245
serious health problems as result of, 100
smoking tobacco, 98–99
spectrum of, 96
and substitution therapy, 312–313
and supervised consumption sites, 117
tracking your own, 118
varieties and methods of, 95
and withdrawal, 99, 106, 109, 244. *See also* alcohol use; drug use; withdrawal
substance use disorder, 86–88, 99
substitution therapy, 312–313
suicidal behaviour, 318, 322, 326
suicide
among Indigenous Peoples, 179–180, 181, 389
and anomie, 56
of children, 360
of LGBTQ2+, 150, 155
by men, 154–155
as a mental health emergency, 242–243
in Nunavut, 18
by older adults, 219
and political/economic conditions, 58, 61
prevention, 388–389
supervised consumption sites, 117
supply distribution and disposal programs, 117
supported self-management (SSM), 317, 367
sweat lodge ritual, 10–**11**
Szasz, Thomas, 288

task-sharing, 363, 367–368
technology, 57
testosterone, 42
thalidomide, 314
Theatre for Living, 379
tic disorders, 207
tobacco, 98–99, 103–104, 116
Toronto Addis Ababa Psychiatry Project (TAAPP), 367–368

Toronto Mad Pride, 77–78
transcranial magnetic stimulation (TMS), 315
trans
defined, 145
end of classification as mental disorder, 146
mental health concerns of, 155–156
numbers of, 146
suicide and self-harm of, 150, 155
treatment for gender incongruence/dysphoria, 146. *See also* LGBTQ2+
transinstitutionalization, 16, 255
trauma
connection to mental health problems, 132
described, 126
as determinant of substance use, 115–116
factors associated with, 126, 127
and framework for TVIP, 135–136
historical events shaping, 129–131
and Inuit suicide, 389
and public health emergencies, 246
treatment approaches for, 133–134
treatments for, 319
vicarious, 132–133
Trauma and Violence Informed Practice (TVIP), 125–126, 135–136, 167, 303
Trauma-Focused CBT, 319
tricyclic antidepressants (TCAs), 311
trigeminal nerve stimulation (TNS), 315, 316
Trudeau, Justin, 178
Truth and Reconciliation Commission (TRC), 177, 179
Tseshaht, 175
TVIP (Trauma and Violence Informed Practice), 125–126, 135–136, 167, 303
Two Continua Model, 2
Two-Spirit identity, 146–147

unconscious mind, 50
United Nations Committee Against Torture, 271
universal prevention, 386

vagus nerve stimulation (VNS), 315–316
vicarious trauma, 132–133
Vietnam, 367
violence
defined, 126
examples of, 127–128
experience by people with mental health problems, 132
and mental illness, 255–256
structural, 128, 129, 132, 166
against women, 153
virtual services, 348
vitamins, 40

Waddell, Charlotte, 198
well-being budgets, 385
wellness, 163
withdrawal
    from caffeine, 106
    and GHB, 110
    from opioids, 109
    as part of substance use emergency, 244
    from substance use, 99
    and substitution therapy, 312–313
withdrawal management, 241–242
World Health Organization (WHO), 358, 364, 378–379
worry management, 330–331

Years Lived with Disability (YLD), 18
Years of Life Lost (YLL), 18
yogic practices, 32